The Politics of Mental Health and Illness

Series Editor
Bruce M. Z. Cohen
Sociology
University of Auckland
Auckland, New Zealand

The Politics of Mental Health and Illness conceptualises the western mental health system as a social, economic, political, and cultural project which cannot be adequately theorised without considering wider societal and structural issues such as professional power, labelling and deviance, ideological and social control, consumption, capital, and self-governance. Engaging with both social theory and empirical evidence, and situated at the intersections of critical psychiatry, sociology, anthropology, social psychology, social work, history, media studies, and the health and education sciences, the series offers academics, researchers, postgraduate students, and practitioners new and innovative monographs and edited collections with which to contest and challenge the taken-for-granted understandings of psychiatry and the mental health system currently progressed in western society. Research topics for the collection may include: aspects of the medicalisation and/or pharmaceuticalisation of everyday life; psy-professional power and knowledge production; psychopolitics and the expansion of talk therapies; the biomedical model and the future of psychiatric nosology; the marketisation of mental health discourse; social media and self-diagnosing behaviour; capitalism and psychiatric violence; and specific analyses of psy-professionals and their practices from a variety of locations (including prisons, workplaces, addiction clinics, the military, schools, the home, and general hospitals). As the first book series to explicitly encourage critical contributions in the area of mental health and illness, we welcome scholarship from a wide range of different theoretical and empirical perspectives.

If you would like to discuss a book idea prior to submitting a proposal please contact the Series Editor, Dr Bruce M. Z. Cohen, via the Commissioning Editor, Beth Farrow (beth.farrow@palgrave.com).

Bruce M. Z. Cohen
Martin Harbusch • Jo Reichertz
Editors

Addiction and the Medicalisation of Conspicuous Behaviour

New Critical Perspectives

Foreword by Peter J. Adams

palgrave
macmillan

Editors
Bruce M. Z. Cohen
University of Auckland
Auckland, Auckland, New Zealand

Martin Harbusch
Social Sciences
University of Siegen
Siegen, Nordrhein-Westfalen, Germany

Jo Reichertz
Institute for Advanced Study in the Humanities
Essen, Nordrhein-Westfalen, Germany

Foreword by
Peter J. Adams
School of Population Health
The University of Auckland
Auckland, New Zealand

ISSN 2731-5266 ISSN 2731-5274 (electronic)
The Politics of Mental Health and Illness
ISBN 978-3-032-06312-0 ISBN 978-3-032-06313-7 (eBook)
https://doi.org/10.1007/978-3-032-06313-7

Cover illustration: Farhan Baig

This Palgrave Macmillan imprint is published by the registered company Springer Nature Switzerland AG.
The registered company address is: Gewerbestrasse 11, 6330 Cham, Switzerland

This book is warmly dedicated to Howard S. Becker (1928–2023),
inspirational jazz pianist and sociologist

Foreword

Ideas about addiction sure attract their fair share of attention. Discussion of it commonly appears in printed and online news bulletins, in broadcasts on radio and TV, in academic and medical publications, and in diverse forms of media that include popular paperbacks, films, social media posts, and blogsites. Addiction is variously described as a brain disease, a spiritual affliction, a disordered mental condition, or some form of social dysfunction. Those who qualify under its label are often characterised as consuming irrationally, using to excess, lacking self-control, or acting in antisocial ways. These ideas, now so familiar, cast mainly a negative light on addiction that, through constant repetition, fixes this negativity in our minds as an obvious given.

However, when taking time out to examine the concept of addiction more closely, a more complex and diverse picture emerges. Addictions are associated with both pain and pleasure; they intersect with social relations at home, in neighbourhoods and within society; they connect with commercial and industrial interests, and they are intimately entangled with patterns of conformity and deviance with respect to established social norms and cultural practices. Indeed, addictions intersect boundlessly with many of the subjective, social, political, and cultural aspects of our being.

This book is made up of a series of unique and stimulating essays shining a light on ways social science research and theory are contributing to emerging directions in thinking and speaking about addictions. Each essay offers cutting-edge insights into the dilemmas and complexities posed by approaching addiction through a sociological lens. They draw on social theory from the many branches of the social sciences including Marxism, social constructionism, poststructuralism, critical rhetoric studies, and postcritical theory (including affect theory and new materialism). As I read them, I found my mind shooting out in many directions and prompting me to imagine new opportunities for enquiry.

In reflecting on why I found this book so stimulating, I was able to tease apart five major themes, or threads of ideas, that weaved their way in and through the four different parts of the book and each of their chapters. Not all chapters focused directly on all threads but, when not directly discussed, the threads are hinted at in related themes. At the risk of pre-empting how readers will respond, I thought it might be helpful to briefly describe the threads that unravelled for me.

The first thread concerns the dominance of biomedical and psychological approaches that draw on individualised and linear understandings of addiction with an emphasis on neuro-cognitive processes. The criticisms here are not new and echo similar critiques delivered by others in the field, but they differ in the way they focus on the mechanics and tactics employed to achieve such dominance. For example, Matilda Hellman (Chap. 12) analyses the 'neurohype' messages and 'spinning' techniques used in promoting neuroscience in social and online media. Similarly, Martin Harbusch (Chap. 3) explores the interactional processes involved in the medicalisation of what he calls 'passionate behaviours'.

The second thread involves taking a closer look at discourses around 'behavioural addictions' such as sex, work or gambling addictions. Much of addiction theory springboards off ideas derived from substance addictions such as tobacco, alcohol, and illicit drugs. However, with behavioural addictions involving less emphasis on biological processes, the socially constructed and culturally imbued aspects of addiction become more obvious. For example, Baptiste Brossard, Emmanuelle Larocque, Nicolas Moreau, Dahlia Namian, and Mélissa Roy (Chap. 2) provide a conceptual framework for understanding the emergence of representational landscapes that underpin popular discourses on sex, exercise, and work addictions. Later in the book, Baptiste Brossard and Benjamin

Hemmings (Chap. 15) build on this by taking a more specific look at pathologising depictions of sex addiction in movies. Similarly, Kris Taylor (Chap. 8) explores the construction of pornography addiction as a discursive tool that reinforces the language of medicalisation.

The third thread weaving through several chapters focuses on ways in which risk and dangerousness are conceptualised. Addictions, undoubtedly, are linked to risk-taking through aspects such as intoxication and disorderly behaviour, but this does not always need to be interpreted negatively. Lars Arntsen and Nancy Campbell (Chap. 10) investigate what they call 'risk regulatory societies' and examine the practices of cultivating and curating risk in extreme sports such as skydiving and rock-climbing. They draw a parallel between the managed 'edgework' of extreme sports with similarly curated (not 'disorderly') spaces associated with addictive consumptions such as gambling. Jo Reichertz (Chap. 4) also explores the passionate 'edgework' involved with gambling and argues that it offers an alternative communicative construction to that of medicalised notions of gambling addiction.

The fourth and related thread weaves around the morally loaded binaries that we use to talk about addictions. These include positive-negative binaries, such as rational versus disordered, conformist versus deviant, and temperance versus excess. For example, Bruce Cohen (Chap. 5) draws on Marxist theory in exploring the ideological functions for capitalism of casting addiction as a 'deviant consumption practice'. Similarly, Mark Elam (Chap. 7) draws on new materialist theory in exploring what he labels as 'disarming innovations', or affordances in the social and material configuration of things, that allay fears about the impacts of addictive products which he illustrates with nicotine replacement products and behavioural tracking with gambling.

The final thread, and one close to my heart, concerns the exploitation of addiction discourses by corporates interested in both increasing and protecting their profits. These profits provide both the incentive and the capacity for corporations and businesses to invest in tactics of language manipulation that generate more favourable sales environments for their products. For example, Gerd Möll (Chap. 14) focuses on 'gambling friendly' discourses used in the German Parliament to anchor gambling harm as a medical-psychiatric problem. Similarly, Cherie Lacey, Ian

Goodwin, and Antonia Lyons (Chap. 13) explore ways in which designers implant 'dark patterns' into social media that induce affective-cognitive states that advance sales on their online platforms.

While manipulating meanings in common addiction discourses might appear peripheral and ephemeral, several chapters illustrate how these efforts can have dramatic impacts on addictive consumptions. For example, Thaddeus Müller (Chap. 6) tracks the emergence of narratives in popular and medical publications that differentiate 'good' (dependent) from 'bad' (addicted) opioid users and explores how this has contributed to de-stigmatising and legitimising the prescribing of opioids for chronic pain which then prepared the ground for the opioid epidemic. Similarly, Tehseen Noorani (Chap. 11) explores the power of language in his analysis of pro-medicalising discourses that are currently shifting attitudes towards psychedelics as their status moves from a prohibited devil to a celebrated angel for use in treating mental health concerns.

I anticipate that other readers with an interest in addiction will, like me, find the novelty and diversity of what appears in these chapters engaging and challenging. I strongly recommend reading through chapters in all four parts of this book. They will help in shifting ways of thinking about, conceptualising, and developing responses to addiction.

Auckland, New Zealand

Peter J. Adams

Acknowledgements

The editors would like to thank all the authors featured in this volume for their generosity in accepting our invitation to contribute, responding so positively to our feedback, and producing the excellent analyses profiled in the book. Our thanks also to Beth Farrow at Palgrave Macmillan who supported this project from the very beginning and has efficiently worked behind the scenes to ease the path of the collection to publication.

Bruce would like to acknowledge his family in Aotearoa New Zealand—Jessica, Maeby and Milo—who he loves very much despite curtailing their summer with the constant refrain of "just finishing off the addiction collection"! Much love also to family and friends in the London, Colchester, Birmingham, Berlin, Auckland and various other locations. I continue to thrive on the amazing support of sociology colleagues, both home and away, including from the beautiful Sociological Association of Aotearoa New Zealand (SAANZ). Additionally, a big thank you to my co-editors Martin and Jo, who came up with the original idea for this book—I hope I haven't driven them completely crazy with my endless spreadsheets! Lastly, I wanted to thank all the postgraduates who turn up to my critical mental health reading group; it is just one hour a month, but our discussions always invigorate and inspire me, giving me a glimpse of what learning and research can look like beyond the point-scoring insanity of the current neoliberal education system.

Martin would like to acknowledge his sociological family around the globe in Aotearoa New Zealand, Germany, Jordan, the USA, Canada and Europe. Particularly he thanks all members of the Society for the Study of Symbolic Interaction, who never tired of hearing his lectures, his students, who always gave him food for thought in good discussions and with good questions, his brother and his friends in Kassel, who repeatedly endured tiresome sociological discussions with a friendly and interested face and who were always there to support him even in difficult times. He loves you, guys. He thanks Jo Reichertz, who has become more of a friend than a good colleague for him in recent years. And especially he wants to acknowledge Bruce Cohen, without whose structured and motivating way of working this book would certainly not have been written in such a short time. Last but not least, his acknowledgement goes to Jessica Terruhn, whose optimism and mental support must certainly be seen as one of the greatest pillars of this project.

Jo's thanks go first and foremost to the person whose generosity made it possible for him to enter the field of slot machine players, and who was fired precisely because of this generosity. Then my thanks go to the team with whom we have spent a long time familiarising ourselves with the strange world of slot machine players, with great pleasure but also with great profit, namely Miriam Gothe, Ronald Hitzler, Gerd Möll and Arne Niederbacher. I would also like to thank Jessica Terruhn and Bruce Cohen, not only for the wonderful time in Aotearoa New Zealand, but also for their hospitality and solidarity. And of course, thanks to Martin Harbusch, who built the bridge that made it all happen.

Praise for *Addiction and the Medicalisation of Conspicuous Behaviour*

"We desperately need a more intelligent, thoughtful and sociologically literate conversation about addiction, and this important book is a significant part of that."

—Johann Hari, author of *The New York Times*' best-seller, *Chasing the Scream: The First and Last Days of the War on Drugs*

"This is an outstanding collection. Through a series of dazzling individual essays, it illuminates key aspects of addiction, challenging conventional thinking about the field and, ultimately, laying the groundwork for a bold new agenda for critical sociological addiction research.

"An essential volume for anyone interested in critical understandings of addiction—and, indeed, in the wider application of cutting-edge sociological thought to urgent social issues in general.

"I absolutely loved this book! Hugely impressive project; it's going to be a fantastic contribution to the field."

—Gerda Reith, Professor of Social Science, University of Glasgow, UK

"This timely book brings together a thought-provoking collection of theoretical and empirical analyses, demonstrating the unique value of sociological approaches to addiction in its contemporary and multiplying forms. With topics ranging from the cultivation of risk in extreme sports to the technical mediation of nicotine consumption and gambling, the volume rigorously challenges reductive psychiatric frameworks. Moving beyond critique, it offers an expanded and generative conceptual vocabulary to better understand experiences of over-attachment, passionate involvement and boundary transgression."

—Helen Keane, Professor of Sociology, Australian National University

"The critical perspectives articulated in this book demand an answer to the question 'does addiction science cause unintended harm by reinforcing historic power inequalities?'. The book will help addiction researchers across all disciplines to navigate the uncertainties raised by these questions."

—Lee Hogarth, Associate Professor of Psychology at the University of Exeter, UK

The original version of the book has been revised. A correction to this book can be found at https://doi.org/10.1007/978-3-032-06313-7_16

Contents

Notes on Contributors

Lars Arntsen is currently completing his Biomedical Engineering degree at Rensselaer Polytechnic Institute. He aims to pursue a career leveraging technology in psychological intervention, fuelled by his passion for helping others.

Baptiste Brossard is Senior Lecturer in Sociology at the University of York. His research areas are critical mental health and historical sociology. He is the co-author of *Explaining mental illness: Sociological perspectives* (with Amy Chandler, Bristol University Press, 2022).

Nancy D. Campbell is Professor of Science and Technology Studies at Rensselaer Polytechnic Institute in Troy, New York. She is the author of *OD: Naloxone and the politics of overdose prevention* (MIT Press, 2020); *Discovering addiction: The science and politics of substance abuse research* (University of Michigan Press, 2007); *Gendering addiction: The politics of drug treatment in a neurochemical world* (co-authored with Elizabeth Ettorre, Palgrave, 2011); *The narcotic farm: The rise and fall of America's first prison for drug addicts* (co-authored with JP Olsen and Luke Walden, Abrams, 2008); and *Using women: Gender, drug policy, and social justice* (Routledge, 2000).

Bruce M. Z. Cohen is Associate Professor of Sociology at Waipapa Taumata Rau/University of Auckland and current President of the Sociological Association of Aotearoa New Zealand (SAANZ). He is the author of *Mental health user narratives: New perspectives on illness and recovery* (Palgrave Macmillan, 2008) and *Psychiatric hegemony: A Marxist theory of mental illness* (Palgrave Macmillan, 2016), as well as editor of the *Routledge international handbook of critical mental* *health* (Routledge, 2018) and the Palgrave Macmillan book series, *The politics of mental health and illness* (see: https://link.springer.com/series/16854).

Mark Elam is Professor of Sociology at the University of Gothenburg, Sweden. He researches at the interface between sociology and science and technology studies (STS) on a variety of medical and environmental issues. His recent publications include the co-edited volume, together with Åsa Mäkitalo and Todd Nicewonger, *Designs for experimentation and inquiry: Approaching learning and knowing in digital transformation* (Routledge, 2019).

Ian Goodwin is Associate Professor of Communication at Waipapa Taumata Rau/University of Auckland. With a background in cultural studies, Ian's research has been wide ranging and inter-disciplinary yet centres on understanding the societal changes associated with the rise of digital media technologies. In the last few years, he has focused particularly on social media. He is currently interested in exploring intersections between algorithmic culture, health and well-being, alcohol consumption, unhealthy product marketing, consumer activism, citizenship, and media policy.

Richard Hammersley is Emeritus Professor of Health Psychology in the School of Psychology and Social Work at the University of Hull. Over his career his interests moved from eyewitness research to the psychology of crime, and then addictions, where political, economic, and sociological forces rampantly affect how substance use problems are thought about, regulated, researched, and intervened against. He has authored four books on drugs, as well as writing 160 academic papers, and consulting for Scottish, Welsh, and UK governments during their occasional lucidity about drug problems. Having left the academy, he practises privately as a health psychologist.

Martin Harbusch is current Professor of Research Methods at the University of Siegen. His research and teaching focus on the sociology of knowledge and the sociology of psychiatry. His previous edited volumes include the highly successful collection *Troubled persons industries: The expansion of psychiatric categories beyond psychiatry* (Palgrave Macmillan, 2022).

Matilda Hellman is a sociologist who specialises in representation and social constructions regarding lifestyles, mental health, addictions, social policy, and the welfare society. She holds a Chair at Uppsala University and is an associate professor at the University of Helsinki.

Benjamin Hemmings is a PhD candidate at the Australian National University in the School of Sociology.

Cherie Lacey is a member of the Centre for Addiction Research at Waipapa Taumata Rau/University of Auckland, Aotearoa New Zealand. Cherie has a background in film and media studies and has long been interested in the ways in which our affective and emotional lives are entangled with digital technologies. In recent years, Cherie's research has turned to behavioural designs, in particular 'dark patterns', and how these feed into our contemporary addictogenic culture.

Emmanuelle Larocque is a professor in the Department of Social Work at the Université du Québec en Outaouais (UQO) in Canada. Her research merges her key interests of critical mental health, ecological justice, and nature-based therapy to create links between human and planetary health and well-being.

Antonia Lyons is a professor and the Director of the Centre for Addiction Research at Waipapa Taumata Rau/University of Auckland, Aotearoa New Zealand. She brings a critical health psychology perspective to her work in multidisciplinary teams. Her research has focused on the social and embodied contexts of behaviours related to well-being and developing pathways towards improving outcomes. Her work has explored identities, digital media, drinking practices, drinking cultures and alcohol consumption at different life stages.

Gerd Möll is a sociologist and has been conducting empirical research in the field of gambling for more than ten years. He is the author of *Mit Geld spielt man nicht! Glücksspiel und »Glücksspielsucht« im parlamentarischen Diskurs* [You don't gamble with money! Gambling and 'gambling addiction' in parliamentary discourse] (Transcript Verlag, 2021).

Nicolas Moreau is a professor at the University of Ottawa in Canada. His research focuses on sport as a psychosocial development tool for troubled youths and problematic sporting behaviour (doping, addiction), as well as the challenges of using self-measurement instruments, such as watches and connected applications.

Thaddeus Müller is Reader in criminology at the Law School of Lancaster University. He was the President of the Society for the Study of Symbolic Interaction (2023–2024) and is the current President of its European counterpart. He has researched a range of topics within the symbolic interactionist field of crime, transgression, and stigma, such as the criminalisation and normalisation of drugs, the criminalisation of young immigrant men hanging around in public spaces, and territorial stigma. Within these themes, he focuses on the effects of stigma/labelling, and resisting stigma/labelling (and its effects) through the (collective) construction of empowering (counter-)narratives. He has published in a wide range of journals, such as *Symbolic Interaction*, the *Qualitative Sociology Review*, *Critical Criminology*, *Deviant Behaviour*, the *Journal of Contemporary Ethnography*, and the *British Journal of Criminology*.

Dahlia Namian is Professor of Sociology at the University of Ottawa. Her areas of expertise include social problems, homelessness, and social and health inequalities.

Tehseen Noorani researches the phenomenologies, epistemics, and therapeutics of extreme experiences, including how they are understood through first-person inquiry, traditional knowledges, and contemporary scientific investigations. This is occurring at a time when, across many countries in the Global North, psychedelic experiences are being rapidly medicalised, and psychotic experiences are being reclaimed—and even celebrated—through Mad Pride and neurodiversity movements and the growing discipline of Mad Studies. Tehseen has trained and taught in, and collaborated across, a range of disciplines, informing his interests in the epistemological, ethical, and methodological challenges that arise in attempts to conduct meaningful cross-disciplinary and participatory research. He currently co-leads the project, 'Community strategising about psychedelic therapy in Aotearoa' as Senior Research Fellow at Waipapa Taumata Rau/University of Auckland, and convenes the international and multi-disciplinary 'Reimagining psychedelic trials' working group.

Jo Reichertz is Emeritus Professor of Sociology and Communicative constructivism at the Institute for Advanced Study in the Humanities, University Duisburg-Essen. His extensive published work in the sociologies of communication, science, research methods, and gambling includes over 20 monographs and 25 edited collections. The latter includes the sole-edited collection *Grenzen der Kommunikation—Kommunikation an den Grenzen* [Boundaries of communication—Communication at the boundaries] (Velbrück, 2020), *Braucht die Mediatisierungsforschung den Kommunikativen Konstruktivismus?* [Does mediatisation research need communicative constructionism?] (Springer, 2018) with Richard Bettmann (Institute for Advanced Study in the Humanities, University Duisburg-Essen), and *Emotion. Eskalation. Gewalt. Wie kommt es zu Gewalttätigkeiten vor, während und nach Fußballspielen?* [Emotion, escalation, violence: How does violence happen before, during and after football matches?]

(Juventa, 2018) with Verena Keysers (Institute for Advanced Study in the Humanities, University Duisburg-Essen).

Mélissa Roy is a professor in the School of Social Work of the Université du Québec à Montréal, specialising in theories and contemporary issues in social work. Her work focuses on social problems qualified as 'crises', narratives constructed on these crises, as well as conflicts of knowledge, regimes of truth, and othering processes that emerge during these 'crises'.

Kris Taylor is a researcher, lecturer, and member of the Centre for Addiction Research at the School of Population Health, Waipapa Taumata Rau/University of Auckland. He has worked, taught, and published across multiple fields including social psychology, health psychology, sociology, and history.

Abbreviations

AA	Alcoholics Anonymous
APA	American Psychiatric Association
ARC	advanced responsibility and care system
BAT	British American Tobacco
BDMA	brain disease model of addiction
BDSM	bondage, discipline, dominance, submission
CBD	cannabidiol
CDOH	commercial determinants of health
CTE	chronic traumatic encephalopathy
DSM	*Diagnostic and statistical manual of mental disorders*
EGM	electronic gaming machine
fMRI	functional magnetic resonance imaging
GA	Gamblers Anonymous
GD	gambling disorder
GP	general practitioner
ICD	*International classification of diseases*
ICER	Institute for Clinical and Economic Review
IGT	International Gaming Technology
LSD	lysergic acid diethylamide
MDMA	3,4-methylenedioxymethamphetamine (ecstasy)
MME	morphine milligram equivalents
MMT	methadone maintenance treatment
NGO	Non-governmental organisation

NICE	National Institute for Health and Care Excellence
NIDA	National Institute on Drug Abuse
NRT	nicotine replacement therapy
OCD	obsessive-compulsive disorder
OST	opioid substitution treatment
PET	positron emission tomography
PMI	Philip Morris International
PTSD	post-traumatic stress disorder
QDA	qualitative document analysis
SNS	social networking site
STS	science and technology studies
SUD	substance use disorder
TAS	thrill and adventure seeking
THC	tetrahydrocannabinol
UK	United Kingdom
UNODC	United Nations Office on Drugs and Crime
US	United States
UX	user-experience design
WHO	World Health Organization

List of Figures

1

Introduction: Pathologising Pleasure?

Bruce M. Z. Cohen, Martin Harbusch, and Jo Reichertz

Currently, the dominant medical and scientific discourse on addiction tells us that drug, alcohol and related addictions are on the rise and will continue to affect an increasing number of people (Park, 2024). Though some groups are more likely to become addicts than others, we are told that addiction shows no respect for class location, identified gender, ethnicity, or age group. In the words of Park (2024, p. 1, emphasis added), the addiction experts,

B. M. Z. Cohen (✉)
Waipapa Taumata Rau/University of Auckland, Auckland, New Zealand
e-mail: b.cohen@auckland.ac.nz

M. Harbusch
University of Siegen, Siegen, Germany
e-mail: martin.harbusch@uni-siegen.de

J. Reichertz
Institute for Advanced Study in the Humanities, Essen, Germany

B. M. Z. Cohen et al. (eds.), *Addiction and the Medicalisation of Conspicuous Behaviour*, The Politics of Mental Health and Illness,
https://doi.org/10.1007/978-3-032-06313-7_15

> insist that addiction is a predictable, even natural, response of the human being to what now so often surrounds us, namely, an ample and sure supply of potent thrills and pleasures. On such a view, *the root of addiction is simply human nature.*

As the science improves, so more addictions are being identified and established as official 'mental disorders' in the American Psychiatric Association's (APA) *Diagnostic and statistical manual of mental disorders* (DSM). The media has also become more active in portraying the many lives which have been negatively affected by 'addictive behaviours' and the need to be observant for the early signs of dependence in our own behaviour and those of our friends and family. As a result, people have become more involved than ever before in help-seeking behaviour and in recognising when they might have a potential addiction themselves. While addiction to alcohol, opiates, and illicit substances are still represented as very serious issues, new and emerging forms of addiction associated with gambling, shopping, sex, online gaming, and social media use are becoming more readily recognised in everyday life (Petry, 2016), and has led in turn to an increase in the number of psy-professionals (including counsellors, psychologists, and therapists) who are required to 'treat' such problematic behaviours.

However, in contrast to the above official and often repeated narrative, the 14 contributions which follow in this book will challenge such assumptions regarding the nature of addiction. Surprisingly, the very idea of addiction as a distinct and identifiable disease remains highly contested within medical science (for an overview, see for example, Cohen, this volume; Hall et al., 2015): definitions of what addiction is remain contested (Adams, 2008; Keane, 2002; Room, 1998); theories of aetiology, including the dominant brain disease model of addiction (BDMA), continue to lack rigorous scientific evidence (Campbell, 2007; Clarkson & Kopaczewski, 2013; Hammersley & Reid, 2002); and the 'treatments' offered, whether pharmacological or psychotherapeutic, lack efficacy and may often prove harmful to the user (Bennett, 2011; Bourgois, 2000; Campbell, 2012; Epstein, 2019). On this basis, it is necessary for critical scholars to further investigate a medical, media, and public discourse which has proliferated *despite* a lack of scientific and clinical progress in the area. This collection provides such critical analysis of a variety of forms of conspicuous behaviour either currently labelled as an 'addiction' or potentially vulnerable to that label in the future.

Boundless Addiction: On the Medicalisation of Conspicuous Behaviour

The question of order in a society has been driving sociology since its inception; significant is the question of how order, if necessary, can be established to enable and guarantee the coordination of action of its members. *Culture* is essentially responsible for the fact that the members of a society know what they have to expect from others and how they have to behave themselves; this is the result of not only its history but also of a power-structured societal or communicative construction. Not everyone can participate in this social construction in the same way; some groups are able to assert their interests more, others less. Knowledge is therefore the medium through which social order is produced, transmitted and justified (Berger & Luckmann, 1967)—a critical sociology is thus always a sociology of knowledge, and a sociology of knowledge is always critical (Foucault, 1970). Within this volume we talk about addiction sociologically—as a form of knowledge which is used to focus on forms of behaviour of people, who act in ways which are interpreted as 'deviant'. What 'deviance' is and is not already points to the very fruitful sociological question regarding which behaviours are seen as 'normal' in a society, and who has the power to label others as 'abnormal' and under what terms.

In all societies, tradition, religion, magic, education, science, medicine, laws, and, of course, gossip have ensured that people's actions in certain situations at certain times are expectable and thus predictable. But at all times and in all societies it happens that people act differently from what society expects of them; that they sometimes deviate a little but also sometimes very clearly from what the majority of society's members expect and do. This leads to a discourse about which of these unusual or conspicuous behaviours are still within the bounds of what is socially accepted, whether a boundary has been crossed, and whether the persons in question are outside what is perceived to be normal and expected in a society.

When such an unusual action is discursively labelled as conspicuous and outside the norm, then begins:

(1) the search for the reasons—or the discursive construction of the reasons—that cause this behaviour;
(2) the discursive construction of the ways of dealing with this behaviour; and
(3) the discursive construction of the actors who are responsible for dealing with these behaviours.

Depending on whether the society sees itself as more secular, religious, natural philosophical, individualistic or collective, capitalistic or anti-capitalistic, the causes of the conspicuous behaviour—and, of course, the ways of dealing with it and the determination of the groups of people responsible for carrying out these actions—are permeated by the prevailing norms and values of the respective society. For example, religious societies like to see the devil as the cause of conspicuous behaviours, which results in priests being responsible for expelling them, whereas secular societies like to blame the individual and his or her body for particular behaviours (including those labelled as addictive), resulting in professions that make their living restoring functioning bodies (see for example, Henzgen & Meier, 2024).

Western societies use the term 'disease' when attributing the causes of abnormal behaviour. However, this is primarily the case when a person's body becomes dysfunctional and is at risk of diminished functioning or even death. While the concept of illness was initially applied primarily to physical impairments and changes in the body, in the early modern period the view emerged in the Global North that not only the body, but also the disembodied part of a person—the soul or spirit—could be 'sick', and that this illness could be cured by certain measures performed by people trained to do so. Partly due to the lack of clarity about what is meant by the soul or the spirit, the concept of mental health/illness has been significantly promoted in recent decades, particularly by the psychiatric branch of medicine (that is, those professionals who have claimed an expertise and responsibility for the healing of the psyche). In 1965, Ivan Illich (1976) named this process *medicalisation*, and since then a number of studies can be found that show how the process of medicalisation is structured to encompass ever wider areas of human behaviour: for example, anyone who likes to sit at slot machines is a gambling addict, anyone who likes to eat is an eating addict, and anyone who very much enjoys sex is a sex addict. In particular, the concept of *addiction* plays a major role in the process of medicalisation because, due to the vagueness of this term, many behaviours that are pursued with passion, such as the voluntarily taking of risks, are labelled as expressions of addiction, and thus as 'sick' and in need of 'treatment'.

Addiction is understood in this book as a metaphor, a cultural label which communicates certain moral codes regarding the nature of economic and social life in Western society (Reith, 2019). Divided into four parts (involving: theoretical directions in understanding addictions; negotiations with the 'addiction' label; conspicuous behaviours as potential 'addictions'; and engagement with media, political, and public discourse on 'addiction'), this volume demonstrates that addiction is less an area for psychiatric than for sociological analysis, and that when we speak of addiction we need to recognise the discourse as fundamentally political rather than medical in nature. The collection focuses primarily on the recent proliferation of the addiction concept, which includes consideration of how medicalisation processes develop and what the current landscape looks like. At first sight it seems to us that the process of medicalisation is not directed against all social groups in the same way, but rather that the less privileged are much more targeted by 'moral entrepreneurs' (Becker, 1963) who, in a paternalistic manner, want to stigmatise and forbid to some what they let pass and admire as extravagant behaviour in others (namely, the wealthy).

To gain a clearer understanding of addiction, typical sociological questions are raised and discussed here, including who benefits from the labelling of certain conspicuous behaviours as 'addictions' and certain populations as 'addicts'. Together with understanding the socio-historical background of addiction as the capture of this area by medicine and psychiatry (see section below), it becomes clear that what is under examination in this book is varieties of social deviant practice and behaviour by populations sometimes considered as "the dangerous classes" (Campbell, 2007, p. 12). We can therefore better conceptualise addiction as yet another example of the medicalisation of social deviance (Conrad, 2007). These deviant practices have been named in a variety of ways by critical addiction scholars but share a commonality in emphasising *forms of consumption* which have been considered by moral authorities (whether the criminal justice system, the mental health system, a religious body, or a political institution) as morally problematic (for example, illegal drug use, gambling or drinking excessively).

The Purpose of This Collection

In the best tradition of critical studies on addiction, this edited collection challenges commonly understood and widely circulated ideas on 'addiction' and 'addicts'. It is the first anthology in 13 years (see Netherland, 2012) to take up this topic again, and it offers a range of critical contributions which problematise the widely accepted psychiatric discourse that addiction is a proven biomedical disease for which there are established and effective treatments. Involving both established and emerging critical scholars from the US, Canada, the UK, Germany, Sweden, Aotearoa New Zealand, and Australia, the book provides new empirical and theoretical reflections of passionate actions or behaviours that have either already been labelled as an addiction or could potentially be expected to be medicalised in due course. These include the active consumption of social media, pornography, and sport, opioid and psychedelics use, and the passionate involvement in gambling, smoking, and sexual practices. The volume also critically considers media, political, and public discourse which engages with the current labels of 'addiction'. Moreover, it sheds much more light on methodological issues, in turn placing more emphasis on the social construction thesis than previous addiction collections have, thus pursuing a genuinely sociological approach. The aim of the book is not only to enrich the discourse with new studies and new objects for critical addiction research, but also to advance methodological reflections.

In putting together this collection, we were inspired by those critical scholars who have previously disrupted and problematised addiction science (see for example, Becker, 1963; Castellani, 2000; Campbell, 2007; Douglas, 2002; Hammersley & Reid, 2002; Keane, 2002; Netherland, 2012; Peele, 1985; Reith, 2019; Room, 1998; Suissa, 2006; Young, 1971). In critical addiction studies, these scholars have taken different theoretical positions (for example, following a labelling, critical realist, sociology of knowledge, Marxist or Foucauldian perspective) but there remains a commonality in conceptualising addiction as a culturally and historically constituted moral marker. In essence, this is broadly a *social constructionist* approach which considers the socio-political implications of labelling some forms of consumption as 'risky', 'excessive', 'dark', and thus 'addictive', while other forms (such as wellness activities and extreme sport; see respectively, chapters from Hammersley, and Arntsen and Campbell, this volume) escape this designation.

The Social Construction of Reality: Constructivism or Constructionism?

The entire critical discourse on addiction and medicalisation is based on the theoretical premise that both terms are social constructions (see for example, Hammersley, 2017; Levin, 2018; Rowe, 2021; Truan, 1993); this has also been shown by several authors when investigating specific topics on health and addiction (on drugs, see Klaue, 1999; on gambling, see Reith, 2019, and Venuleo & Marinaci, 2017; on illness, see Conrad & Barker, 2010; on working, see Negura et al., 2023). It is therefore no coincidence that many authors in this anthology *explicitly* (see for example, Arntsen and Campbell, Hammersley, Harbusch, Hellmann, Möll, and Reichertz) or *implicitly* (see for example, Lacey et al., Cohen, and Taylor) refer to social constructionism. However, we need to be mindful that there are different versions of constructionism that can be drawn upon, and are indeed taken up by our authors. Therefore, clarification of this central concept of social construction is necessary if we want to better understand the individual contributions. After all, the term *social construction* is very broad and is often used as an umbrella concept. Therefore, in this section we will briefly explain the program of social constructivism and its various currents, and shed some light on the theoretical background of the argumentation for the reader.

Social constructivism (in all its variants; see Eberle, 2019; Hacking, 1999; Pfadenhauer & Knoblauch, 2019) is very much based on early work in the area of the sociology of knowledge (Bluhm, 2010; Mannheim, 1980), which showed that the *knowledge* available to a specific society at a specific time is not a reflection of social reality but instead significantly dependent on social location and available social perspectives. Peter Berger and Thomas Luckmann play a particularly important role within *social constructivism*. In their 1967 book, *The social construction on reality*, they presented a draft *sociological* theory (Berger and Luckmann, 1967) which, based on the aforementioned insights from the sociology of knowledge and in combination with phenomenological (Schutz, 2012), anthropological (Gehlen, 1972) and interactionist (Mead, 1934) concepts, proposed an innovative social theory.

With their new *sociology of knowledge*, Berger and Luckmann (1967) showed that knowledge is developed by society, legitimised by means of institutions and passed on to each new generation via socialisation. The special feature of this approach was that social knowledge was primarily and significantly objectified in *language* and is passed on to the (new) members of society in primary and secondary education via language and *knowledge* about language. This knowledge is safeguarded and legitimised by social institutions developed for this purpose, such as kindergartens, schools, and universities, as well as the police and the judiciary. In this version of social constructivism, knowledge is objectified *with and in language* and finds its way into the minds and bodies of society members via *language acquisition* (see Pfadenhauer & Knoblauch, 2019; Reichertz, 2019).

However, because language and knowledge are central to Berger and Luckmann's (1967) social constructivism, it becomes important for this variant of social constructivism to see the world *through the eyes of the subjects*, to reconstruct the subjective meaning. From this standpoint the world is not objectively given but rather—following the Thomas theorem (Thomas & Thomas, 1928)—what people consider to be reality in their subjective view. The sociology of knowledge then has the task of reconstructing the processes of construction, transmission and the impact of knowledge. Subjects play a minor role in this theory, as they are primarily conceptualised as carriers and transmitters of socially acquired knowledge and not as discoverers or revolutionaries who renew or fundamentally change society and the knowledge of society. In this version of constructivism science plays a prominent role in the creation of new knowledge on addiction (for example), as it is responsible for both the acquisition and legitimisation of knowledge. This kind of social constructivism is used more often in sociology, anthropology, and philosophy than in psychology in the Anglophone world.

Largely initiated by Kenneth Gergen (1991; Gergen & Davis, 1985), in a critical examination of Berger and Luckmann's (1967) social constructivism, the concept of *social constructionism* was developed—and indeed some of the contributors to this volume are more influenced by Gergen than by Berger and Luckmann (see for example, Brossard et al.; Cohen; Lacey et al.; Taylor). Inspired by the work of the Frankfurt School (see for example, Horkheimer et al., 2002) and the writings of Foucault (1990), social constructionism is still widely used in English-speaking countries (Eberle, 2019) and remains a significant approach in psychology, sociology and anthropology. The field of social constructionism (see Reichertz & Zielke, 2008) includes such diverse directions within psychology as Gergen's postmodern, linguistic-pragmatic variant. However, representatives of *critical psychology* and *sociology* (see also Cohen, 2016; Cromby & Nightingale, 1999; Parker, 1999; Rose, 1999, 2007) have also played a significant role in shaping the discourse of social constructionism.

Despite the diversity of approaches, from the perspective of social constructionism *everything*, including addiction, is 'socially constructed'. Accordingly, everything is also socially and culturally variable because it is 'made' and not 'given'. Everything cultural can be broken down into and traced back to power-structured discourses and narratives. Methodologically, the social dimension takes precedence over the internal perspective of the subject; social interactions of all kinds, which are always *communications*—in particular everyday discourse, practices and conversations—come into focus. Analysing these everyday social practices is regarded as the basic operation of constructionist research. This direction of psychology is understood by many scientists as a 'discourse science' in the sense that, primarily, discourse analyses are carried out, the significance of which they illustrate using numerous examples.

In addition to the special features of *social constructionism* outlined above, almost all of the works show a *socio-critical or power-critical* concern in their agenda, which also includes the uncovering and elimination of forms of social inequality and oppression. There is also a fundamental scepticism towards any kind of knowledge that claims to be universally valid. Even the methods and theories of social constructionists are only narratives that move within a field of discourse, and can be replaced by others at any time: as Gergen (2019, p. 261) rightly questions, "[i]s social construction itself not a social construction?"

In a critical dialogue with the social constructivism of Berger and Luckmann (1967), the social constructionism of Gergen (1991), the discourse theory of Foucault (2008), and the actor-network theory of Latour (1993), in German-speaking countries the concept of *communicative constructivism* has recently been developed (Keller et al., 2013; Knoblauch, 2020; Reichertz, 2019, 2024). This new approach sees the most important components for the construction of reality in power-structured *communication* from person to person (Reichertz 2021, 2024) *and* the *power-structured public media debate* (see Keller, 2024; Reichertz, this volume).

Before introducing each chapter in more detail, the following section contextualises these discussions in a socio-historical analysis of the discovery and expansion of the addiction label in Western industrial society.

A Critical History of Addiction

While it is estimated that the human consumption of opiates and alcohol may go back as far as six thousand years, theories of psychological dependence and addiction to such substances does not arise until the emergence of Western industrial society (Conrad & Schneider, 1992, p. 111). Between the sixteenth and nineteenth centuries concerns were noted regarding the potential vices and immoral habits of the population, yet as

Peele (1985, p. 3) notes, they were not configured as forms of dependence per se. More, certain unusual or excessive behaviours such as gambling or drinking were religiously ascribed as *amoral*, ultimately caused by the devil's seductive powers; people were seen as weak and morally questionable in that they could not resist the devil's temptations. However, during the Enlightenment, religious views were slowly replaced by more medical understandings of such immoral practices (Flusser, 2006; Le Goff, 1990).

Benjamin Rush is often credited as the first in the medical profession to suggest alcohol could be 'addictive' and that habitual drunkenness should be considered a disease, a mental illness. He theorised in the 1780s that the key element of this addiction to alcohol was a 'loss of control' of the drinker in which they were unable to make adequate moral distinctions (Peele, 1989, p. 38), with the symptoms including swearing, rudeness, immodesty, and fighting (Conrad & Schneider, 1992, p. 79). Significant to this start of the process of medicalising alcohol use was Rush's understanding that, while alcoholism could potentially effect anyone, it was those with 'defective wills' who were more susceptible to the mental disorder (cited in Conrad & Schneider, 1992, p. 83). Therein the habitual drinker was absolved of moral guilt, and the responsibility for drinking was shifted to the sick body (see Spode, 1991, p. 214; Wiesemann, 2000, p. 34).

Influenced by strong religious and cultural mores, proposes Campbell (2007, p. 13), abstinence and temperance to alcohol were promoted from the very beginning of this disease model of addiction. The temperance movement would promote such a view of alcohol consumption over the next century: namely, that one drink could lead to alcoholism, that alcohol was addictive, and that the 'loss of control' of the drinker led to immoral behaviour (Peele, 1989, pp. 37–38). The solution, as Peele (1989, p. 38) comments, was religious conversion and a commitment to abstinence from alcohol. Rush's conception of alcohol consumption as a 'disease of the will' (Levine, 1978, p. 151; Reith, 2019, p. 39; Valverde, 1998; Wiesemann, 2000, p. 33) and morally corrupting remains a central component of the Alcoholics Anonymous' (AA) philosophy today, with religious overtones including: admissions of powerless; acceptance and declaration that the person is an alcoholic; public confession and repentance; the striving for spiritual rebirth and a new identity; as well as the need to covert others to the AA faith (Peele, 1989, pp. 43–46).

Despite physicians in the US and UK following Rush in "calling self-destructive drug use a disease" (Heyman, 2009, p. 7), the critical mass of the medical establishment remained resistant to idea that consuming alcohol or other drugs could lead to a mental disorder until the official formulation of the 'addition' concept in the late nineteenth century. Peele (1985, p. 4) notes that this period witnessed widespread opiate consumption in the population with few considering it a problematic practice; as Conrad and Schneider (1992, p. 117) have pointed out, opium use was not associated with social deviant behaviour at the time, despite the likelihood that there were greater levels of 'dependency' to opioids than today. Yet from the latter half of the nineteenth century and into the early twentieth century this view of narcotics dramatically changed, with growing concerns from the medical establishment for the potential addictive qualities of opioids and the wider consequences for society. While morphine addiction was first noted in 1877 (Peele, 1985, pp. 3–4), drug addiction did not appear in Eugen Bleuler's popular *Textbook of Psychiatry* until 1916 (Conrad & Schneider, 1992, p. 115). By the mid-1920s, however, opiates were outlawed, 'addicts' were labelled as 'dope fiends', rates of dependency and criminality associated with the procurement of drugs increased, and as Conrad and Schneider (1992, p. 121) note, a subculture of deviant drug users was established (and remains today).

Understanding this dramatic change in perceptions of drug consumption from something as socially acceptable and commonplace to behaviour conceptualised as an addiction and socially abhorrent in society is crucial to identifying the key political and social dynamics which continue to play a significant role in labelling patterns of deviant consumption as 'addictive' today. The formal discovery of addiction in this period has been theorised by critical scholars as the result of a number of elements unrelated to the myth of medical progress as promoted by academic psychiatry and the neurosciences. As summated by Clarkson and Kopaczewski (2013, p. 129), "[t]he modern formulation of addiction emerged as a result of societal fears of potentially dangerous and immoral practices of immigrants in Britain and the United States during the 19th century". Peele (1985, pp. 4–5) has identified three key factors which led to the change in these societal attitudes towards opioid use and users: firstly, a change in the population using narcotics from middle class women (consuming laudanum) to lower class men (using heroin); secondly, an exaggerated response from moral entrepreneurs to such changes in usage; and thirdly, the framing of narcotic use as antithetical to US lifestyle, and users as "debased, immoral, and uncontrollable" (Peele, 1985, p. 5; see also Berridge and Edwards, 1987; Wiesemann, 2000, p. 27).

At the birth of the addiction concept then, it is noted that the construction took place as a moral and political activity against those deemed as part of the 'dangerous classes', typically identified by the medical (and criminal) label as African American and white ethnic working-class males who took drugs not for 'medical treatment' but rather for 'recreation' (Campbell, 2007, p. 12; see also Müller, this volume). As Reith (2019, p. 45) comments, opium came to signify "all that was disorderly or dangerous in working class consumption". In the words of Clarkson and Kopaczewski (2013, p. 130), "[t]he xenophobic, racist, and sexist origins of the concept of addiction should encourage a judicious skepticism about new medical discourses of pathology." In effect, the middle classes were able to successfully generalise its own social norms while stigmatising behaviour that deviated from these. As Berridge and Edwards (1987, p. 28) remark of the emergence of the disease model of conspicuous behaviour, addiction "acted not simply as an agency of social control, but as one of social assimilation, in which the symptoms were defined in terms of deviations of conformity and self-help". In other words, "the disease of the will became a prime example of the threat to bourgeois order" (Wiesemann, 2000, p. 35).

No longer respectable but increasingly prohibited by law, opiate consumption was consequently reformulated as leading to an almost instant lifetime addiction, despite the dubious medical evidence for this view (Conrad & Schneider, 1992, p. 119). While Peele (1985, p. 5) highlights that medicine initially lost out in the criminalisation of opiate use—as such substances could no longer be utilised as a part of treatment—it nevertheless gained from the reframing of narcotic use as a 'disease' (that is, an addiction), which brought the field further credibility and legitimacy in the long run. As Berridge and Edwards (cited in Peele, 1985, p. 5) comment of medicine's capture of the area,

> The profession, by its enthusiastic advocacy of a new and more 'scientific' remedy and method, had itself contributed to an increase in addiction ... The belief in scientific progress encouraged medical intervention in less definable conditions [than that of typhoid or cholera, for example] ... [S]uch views were never, however, scientifically autonomous. Their putative objectivity disguised class and moral concerns which precluded a wider understanding of the social and cultural roots of opium [and later morphine] use.

Informed by Rush's conception of the disease of the will, such moral concerns were also evident in the prohibition movement's successful outlawing of alcohol consumption in the US between 1920 and 1931. "Backed by powerful political, moral, nativist, and capitalist forces", states Peele (1989, pp. 40–41), "prohibition became a movement for preserving the family and the nation and for eliminating sloth and moral dissolution." Just as the criminalisation of opioid use led to higher levels of consumption, Peele (1989, p. 41) notes that the 1920s witnessed a period of heavy alcohol use in the US.

Post-prohibition, medical science began to take more interest in the chronically drunk person (Conrad & Schneider, 1992, p. 86). In 1939, the AA published their bible, the *Big Book*, which formally outlined their 12-step programme, still a bedrock of the organisation today. In it, alcoholism is conceptualised as a lifelong condition; alcoholics are framed as having an 'allergy' to alcohol for which abstinence (rather than temperance) is crucial to potential recovery (Peele, 1989, p. 44). Along with a revivalist Protestant philosophy of personal responsibility and redemption, Peele (1989, pp. 45–46) also notes the growing ties AA developed with medicine and addiction science over time, including fusing their philosophy with biological theories of alcoholism in the latter half of the twentieth century. After it appeared in the addiction section (alongside drug addiction) of the first iteration of the DSM as an official mental disorder in 1952, the American Medical Association finally accepted alcoholism as a disease in 1956 (Peele, 1989, p. 46).

Eager to separate their work in the area from the historical associations with crime, immorality, and social deviance, medical authorities argued in the post-war period for a shift in terminology from the use of 'addiction' to 'dependence' as a more scientifically accurate descriptor for the condition. It was, states Campbell (2012, p. 7), medical science's attempt to 'destigmatise' the field as well as further their own legitimacy as the rightful institution for studying and treating this social problem: "[t]he term 'dependence' was offered by policy-active scientists and public health researchers in the mid-20th century seeking to legitimate medical and scientific authority and overcome the pejorative and moralistic connotations then understood as inherent in the word 'addiction'." Indeed, 'drug dependence' (a mental disorder requiring "evidence of habitual use or a clear sense of need for the drug") replaced 'drug addiction' in the second edition of the DSM in 1968 (American Psychiatric Association, 1952, p. 39, 1968, p. 45).

Medical authority in the field was further extended in 1980 with the release of the third edition of the DSM (the DSM-III; American Psychiatric Association, 1980), which both institutionalised the growing theory of addiction as a biological disorder as well as expanding the range of conditions covered by the label, with the introduction of 'pathological gambling' (American Psychiatric Association, 1980, pp. 291–293). As Castellani (2000) details, this label had a more recent post-war history with the foundation—along similar lines to AA—of Gamblers Anonymous (GA) in 1957, and the establishment of therapeutic programmes by the psychiatrist Robert Custer in the 1970s (who also successfully pushed for the inclusion of the label in the DSM-III). Significant in understanding the expansion of categories in the area, pathological gambling was the first *behavioural* disorder to be marked as an addiction; unlike drugs and alcohol, gambling is not something which involves ingestion (Castellani, 2000, p. 57), however the 'chase' to win in gambling was theorised as involving similar issues of compulsion and dependency as other addictions.

The claims of 'diagnostic creep' and psychiatry's desire to medicalise more aspects of human behaviour as potentially addictive has led Courtwright (2019, p. 224) to exclaim that "[g]iven enough time, every excess will wind up in the *Diagnostic and Statistical Manual of Mental Disorders*." Although the DSM has yet to add any further addiction labels to the main manual, 'internet gaming disorder' remains in the appendix of the latest DSM (the DSM-5-TR; American Psychiatric Association,

2022) awaiting further research evidence (whereas the World Health Organization already added 'gaming disorder' as a fully fledged mental disorder to the eleventh edition of their *International classification of diseases* (ICD-11) in 2018 (Courtwright, 2019, pp. 2–3)). Petry (2016) has profiled the ongoing research on the following behavioural addictions towards possible future inclusion in the DSM: internet addiction, sex addiction, shopping addiction, exercise addiction, eating addiction, and tanning addiction. In following the official APA line, she remains adamant that the current absence of these addiction labels from the DSM "does not mean they are not psychiatric disorders", and that "[a]s science progresses, subsequent versions of the DSM may officially classify some of them as psychiatric conditions" (Petry, 2016, p. 4).

With addiction, then, a new 'disease' and a new population of 'sick' individuals have been 'discovered' by psy-professionals over the past 200 years. Many conspicuous behaviours of everyday life have now been officially labelled as addictions in the DSM, while others inhabit a greyer area, still awaiting official designation but increasingly conceptualised in both public and psychological discourse as morally problematic. Anyone today who pursues something passionately, beyond the normal level, to the neglect of their work, their money and their social relationships, risks being labelled an 'addict' by others. There is a growing potential in the twenty-first century that we can be addicted to love or sex, to work, to fitness, to recognition and fame, but also to leisure and relaxation (see for example, the chapters in this volume from Arntsen and Campbell, Brossard et al., Hammersley, and Lacey et al.). In contrast, areas where one cannot become addicted to some activity or behaviour are diminishing. We are therefore seeing the increase in the medicalisation of a form of social deviance, of conspicuous behaviours, over time. Assessing why we have witnessed such a form of medicalisation, explaining the recent proliferation of addiction discourse, and considering who ultimately benefits from such expansion calls for the sociological analysis which is given in the rest of this book. Below we outline the structure of the volume, and offer a brief summary of each discussion which follows in the book.

About This Book: New Critical Perspectives on Addiction

The first part of the book introduces a range of theoretical analyses which can aid our understanding of the purposes of the addiction discourse and those who are labelled (or self-label) as addicts. Using examples from their fieldwork on sex, exercise and work addictions in North America and Australia, **Baptiste Brossard**, **Emmanuelle Larocque**, **Nicolas Moreau**, **Dahlia Namian, and Mélissa Roy** introduce the reader to 'The ecological niche of behavioural addictions' in Chap. 2. Underpinned by the work of Ian Hacking (2002), the authors present a fascinating explanation for how 'normal' behaviours can become pathologised through 'looping effects', informed by a convergence of professional, institutional, media, and consumer interests. While none of the examples profiled in the chapter currently appear as formal addictions in the DSM, the authors note how they have nevertheless proliferated as meaningful categories in Western society. The theory of ecological niches usefully bridges some key theoretical approaches including Marxist, interactionist, constructionist, and poststructuralist.

Discussion of the complex dynamics through which addiction categories might appear and proliferate as outlined by Brossard and colleagues is continued by **Martin Harbusch** in his consideration of 'The triangle of medicalisation' in Chap. 3. Informed more centrally by symbolic interactionism and drawing on examples from across addiction research, he argues that we should see the labelling of consumption behaviours and experiences as 'addictive' as a process of negotiation between three main forces: namely, medical and psychiatric professionals; associated institutions including pharmaceutical companies, detox clinics, educational institutions, and insurance companies; and lay people, who are labelled or label themselves with the term 'addiction'. Harbusch argues that reductionist, top-down analysis (as seen, for example, in Marxist scholarship) can often ignore the significance of people's own perspectives and constructed lifeworlds, which may help us better explain the growing enthusiasm for self-labelling everyday behaviour as problematic and in need of the 'addict' label. Recognising the bottom-up perspective opens up more analytical space for thinking through the proliferation of addiction discourse in current society. For Harbusch, understanding the potential key drivers of medicalisation is therefore an interactional process that does not take place unilaterally but is instead fluid and situational, involving interactions between lay people, medicine, and addiction-related institutions.

However, towards an explicit sociology of knowledge perspective is **Jo Reichertz**'s discussion in Chap. 4 on 'The communicative construction of addiction'. Reichertz draws on his extensive observations of gamblers to outline the contribution of communicative construction to the field of critical addiction studies. Such an approach allows us to see more clearly the power dynamics which underpin the medicalisation of the activities and behaviours which are more common among the less privileged in society. Contrasting addiction discourse on gambling with extreme sport and wellness activities, Reichertz demonstrates the resonance of psychiatric language as biased and informed by middle class prejudices. He concludes that we should see the activity of gambling on slot machines and pokies as in fact a form of resistance of less privileged populations to capitalism; rather than conceptualising such voluntary risk-taking as 'addiction', then, Reichertz argues that passionate gambling with money should be better understood as 'edgework'.

Bruce Cohen takes up the challenge a structural, top-down analysis in Chap. 5 when he discusses 'A Marxist theory of addiction'. Given the contested nature of addiction science, Cohen argues that the recent proliferation in the addiction discourse can be explained through understanding the demands of neoliberal capitalism for both productive labour as well as increasing surplus value. Using critical research evidence from areas including alcohol and drug use, gambling, smoking, eating, and sex addiction, he demonstrates that while addiction 'treatments' lack efficacy, the groups connected to the troubled persons industries (Harbusch, 2022) who work in the addiction field (including insurance companies, pharmaceutical corporations, new media and biotech businesses, research organisations, and private doctors, therapists and clinics) have been economically very successful. However, Cohen proposes that it is the ideological role played by addiction discourse that has become an increasingly important element in the twenty-first century. Performing an analysis of the official psychiatric discourse given in the DSM, he shows how 'addiction' is constructed through current nosology as the limits of consumption practices in capitalist society; that is, the point at which consumption leads the worker to neglect their primary tasks in being 'productive' for capitalist society. In agreeing with Gerda Reith (2019, p. 68), the assumptions made in the language of the addiction criteria represents "a mirror image of the neoliberal ideal."

The second part of the book considers professional and user negotiations with consumption behaviours which have already been medicalised as addictions or are danger of soon being labelled as such. **Thaddeus Müller** considers the current opioid epidemic via an historical analysis of the official addiction research literature in Chap. 6, on 'The social construction of "good" and "bad" addicts: How relabelling addiction shaped the opioid epidemic'. Müller takes a traditional labelling approach in assessing how medicine cultivated a discourse on opioid use as non-addictive, utilising poor science and morally separating 'good' from 'bad' users. As he argues, 'bad' patients became 'addicted' to opioids because, according to the official narrative, they did not follow the medical guidelines (and thus became labelled as 'addicts'). The core theme of the medical narrative was that the user, rather than the pill, was the problem. Müller's chapter offers a cautionary tale on the power of medicine to define what is and what is not an addiction, based on professional and economic interests rather than good science.

Similarly, Chap. 7 from **Mark Elam** on 'Excessive appetites and disarming innovations: The shifting socio-materialities of nicotine and gambling addiction' is a timely analysis of how technological innovations, and the economic benefits than can accrue from them, tend to precede medical ideas on addiction. For Elam, 'disarming innovations' (such as nicotine replacement technologies, or data-tracking which can exclude high-risk gamblers from online gambling sites) are innovations introduced in response to growing public concerns about the harms of different addictions; they are disarming in the sense of seeking to allay fears regarding the basic safety of addictive technologies, but they can also aim to break and disrupt addictive patterns of consumption. He shows, however, that while doubts remain about the success for consumers of such disarming innovations, they have become deeply entangled with new forms of scientific research and, consequently, the further medicalisation of consumption practices.

Meanwhile, **Kris Taylor** considers user negotiations with the addiction label in Chap. 8, titled '"Addiction" and agency at the threshold of infinite pornographic access'. Drawing on firsthand accounts of self-identified pornography addicts, Taylor critically reflects on the point at which 'normal' behaviour in this area is perceived to have become pathological or 'addictive'. Critical addiction studies has long noted that there are no reliable measures to separate normal from abnormal levels of consumption, instead the psychological sciences rely on self-reports of user distress. Taylor's chapter investigates the issue in more depth by illuminating at which point pornography viewing becomes problematic, and what exactly for the viewer qualifies as an addiction attribution. A compelling and thought-provoking contribution, Taylor aids our understanding of the ways in which the concept of 'addiction' can stand in for more complex and difficult questions about how we are able to make sense of pornography viewing as personally problematic.

The third part of the collection investigates conspicuous behaviours which have currently or previously escaped the addiction label, and the reasons why this might be the case. In Chap. 9, **Richard Hammersley** problematises the common sense view of addiction with his consideration of 'Wellness, addiction and temperance'. While the excessive consumption of alcohol and illegal drugs are seen as the moral opposite of 'wellness' (as ill-defined as this concept is), Hammersley argues that, in fact, addictions can be considered as a residual problem of the accepted and encouraged use of substances, and the widespread general message that pharmaceuticals, vitamins and 'health' foods can enhance wellness. He proposes that attempts to separate out alcohol, caffeine, nicotine, medicines, over-the counter analgesics, vitamins, and supplements from addictive drugs on the basis of their psychopharmacology does not work because drug harms depend not just on the drug but also on the mindset of the user and the socioeconomic, legal and political settings of usage. In contrast, the multi-billion dollar wellness industry can be better understood as pushing a highly inducing set of consumption practices which are inherent with the same dangers and benefits as those which have already been labelled as 'addictions'.

Lars Arntsen and **Nancy D. Campbell**'s discussion on 'Using sports: Constructing extremity as addiction' in Chap. 10 continues this problematisation of what might be seen as morally affirming consumption practices. More specifically, the authors consider the tension between extreme sports (including BASE jumping, kite surfing, wingsuiting, snowboarding, and big wave surfing) as 'edgework' (Lyng, 1990) as opposed to other 'risky' consumption activities labelled as 'addictive' (such as excessive drug use). Drawing on interviews with extreme sport enthusiasts, alongside Giddens' (1991) and Beck's (1992) discussions of 'risk', Arntsen and Campbell argue that using the term 'addiction' around such activities is growing due to the heightened emphasis on safety, compliance, and insurance to anchor social norms and routines of risk avoidance in everyday life.

In Chap. 11, 'From medicalisation to cultural embrace: Drug foundationalism versus techné in the psychedelic revival', **Tehseen Noorani** continues with the focus on contemporary consumption practices by providing a critical discussion of the changing medical and cultural construction of psychedelics. As previously outlawed hallucinogenic drugs, psychedelics are experiencing a renaissance in which they have been reconstituted by medicine and the psy-sciences as 'therapeutic' rather than 'addictive'. In other words, notes Noorani, we are currently witnessing the global medicalisation of psychedelics. In a nuanced analysis which considers the implications of such a change, he suggests that psychedelic therapy offers a 'post-critical gesture', at once revealing and challenging the traditional addiction discourse. Noorani's chapter has some very interesting similarities to Thaddeus Müller's chapter (see above) in that it considers the way in which a growing research literature—in contrast to previous views of such drug taking—is currently proposing that psychedelics are 'non-addictive' and can be safely used in medically controlled environments.

Part four, the final part of the volume, considers addiction discourse in the public space, which includes discussions of cinema, online and social media, and parliamentary debates. **Matilda Hellman** considers how brain research is portrayed in popular online news as a superior form of knowledge in Chap. 12, on 'Addiction discoveries: Hyping and spinning the superiority of neuroscience'. She proposes that using the concepts of *hype* and *spin* in assessing such news reporting (namely, assessing the packaging of media references to 'what is' in a wrapping of 'what it means') helps us achieve a clearer understanding of this genre as a force of (bio)medicalisation. Strongly informed by science and technology studies, Hellman's analysis demonstrates how the presentation of neuroscientific research on addiction is cast in the language of scientific progress and major breakthroughs; the messiness of the continuing knowledge gaps in the addiction area are overlooked in favour of the more 'clean' biomedically informed solutions. Hellman concludes that a central function of this reporting genre appears to be to convey, upkeep and strengthen humanity's belief in science- and technology-based outsmarting of its many challenges.

At a time when governments are considering the banning of social media to young people (see for example, Sullivan, 2024), in Chap. 13 **Cherie Lacey**, **Ian Goodwin, and Antonia Lyons** provide a timely discussion on 'Social media, dark patterns and contemporary discourses of addiction'. While the technology may be relatively new, Lacey and colleagues argue that the central debates surrounding the idea of 'social media addiction' reflect ones that we have seen in this area before; in this case, an underlying tension between those who position addiction as an individual problem, and those who see it as a deliberate and malicious business model built on 'dark patterns' of interface design. The chapter offers the reader a sociological analysis which considers the potential benefits and interests on both sides of this 'ideological battlefield', including reflections on the power of Big Tech as well as the concerns of public legislators. The authors conclude their analysis by suggesting that current individualising discourses on social media addiction are effectively working ideologically to obscure the wider economic, political, and technological systems that underpin all social media platforms. Going forward, the latter requires much more attention in critical addiction studies.

In Chap. 14, **Gerd Möll** provides a further example of the political utilisation of the individualising discourse of addiction, when he discusses 'The instrumentalization of the concept of "gambling addiction": A discourse analysis of German parliamentary debates'. While the state can serve an important role in regulating consumption practices and responding to public and media concern regarding potential 'addictive' behaviour, what Möll demonstrates here is the state's use of the dominant psychiatric discourse on deviant consumption practices to maintain economic and political control over the gambling sector. Through a discourse analysis of parliamentary documents in Germany, the author argues that, under the pretext of addiction prevention and consumer protection, measures have been propagated that justify attempts to solve urban planning problems, to guarantee gambling as a source of state revenue, and to legitimise the existence of legal gaming halls in urban centres. Rather than protecting the player from the risks of gambling, Möll summarises, such parliamentary discourse and the resulting policy initiatives can be considered as a form of social control which seeks to protect society from the so-called problem of 'addictive gamblers'.

Completing the book is **Baptiste Brossard** and **Benjamin Hemmings**' discussion on 'Aesthetic pathologisation: Cinema, psychiatry and sex addiction' in Chap. 15. Taking a cultural studies approach to exploring representations of sexual excess (of which 'sex addiction' is argued to be a recent form) in Western films since the 1930s, the authors identify five ideal-typical narratives of sexual excess: namely, self-serving women and idealists (1930s); nymphomaniacs and reasonable men (1950s); emancipated people and 'squares' (1970s); one-sided and multi-faceted characters (1990s); and self-deceptive addicts and healthy people (2000s–2010s). Each ideal type is reflected upon in relation to psychiatric classifications of the period. What is noticeable in Brossard and Hemmings' analysis is not only the change in dominant attitudes to sexual activities portrayed on screen (as often reflective of, and in, the DSM), but crucially, changing gender roles in society which see a decline in 'screenwriting punishments' against women and the rise in the pathologising of (often) men as sex addicts. Yet this discussion should not be read as a 'progressive' narrative on the increasing medicalisation of sexual practices, rather the authors conclude that the Western cinematographic treatment of sexual excess has shifted over the twentieth century from *scripting* the negative *consequences* of excessive sexuality to *framing* the *anticipation* of sexual activities—that is, developing an aesthetic that problematises *desire itself*.

References

Adams, P. J. (2008). *Fragmented intimacy: Addiction in a social world.* Springer.

American Psychiatric Association. (1952). *Diagnostic and statistical manual: Mental disorders.* American Psychiatric Association.

American Psychiatric Association. (1968). *Diagnostic and statistical manual of mental disorders* (2nd ed.). American Psychiatric Association.

American Psychiatric Association. (1980). *Diagnostic and statistical manual of mental disorders* (3rd ed.). American Psychiatric Association.

American Psychiatric Association. (2022). *Diagnostic and statistical manual of mental disorders* (5th edn. text Rev). American Psychiatric Association.

Beck, U. (1992). *Risk society: Towards a new modernity.* Sage.

Becker, H. S. (1963). *Outsiders: Studies in the sociology of deviance.* Free Press.

Bennett, C. (2011). Methadone maintenance treatment: Disciplining the 'addict'. *Health and History, 13*(2), 130–157. https://doi.org/10.1353/hah.2011.0019

Berger, P., & Luckmann, T. (1967). *The social construction of reality: A treatise in the sociology of knowledge.* Bantam.

Berridge, V., & Edwards, G. (1987). *Opium and the people: Opiate use in nineteenth century England.* Yale University Press.

Bluhm, H. (Ed.). (2010). *Karl Marx/Friedrich Engels: Die deutsche Ideologie.* Akademie Verlag GmbH.

Bourgois, P. (2000). Disciplining addictions: The bio-politics of methadone and heroin in the United States. *Culture, Medicine and Psychiatry, 24*(2), 165–195. https://doi.org/10.1023/A:1005574918294

Campbell, N. D. (2007). *Discovering addiction: The science and politics of substance abuse research.* University of Michigan Press.

Campbell, N. D. (2012). Medicalization and biomedicalization: Does the diseasing of addiction fit the frame? In J. Netherland (Ed.), *Critical perspectives on addiction* (pp. 3–25). Emerald Group Publishing.

Castellani, B. (2000). *Pathological gambling: The making of a medical problem.* State University of New York Press.

Clarkson, J., & Kopaczewski, S. (2013). Pornography addiction and the medicalization of free speech. *Journal of Communication Inquiry, 37*(2), 128–148. https://doi.org/10.1177/01968599134823

Cohen, B. M. Z. (2016). *Psychiatric hegemony: A Marxist theory of mental illness.* Palgrave Macmillan.

Conrad, P. (2007). *The medicalization of society: On the transformation of human conditions into treatable disorders*. John Hopkins University Press.
Conrad, P., & Barker, K. K. (2010). The social construction of illness: Key insights and policy implications. *Journal of Health and Social Behaviour, 51*(1_suppl), S67–S79. https://doi.org/10.1177/0022146510383495
Conrad, P., & Schneider, J. (1992). *Deviance and medicalization: From badness to sickness* (2nd ed.). Temple University Press.
Courtwright, D. T. (2019). *The age of addiction: How bad habits became big business*. Harvard University Press.
Cromby, J., & Nightingale, D. (Eds.). (1999). *Social constructionist psychology*. Open University Press.
Douglas, M. (Ed.). (2002). *Constructive drinking*. Taylor & Francis.
Eberle, T. (2019). Variations of constructivism. In M. Pfadenhauer & K. Knoblauch (Eds.), *Social constructivism as paradigm* (pp. 131–151). Routledge.
Epstein, W. M. (2019). *Psychotherapy and the social clinic in the United States: Soothing fictions*. Springer Nature.
Flusser, V. (2006). *Die Geschichte des Teufels* [The history of the devil]. European Photography.
Foucault, M. (1970). *Die Ordnung des Diskurses*. Ullstein.
Foucault, M. (1990). *The history of sexuality: An introduction* (Vol 1). Vintage.
Foucault, M. (2008). *The birth of biopolitics*. Palgrave Macmillan.
Gehlen, A. (1972). *Die Seele im technischen Zeitalter: Sozialpsychologische Probleme in der industriellen Gesellschaft*. Rowohlt.
Gergen, K. G. (1991). *The saturated self: Dilemmas of identity in contemporary life*. Basic Books.
Gergen, K. G. (2019). The social construction of reality. In M. Pfadenhauer & K. Knoblauch (Eds.), *Social constructivism as paradigm* (pp. 259–272). Routledge.
Gergen, K. G., & Davies, K. E. (1985). *The Social Construction of the Person*. Springer VS.
Giddens, A. (1991). *Modernity and self-identity: Self and society in the late modern Age*. Stanford University Press.
Hacking, I. (1999). *The social construction of what?* Harvard University Press.
Hacking, I. (2002). *Historical ontology*. Harvard University Press.
Hall, W., Carter, A., & Forlini, C. (2015). The brain disease model of addiction: Is it supported by the evidence and has it delivered on its promises? *The Lancet Psychiatry, 2*(1), 105–110.

Hammersley, R. (2017). How and why addiction is socially constructed. *Sociology of Addiction, 2*, 1–18.
Hammersley, R., & Reid, M. (2002). Why the pervasive addiction myth is still believed. *Addiction Research & Therapy, 10*(1), 7–30. https://doi.org/10.1080/16066350290001687
Harbusch, M. (Ed.). (2022). *Troubled persons industries: The expansion of psychiatric categories beyond psychiatry*. Palgrave Macmillan.
Henzgen, D., & Meier, D. (2024). *Der Mensch, das Spiel und der Zufall: Eine historisch systematische Untersuchung*. Springer.
Heyman, G. M. (2009). *Addiction: A disorder of choice*. Harvard University Press.
Horkheimer, M., Adorno, T. W., & Noeri, G. (2002). *Dialectic of enlightenment*. Stanford University Press.
Illich, I. (1976). *Limits to medicine: Medical nemesis—The expropriation of health*. Marion Boyars Publishers Ltd..
Keane, H. (2002). *What's wrong with Addiction?* Melbourne University Press.
Keller, R. (2024). *The sociology of knowledge approach to discourse*. Springer.
Keller, R., Knoblauch, H., & Reichertz, J. (Eds.). (2013). *Kommunikativer Konstruktivismus: Theoretische und empirische Arbeiten zu einem neuen wissenssoziologischen Ansatz*. Springer VS.
Klaue, K. (1999). Drugs, addiction, deviance and disease as social constructs. *Bulletin on Narcotics, 51*(1/2).
Knoblauch, H. (2020). *The communicative construction of reality*. Routledge.
Latour, B. (1993). *We have never been modern*. Harvard University Press.
Le Goff, J. (1990). *Die Geburt des Fegefeuers*. DTV.
Levin, L. G. (2018). Addictions as a social construction: Knowledge's, public positioning, and state implementation of treatments. *Addiction Medicine & Therapy, 5*(3), 106–120.
Levine, H. G. (1978). The discovery of addiction: Changing conceptions of habitual drunkenness in America. *Journal of Studies on Alcohol, 39*(1), 143–174. https://doi.org/10.15288/jsa.1978.39.143
Lyng, S. H. (1990). Edgework: A social psychological analysis of voluntary risk taking. *American Journal of Sociology, 95*(4), 851–886.
Mannheim, K. (1980). *Structures of thinking*. Routledge & Kegan Paul.
Mead, G. H. (1934). *Mind, self, and society from the standpoint of a social behaviorist*. University of Chicago.
Negura, L., Plante, N., & Namian, D. (2023). The social construction of workaholism as a representational naturalization. *Heliyon, 9*(6), e17447.
Netherland, J. (Ed.). (2012). *Critical perspectives on addiction*. Emerald Publishing Limited.

Park, J. (2024). *Addiction becomes normal: On the late-modern American subject.* University of Chicago Press.
Parker, I. (1999). *Social constructionism, discourse and realism.* Sage.
Peele, S. (1985). *The meaning of addiction: An unconventional view* (Rev. edn.) Jossey-Bass Publishers.
Peele, S. (1989). *Diseasing of America: How we allowed recovery zealots and the treatment industry to convince us we are out of control* (Rev. edn.) Jossey-Bass Publishers.
Petry, N. M. (2016). Introduction to behavioral addictions. In N. M. Petry (Ed.), *Behavioral addictions: DSM-5® and beyond* (pp. 1–5). Oxford University Press.
Pfadenhauer, M., & Knoblauch, K. (Eds.). (2019). *Social constructivism as paradigm? The legacy of the social construction of reality.* Routledge.
Reichertz, J. (2019). From understanding to impact: Communicative power. In M. Pfadenhauer & K. Knoblauch (Eds.), *Social constructivism as paradigm* (pp. 292–310). Routledge.
Reichertz, J. (2021). "Wer mehr sieht, hat mehr Recht": Über die Notwendigkeit und die Grenzen der Säkularisierung von Forschung. In G. Betz, M. Halatcheva-Trapp, & R. Keller (Eds.), *Soziologische Experimentalität* (pp. 274–290). Juventa.
Reichertz, J. (2024). *Kommunikationsmacht: Wirkungen und Potentiale kommunikativen Handelns* (2nd ed.). Springer VS.
Reichertz, J., & Zielke, B. (2008). Theories that matter: On some pragmatic aspects of social constructionism. *Forum Qualitative Sozialforschung / Forum: Qualitative Social Research*, *9*(1).
Reith, G. (2019). *Addictive consumption: Capitalism, modernity and excess.* Routledge.
Room, R. (1998). Alcohol and drug disorders in the International Classification of Diseases: A shifting kaleidoscope. *Drug and Alcohol Review, 17*(3), 305–317. https://doi.org/10.1080/09595239800187141
Rose, N. (1999). *Governing the soul: The shaping of the private self* (2nd ed.). Free Association Books.
Rose, N. (2007). *The politics of life itself: Biomedicine, power, and subjectivity in the twenty-first century.* Princeton University Press.
Rowe, H. (2021). *Exploring the social constructions of 'addiction' and the consequences of their application within discursive practice through critical discourse analysis.* (Doctoral thesis), University of East Anglia. https://ueaeprints.uea.ac.uk/id/eprint/82239/

Schutz, A. (2012). *Collected papers I. The problem of social reality* (Vol. 11). Springer Science & Business Media.

Spode, H. (1991). Krankheit des Willens: Die Konstruktion der Trunksucht im medizinischen Diskurs des 19. Jahrhunderts. *Soziologica Internationalis, 29*, 207–234.

Suissa, A. J. (2006). Gambling addiction as an individual pathology: A commentary. *International Journal of Mental Health and Addiction, 4*, 195–199. https://doi.org/10.1007/s11469-006-9029-5

Sullivan, H. (2024). Australia passes world-first law banning under-16s from social media despite safety concerns. *The Guardian*. https://www.theguardian.com/media/2024/nov/28/australia-passes-world-first-law-banning-under-16s-from-social-media-despite-safety-concerns.

Thomas, W. I., & Thomas, D. S. (1928). *The child in America: Behavior problems and programs*. Alfred A. Knopf.

Truan, F. (1993). Addiction as a social construction: A postempirical view. *The Journal of Psychology, 127*(5), 489–499. https://doi.org/10.1080/00223980.1993.9914886

Valverde, M. (1998). *Diseases of the will: Alcohol and the dilemmas of freedom*. Cambridge University Press.

Venuleo, C., & Marinaci, T. (2017). The social construction of the pathological gambler's identity and its relationship with social adaptation: Narratives from members of Italian Gambling Anonymous and Gam-Anon gamily groups. *Journal of Gambling Issues, 36*, 138–163. https://doi.org/10.4309/jgi.2017.36.7

Wiesemann, C. (2000). *Die heimliche Krankheit: Eine Geschichte des Suchtbegriffs*. Frommann-Holzboog Verlag.

Young, J. (1971). *The drugtakers: The social meaning of drug use*. MacGibbon & Kee.

Part I

Theoretical Perspectives

2

The Ecological Niche of Behavioural Addictions

Baptiste Brossard, Emmanuelle Larocque, Nicolas Moreau, Dahlia Namian, and Mélissa Roy

How can we explain that some people, in some societies, come to experience their own desires through the prism of 'addiction'? As the metaphor of addiction has permeated Western cultures since the late twentieth century (Fraser et al., 2014), such an expansion has not only generated new

B. Brossard (✉)
University of York, York, UK
e-mail: baptiste.brossard@york.ac.uk

E. Larocque
Université du Québec en Outaouais, Gatineau, QC, Canada
e-mail: emmanuelle.larocque@uqo.ca

N. Moreau • D. Namian
University of Ottawa, Ottawa, ON, Canada
e-mail: nicolas.moreau@uottawa.ca; dahlia.namian@uottawa.ca

M. Roy
Université du Québec à Montréal, Montréal, QC, Canada
e-mail: roy.melissa.3@uqam.ca

B. M. Z. Cohen et al. (eds.), *Addiction and the Medicalisation of Conspicuous Behaviour*, The Politics of Mental Health and Illness,
https://doi.org/10.1007/978-3-032-06313-7_1

ways of talking about certain issues; it has also produced a pattern of subjectivation that concerns how individuals can feel, embody, rationalise, and live.

In the social sciences and humanities, several theories can help understand these generative processes. Some highlight the diffusion of psy-expertise and how it shapes human emotions and conducts (Rose, 1998); others focus on the production and circulation of labels (Scheff, 1966); some underscore the interests at play in the cultural domination of psychiatry (Cohen, 2016); others point to the unequal production of stress in societies (Pearlin, 1989). In the middle of these perspectives resides Ian Hacking's theory of ecological niches (Brossard & Chandler, 2022, pp. 110–115). This theory provides solid epistemological ground to approach mental disorders as both constructed artefacts and experienced realities; and it integrates issues related to inequalities, categorisation, culture and emotions, within a coherent explanatory model of the emergence of mental disorders at certain points of history. After introducing Ian Hacking's perspective, this chapter will draw on an extensive multi-sited study of behavioural addictions in Australia and North America, to analyse the diffusion of so-called addictions to sex, work and exercise through the theory of ecological niches.

Making up People

When a set of emotions, behaviours and thoughts is encapsulated by a category, such categorisation will influence what it designates, which in turn fashions the development of this category, which will impact what this category captures, and so forth. This observation applies well to mental health conditions. For instance, the category 'depression' was originally designed to capture a set of symptoms—sadness, numbness, and so on—but in channelling the production of related knowledge, through diagnoses, treatment methods, institutions and identities, this categorisation and the activities it orchestrated, transformed what depression actually 'is'. What was understood and experienced as depression in the nineteenth century differs from depression today, with contemporary experiences increasingly relating to a lack of motivation, productivity or autonomy (Moreau, 2009; Otero, 2012). Ian Hacking (1996) names these processual relationships between certain classifications and certain human realities as 'looping effects'.

Hacking (2002, p. 2) sometimes described himself as a "dynamic nominalist interested in the way in which naming practices interact with named things". 'Historical ontology' is another way to characterise his work on looping effects, taken as the interplay between historical changes in classifications and the impact of these changes on behaviours, perceptions, and identity, which then feed back into the classification system (Hacking, 2007). In other words: categories emerge and gain meaning in a specific historical context, influencing the way in which categorised people understand themselves and lead their lives.

In these reflections, Hacking's primary influence remains Michel Foucault. This is evident in his 2004 article 'Between Michel Foucault and Erving Goffman', as well as in the collection of texts *Historical Ontology* (Hacking, 2002). The very notion of the looping effect owes much to the Foucauldian focus on how knowledge, discourses, and institutions shape subjectivities. However, it would be reductive to interpret Hacking's work as merely a continuation of this research programme. His initial affiliations leaned towards the philosophy of science and language, and later he became interested in microsociology—claiming to be Goffmanian (Hacking, 2004, 2007) and sometimes referring to labelling theories, from which he adopts the idea that categorisations tend to become second nature for the categorised (Hacking, 1996, pp. 369–370, 1998, p. 70).

Furthermore, Hacking's work pays constant attention to the actors and processes through which looping effects concretely take place. This is why he inquired into the multiple—social, historical, concrete, material, symbolic—conditions in which looping effects can thrive, notably by analysing case studies such as multiple personality disorders, pathological fugue, autism or trauma. According to Hacking (2007, p. 298), for a looping effect to occur, classifications, classified people, classifying institutions and associated knowledge and experts must all interact. They do so through various ideal-typical activities: quantifying and classifying populations and their problems, creating norms, correlating certain issues with other variables, medicalising these issues, looking for their genetic and biological bases, sometimes normalising them, bureaucratizing them, labelling or claiming an identity for them (Hacking, 2007, pp. 305–306).

The Theory of Ecological Niches

The search for the social conditions of successful looping effects takes its most refined and complex form in the theory of ecological niches, formulated in Hacking's study on pathological fugue (1999). This theory seeks to explain the emergence of 'transient mental illnesses'; that is, mental illnesses that temporarily appear at a given moment in the history of a society before disappearing. Hacking (1999) explored the historical development of 'fugue states', a type of dissociative disorder characterised by sudden and unexpected travel away from home, accompanied by amnesia. Transient mental illnesses are influenced by the social and cultural milieu in which they occur and thrive, and more specifically, they take shape in 'ecological niches'; that is, cultural narratives, medical practices, and institutional responses shaping experiences and behaviours within these contexts. As outlined below, an ecological niche is composed of four 'vectors', which, when converging, offer a favourable socio-historical terrain for the emergence of a new mental illness:

Medical taxonomy: the behaviours and emotions attributed to the illness must fit into the medical conceptions of the time, such as psychiatric classifications. In a previous article, we contend that this vector should be extended to account for situations in which a category is not durably included in a medical classification, but still circulates widely in cultures (Brossard et al., 2023).

Observability: the disorder must be visible and interpreted as a problem. It must be caught by the police (as multiple personality disorders, involved in some public disturbances or crime; Hacking, 1996), customs (as is the case with pathological fugue; Hacking, 1998) or informal actors such as families (as with anorexia; Pestaña, 2006).

Cultural polarity: "the illness must be situated between two elements … of contemporary culture, one romantic and virtuous, the other vicious and tending towards crime" (Hacking, 1998, p. 2). For instance, eating disorders stand between the ideal of thinness and the disturbing figure of the self-destructive youth.

Release: "illness, despite the pain it produces, should also provide a certain release that is not available elsewhere in the culture … in which it develops" (Hacking, 1998, p. 2). In the case of pathological fugue, the condition seemed to provide individuals with one of the only possible opportunities to travel and escape their daily lives.

To enhance and extend this theory, we will present two arguments. First, instead of focusing on 'transient mental illness', we propose applying this theory to *any* category of mental illness, primarily because it is not possible to ontologically differentiate between illnesses that would be transient and others that would be permanent (Brossard, 2019). Second, we can also use this theory to analyse the emergence of mental issues in individuals. To do so, Pestaña (2006) suggested turning vectors into *thresholds*. While vectors delineate a space of sociohistorical possibilities, thresholds consist of biographical conditions for individuals to 'fall into illness'. Thus individuals have to: (1) be exposed to a label and endorse it, or be diagnosed with it; (2) be observed by someone, or by themselves, so that a problem is declared; (3) stand between several images or stereotypes; and (4) find in the disorder some relief, release, freedom or permissiveness not available elsewhere.

Methodology

Drawing on Hacking's approach, we collected and analysed data on the history, appropriations, and experiences related to sex, exercise, and work addictions in Australia and North America. This collective project involved a team of researchers, with each addiction being studied by a primary investigator—Baptiste Brossard for sex addiction, Nicolas Moreau for exercise addiction, and Dahlia Namian for work addiction—supported by graduate students and overseen by research coordinators, Melissa Roy and Emmanuelle Larocque.

Between September 2019 and April 2022, we conducted 26 interviews with key actors in the field of behavioural addictions, including specialised therapists, influential authors, researchers, and self-designated addicts (17 for sex, 17 for exercise, and 11 for work). The interview protocol for key actors was inspired by Hacking's 'vectors' and focused on several main themes: namely, their professional trajectory, theoretical perspectives and orientation; the historical development of the addiction; their views on the addiction category; the category's impact on their career; and the strategies used to promote specific representations of the addiction.

In addition, interviews with self-designated sex and work addicts were conducted both face-to-face and online, particularly during the COVID-19 pandemic, using traditional qualitative interviewing methods. The exercise addiction team employed a mobile interviewing method, which aimed to capture the embodied experiences of participants as 'bodies in context' (Moreau et al., 2023). A semi-structured interview grid was designed to explore the experiences and trajectories of the studied addictions, also inspired by Hacking's four vectors. This method aimed to better understand how individuals came to identify as addicts, their interpretations and understanding of the addiction category, the effects of the label on their self-concept and behaviours, and the strategies they used to manage their addiction. Note that the lack of scientific consensus on defining non-substance addictions complicated recruitment: many individuals self-identify as addicts without ever seeking advice from health professionals, who are, we have observed, often reluctant to 'diagnose' these controversial conditions—which is why we study 'self-designated' addicts and not 'diagnosed' addicts. Given that many individuals with behavioural addictions do not seek help from health professionals, we recruited participants through social networks, discussion forums, and addiction support groups (Larocque et al., 2022; Negura et al., 2023).

We also performed extensive literature reviews on the evolution of the specific conceptualisations of the three addictions (on sex addiction, see Brossard et al., 2023; on exercise addiction, see Larocque & Moreau, 2023; on work addiction, see Negura et al., 2023). Depending on the addiction, data collections included other sources such as clinical assessment or screening tools, as well as media analyses of newspaper articles. Moreover, in the case of sex addiction, self-help books, tabloids, court reports, online spaces (see Brossard et al., 2023) and cinematographic productions (see Brossard and Hemmings, this volume) were analysed. These complementary analyses aimed to capture data beyond traditional medicalisation processes (for example, those usually focusing on psychiatric professionals or pharmaceutical corporations) (Conrad, 2005) and examine the diverse fields where the addictions are unfolding and taking shape. Data were compiled in *NVivo* and analysed primarily through Hacking's theory of ecological niches. An inductive thematic analysis method (Braun & Clarke, 2006) was applied to each dataset to further account for emerging themes and unexpected findings.

Vector 1: The Production of Categories

For a mental illness to emerge in a given society, it has to be categorised as such. Focusing on the medical apparatus, Hacking called this vector 'medical taxonomy'. However, apart from sex addiction, which was shortly included in the *Diagnostic and Statistical Manual of Mental Disorders* (DSM), neither exercise addiction nor work addiction have been featured in the American Psychiatric Association manual (American Psychiatric Association, 1987, 1994, 2013, 2022) or the *International Classification of Diseases* (see World Health Organization, 2019). Beyond psychiatry, the diffusion of these categories relied on other actors and disciplines—the 'troubled persons industries' (Harbusch, 2022) that include the self-help movement and are bolstered by a significant presence in popular culture.

Sex addiction: While multiple notions existed to medicalise sexualities deemed excessive, the term ‘sex addiction’ was used sporadically in the 1950s and 1960s before gaining traction in the 1970s and 1980s, primarily through self-help groups that adapted the Alcoholics Anonymous model (Irvine, 1995). Its brief inclusion in the DSM, between 1987 and 1994 (American Psychiatric Association, 1987, 1994), did not grant it substantial medical legitimacy (Reid & Kafka, 2014), however it has become and remained the most popular category of sexual excess in the Global North since the 1980s (Reay et al., 2013). Despite this lack of medical recognition, the term ‘sex addiction’ has been increasingly used in academic literature since the 1990s, particularly supported by psychologists, therapists, and counsellors. The US-based centre, The Meadows, offering tailored treatment programmes for this ‘condition’, became the epicentre of such diffusion, notably through creating its own microcosm including signs of recognition (for instance, the Patrick Carnes Award for the lifetime contribution of researchers and practitioners) and scholarly outlets such as the journal *Sexual Addiction and Compulsivity*, which was founded the same year sex addiction was removed from the DSM; 43 percent of all scientific articles we collected in our research were published in this journal (Brossard et al., 2023). Also, figures such as Patrick Carnes, Clinical Director (1996–2004) of Sexual Disorder Services at The Meadows and founder of the Gentle Path programme, played a central role. Originally published in 1983, his book *Out of the Shadows* (2001) became both a cultural and professional reference, legitimising sex addiction as a clinical category.

Exercise addiction: While sport has been considered a healthy practice since at least the nineteenth century (Carney et al., 2018), the concept of ‘exercise addiction’ appeared in academic literature in the 1970s (Larocque & Moreau, 2023). Despite growing scientific interest, the category has never been included in the DSM. William Glasser (1976), a medical doctor, first described addiction to running by emphasising joy, elation and healthier living, while also noting possible symptoms of withdrawal and increased tolerance. In 1979, kinesiologist William Morgan (1979) compared exercise addiction to drug addiction—a comparison that became increasingly complex and frequent in the 2000s as the drug-like effects of exercise were examined in neurobiological terms (Larocque & Moreau, 2023). Nevertheless, as with sex addiction, the field of psychology has held the greatest authority over the diffusion of this label, producing psychological models to frame exercise addiction. From 1979 to 2017, over one-third of articles on exercise addiction were published in psychological journals (Larocque & Moreau, 2023). The launch of the *Journal of Behavioural Addictions* (2012) increased this category's exposure (Beaudoin, 2023).

Work addiction: The term 'workaholism' first appeared in the late 1960s. Wayne Oates (1968), an American psychologist and pastor, defined it as a compulsive, uncontrollable need to work, building on the Protestant ethic in which work was seen as a key virtue leading to grace, while leisure time was regarded as a source of guilt. Over time, religious interpretations diminished in favor of clinical perspectives from psychologists and health professionals, who began to consider workaholism a form of 'work addiction' (Di Stefano & Gaudiino, 2019). The category gained increasing traction in the 1990s, particularly after the publication of a widely cited article by Spence and Robbins (1992), which presented workaholism as the end of a continuum of work engagement, no longer including positive manifestations of hard work (Negura et al., 2023). As with sex and exercise addiction, although work addiction is excluded from diagnostic manuals such as the DSM-5-TR (American Psychiatric Association, 2022) and ICD-11 (World Health Organization, 2019), our literature review revealed that the concept of workaholism has had a significant impact on popular culture and everyday discourse. Movies, television shows, radio programmes, novels, and the media have largely contributed to make this category a plausible 'identity trait' for Western workers.

In summary, the concepts of sex, exercise, and work addiction emerged during the same historical period and have attracted growing scientific interest, particularly within psychology. These categories exist not only in academic publications but also in popular culture, despite lacking formal medical recognition. This highlights the need to consider, following Hacking, that an ecological niche may not necessarily require a condition to be included in medical taxonomy, but can arise from any large-scale, potentially decentralised, matrix of categorical production.

Vector 2: Observation Networks

For a mental illness to emerge, the behaviours and emotions it encompasses must be observed and framed as a problem. In this regard, all three studied addictions are identified and deemed problematic not only by consulted professionals but also by a diverse range of individuals, such as relatives, and 'addicts' themselves.

Sex addiction: The issues that lead to grasping the category of sex addiction are often detected in the domestic sphere. Both Canadian and Australian therapists reported that a significant part of their clients were heterosexual couples—typically, a woman asking for help after discovering her husband's infidelity or pornography-watching habits. By the same token, one-third of the court trials dealing with sex or porn addiction in Australia and Canada referred to child custody—wives questioning their ex-husband's ability to care for children after catching them watching pornography at inappropriate times or places (see Brossard et al., 2023). In all these accounts, the home becomes a space of scrutiny. Further, technologies of communication such as mobile phones and social media has become means of monitoring sexual conducts. In the case of singles who come out as addicted to sex, self-scrutiny is a major element: feeling that something is 'wrong', or concern over the amount of time spent watching pornography. This corroborates a trend we noticed in clinical tests—that is, around the mid-2000s, the decrease in attempts to detect sexual addiction via quantitative indicators, such as the frequency of sexual behaviours or thoughts, in favour of qualitative evaluations of individuals' relationship with sexuality (for instance, whether they use sex as a 'coping strategy'). This latter criteria can only be asserted as the result of a self-reflective process, involving *oneself* as the main observer of the healthiness, the motives and the meaning of one's sexual practices and thoughts.

Exercise addiction: Interestingly, while the field of psychology holds dominance in the diffusion of exercise addiction as a clinical category, psy-professionals are rarely involved in diagnosing the problem. Rather, training injuries often serve as a key moment revealing to an individual that their sport practice might be problematic: when forced to stop exercising, they often experience distress and symptoms akin to withdrawal. As one participant explained, "if you don't have your 'fix', you can be unpleasant, like any other addiction. If I wasn't addicted, perhaps I would have better control of my mood and perhaps I wouldn't miss it as much when [I can't train]". The possibility of addiction becomes more likely as, when injured, the individual seeks ways to keep exercising at the expense of their physical health. Moreover, the 'addict's' social network, including spouses, partners, parents and colleagues, often express concern about their close one's exercise habits. Exercise 'addicts' then tend to develop effective techniques to remain highly functional and attempt to evade this observation network's negative judgement. For example, they may alter their schedules to incorporate excessive exercise into their routine without arousing suspicion (such as exercising during the workday, finding a community with shared habits, or cutting back on sleep). This thus situates the site of observability within the individuals themselves.

Addiction to work: Unlike burnout or depression, self-designated work addicts do not suffer as much from fatigue and overwork as from the guilt, or sometimes status anxiety, tied to a perceived lack of productivity or the stigma of not being 'sufficiently performant'. People who self-identify or have been identified as workaholics report fighting, intensely and at length, against fatigue and manifestations of tiredness, faced with the fear of having to stop working. They thus neglect their health to continue working, in a pattern similar to exercise addicts. Moreover, the disinvestment from social roles outside work appears problematic to their family and friends. This establishes a spiral: the disapproval from family and friends reinforces the perceived need to invest oneself at work, which then nurtures this disapproval. As a consequence, family members or friends who feel neglected are the main observers of work addictions, along with workers themselves, when they feel that they are no longer able to experience pleasure and fulfilment in their non-work life, to the point of losing the very meaning of their existence beyond work.

To summarise, the observability of the three studied addictions is characterised by the relatively minimal role of health professionals and the importance of self-scrutiny. Although the identification of problematic behaviour by one's social network (family members and friends) is common in cases of work and sex addiction, exercise addicts often devise effective strategies to obscure the effects of their behaviour on those around them, thereby complicating the process of observation.

Vector 3: Representational Landscapes

For a mental illness to emerge in a given society, the behaviours and emotions it encompasses must fall between two cultural poles, figures, or stereotypes: one positive, or 'virtuous', and the other 'vicious' or negative (Hacking, 1998, p. 2). Drawing on Hacking's 'cultural polarity' vector, we will demonstrate that each of the studied addictions thrives in a representational landscape that spans a continuum between these poles, rather than a clear-cut division between the positive and the negative. This difficult positioning explains why the behaviours and emotions in question elicit social reactions often marked by misunderstanding. Individuals labelled as sex, exercise, or work 'addicts' are seen as ambiguous because their lifestyles straddle conflicting images, stereotypes, and representations.

Sex addiction: The cultural polarity vector applies effectively to sex addiction, situated somewhere between the figure of the pervert and that of the seducer. On the one hand, 'sex addicts', through their intense sexual lives, could be regarded as 'womanizers', or, in the case of those who watch porn or engage with sex work, as open-minded sexual beings; however, the suffering that accompanies their action challenges this interpretation. On the other hand, they could be labelled as 'perverts', 'sex maniacs', or 'lechers', but the deep suffering they experience prevents such judgments, particularly when, as psychological literature suggests, their behaviour is considered as resulting from childhood trauma (see for instance, Hughes, 2010). The ambivalence surrounding the social image of sex addicts is evident in the evolution of media and tabloid portrayals. In the 1980s and 1990s, the US magazine *People* used to depict sex addicts as "players", and the 'addiction' itself was contemptuously dismissed as a "fashionable disorder". This tone shifted in the mid-2000s when articles began to focus on celebrities disclosing their struggles with infidelity, tragically destroying marital relationships and entering rehabilitation facilities—such as the cases of Tiger Woods and David Duchovny (see Brossard et al., 2023). The figure of the sex addict made its way in Western cultures through a 'redemption narrative'.

Exercise addiction: Until recently, the academic literature focused primarily on the benefits of exercise, and the long-standing cultural infatuation with intensive exercise makes this positive pole much more visible than potentially negative ones. In this context, exercise addicts might appear as socially acceptable figures, as they embody normative health, attractiveness, productivity, and performance standards (Moreau et al., 2023). They are often portrayed as "type-As", "over-achievers" or "extroverts", embodying personality traits aligned with contemporary bodily culture and the valorisation of fitness, sometimes referred to as "fitspiration" (Holland & Tiggemann, 2017). In opposition to these virtuous interpretations of the excessive behaviour, exercise addiction is also sometimes associated with pejorative personality traits such as narcissism, neuroticism, perfectionism, and obsessive-compulsiveness—characteristics that can be interpreted as negative poles of psychological weakness or rigidity (Larocque & Moreau, 2023). In the case of self-proclaimed exercise addicts who have struggled with other types of addictions (through "addiction transfer" or "cross addiction"), this form of addiction remains perceived as the less destructive option: "it remains much healthier than not listening to the signals when drinking alcohol" (Moreau et al., 2024, p. 114). Ultimately, these ambivalences position exercise addiction as an in-between category—what one psychologist described as a "razor's edge", akin to a "yin and yang" phenomenon.

Addiction to work: Similar to exercise addiction, work addiction is marked by ambivalence due to the largely positive cultural representation of work in our society. Aligned with neoliberal ideals and the associated expectation to 'freely' commit to labour, encouraging workers to subject themselves to long working hours as a measure of personal value and merit, participants reported being "addicted" to the pleasant feeling associated with being recognised as high-performing and "ahead of the pack" (Namian et al., 2022, p. 31): "You're like addicted to the recognition that comes with [it]. You're addicted, let's say, to being told that you're better than your peers, to … [earning] recognition." So-called workaholic employees are perceived as highly and intrinsically motivated, efficient, satisfied with their approach to work, happy to exceed work requirements and, generally speaking, professionally rewarded. Furthermore, contemporary forms of management promote the idea that work should be enjoyable and fulfilling. However, while behaviours and attitudes typical of workaholics are encouraged in many workplaces, psychologists warn that they also pose a risk of leading to health and family problems—becoming 'bad' partners or parents—as well as eventual declines in performance and productivity—becoming 'bad' workers (Clark et al., 2014; Gorgievski et al., 2010; Shimazu et al., 2015; Sussman, 2012).

Thus, all three addictions exist within a cultural polarity: between the figure of the seducer and the pervert in the case of sex addiction, between the high-achiever and the rigid personality in exercise addiction, and between the model worker and the work junkie in work addiction.

Vector 4: Release

For a mental illness to emerge, its manifestations, or symptoms, must provide a form of release from otherwise inescapable social norms and constraints. In other words, the condition offers an escape that is unavailable by other means.

Sex addiction: Professional literature mostly emphasises the psychological aspect of release, in the sense of framing sexuality as an 'unhealthy coping mechanism'. For instance, Dew and Chaney (2004, p. 101) suggest that sex "has the potential to provide a temporary emotional or mental escape from the pressures and strains of real life." Through sexual activities and fantasising, 'addicts' appear to temporarily evade personal, domestic or professional challenges, with a momentaneous pleasurable activity. However, this relief is fleeting. Indeed, what might initially seem like sexual curiosity or a lifestyle choice (as a 30-year-old participant from Australia explained about soliciting services from sex workers, "I thought it was what guys do") tends to be reinterpreted as a pathological inability to conform to a certain—healthy and fulfilling—model of relationships and domestic life. Sex addicts generally seem to suffer from the challenge of embodying the ideal of a stable family life, characterised by sexual restraints such as monogamy, but also broader responsibilities, including maintaining a stable routine, making oneself available to family members, participating in household chores and financial management. Interestingly, the release from social pressures briefly allowed by sexual practices is linked to the participants' frustration at not being able to 'fit in'. As the aforementioned participant concluded, "I just want a normal life."

Exercise addiction: The reported motives for 'intensive' exercise provide insight into the constraints and norms from which addicts seek to escape. Exercise addicts expressed a need for "freedom", "liberation," and "connection" in a world where they feel both over-connected (to work, to technology) and disconnected (from themselves, others, and nature). One participant, for example, expressed that sensing her body (sweating, increased heart rate) aroused feelings that cannot be experienced in a home, school or work setting. For many, exercise addiction serves as a way to take control, escape, or slow down amidst the relentless and ever-increasing demands of daily life. Literature also suggests that exercise addiction may be interpreted as a compensatory behaviour to respond to certain social ideals, by compensating for a devalued social identity, whether linked to family, work or gender conformity (Cook et al., 2014; González-Hernández et al., 2021). In this sense, individuals can gain social recognition, and feel validated, 'elevated' through adherence to a valued sport subculture or community (Larocque & Moreau, 2023; Moreau et al., 2024).

Addiction to work: For workaholics, particularly women, work is often seen as an escape from feelings of alienation experienced in the family or domestic sphere. They contrast the dissatisfaction of 'staying at home' with the recognition they receive in the workplace. Routine domestic activities (such as laundry, preparing dinner, and watching television) are viewed as insufficient, meaningless, or boring, and they also lack the social and familial recognition associated with what is frequently termed 'invisible work' (Ciciolla & Luthar, 2019). In contrast, the positive self-image derived from their professional role is a source of gratification, opposed to the feelings of failure, issues or frustrations they can experience in their lives outside of work. The image they project at the office seems more favourable, in their eyes, than the one they project at home. This sense of 'alienation' in the domestic sphere then acts as a self-fulfilling prophecy, reinforcing the idea that it is through work above all else that one can achieve fulfilment and recognition, further weakening family or social ties outside of work.

From this perspective, engagement in sex, exercise, or work addictions reflects a difficulty in finding purpose, recognition, and excitement in one or more traditional spheres of life—whether family, work, or leisure—leading to an excessive investment in activities deemed to provide some sort of compensation, or release.

Enhancing Hacking's Four Vectors

Contemporary applications of Hacking's theory of ecological niches could be enriched by adapting his four vectors to the specific (yet perhaps not uncommon) features of behavioural addictions, as outlined in this chapter.

Firstly, our findings underscore the relevance of broadening Hacking's medical taxonomy and observability vectors. For a mental illness to emerge in a given society, it must be categorised as such: Hacking termed this vector 'medical taxonomy' because, throughout the nineteenth and twentieth centuries, the medical establishment held a near-monopoly on the creation and dissemination of health-related categories in the Global North. However, we observed that the social and cultural presence of the three behavioural addictions we studied extended beyond the medical community's reluctance to adopt these labels. This is why we propose a broader vector: a mental disorder must fit within the prevailing mode of *category production*—whether medical or not—in order to gain recognition and thrive. Similarly, while Hacking's case studies emphasised the role of 'traditional' institutions such as the police, customs, or the judicial system in the observation vector, our findings point to more diffuse networks of observation. These include personal relationships (family and friends), technological tools (for example, self-quantification apps), and self-surveillance. Therefore, it is more precise to speak of an 'observation network'. These adjustments demonstrate the importance of analysing the dynamics of identification and categorisation of problematic behaviours not merely in terms of formal professions, but rather through the lens of expertise, which captures a wider array of actors and forms of knowledge (Eyal, 2010, p. 3).

Secondly, our case studies show the potential to further refine Hacking's cultural polarity and release vectors. In the context of addictive behaviours, the clear two-pole structure observed by Hacking remains valid but less pronounced. This led us to explore the complex set of normative representations, a *representational landscape*, where certain individuals are marked by ambiguity, in the sense that, metaphorically speaking, they 'fall through the cracks' of the existing stereotypes that could label their behaviours and emotions otherwise. Regarding the release vector, our data suggests a tension between inner struggles and social strains—assuming these can be separated. On a subjectively individual level, addiction may 'serve' as an escape from trauma, personal disorders, or situational challenges (for instance, at work, in families). On a subjectively social level, the desire and difficulty to align with cultural expectations of a 'normal life' clash with individuals' so-called addictive behaviours and inclinations. Ultimately, the perceived and structural incompleteness of normative life, shaped by its social context—here exemplified by the strains of the domestic sphere—produces the dissonance between inner struggles and structural constraints. This tension underpins the desire for release and, in this way, extends Hacking's original vector.

Conclusion

As a conclusion, The theory of ecological niches enables capturing, in the same movement, several aspects of social life that are often kept separated by most prevailing social theories in the field of mental health. It incorporates the economic struggles and inequalities central to Marxist approaches (see for example, Cohen, this volume) while integrating elements of governmentality and subjectivity from Foucauldian perspectives (see for example, Taylor, this volume). It acknowledges the social construction of mental illness through labelling processes, as emphasised by interactionist sociology (see for example, Reichertz, this volume), while also addressing 'hard' realities such as suffering and the influence of social institutions. Moreover, it encompasses the impact of representations, as explored in cultural studies, and existential concerns found in phenomenology. In doing so, it offers what contemporary sociology of mental health might lack: namely, a comprehensive framework for understanding the social forces and the social conditions under which looping effects arise; or how, throughout history, certain patterns of thoughts, emotions, and behaviours stand out from the routines of everyday life to be labelled and experienced as 'mental disorders'.

Acknowledgements The research project discussed in this chapter was supported by a 2018 grant from the Social Sciences and Humanities Research Council of Canada (Grant No. 435-2018-0729; principal investigators: Nicolas Moreau, Dahlia Namian and Baptiste Brossard; research coordinators: Mélissa Roy and Emmanuelle Larocque). We are grateful to the many collaborators and assistants who contributed to data collection and literature review, including Jonathan Binet, Julia Brown, Ella Dilkes-Frayne, Emily Faithful, Benjamin Hemmings, Alexandre Larivée, Sarah Lambert, Lilian Negura and Isabelle Vu. Special thanks are extended to the editors of this volume, Bruce Cohen, Martin Harbusch and Jo Reichertz, for their careful revisions.

References

American Psychiatric Association. (1987). *Diagnostic and statistical manual of mental disorders*, 3rd edn. Text revision. American Psychiatric Association.
American Psychiatric Association. (1994). *Diagnostic and statistical manual of mental disorders*, 4th edn. American Psychiatric Association.
American Psychiatric Association. (2013). *Diagnostic and statistical manual of mental disorders*, 5th edn. American Psychiatric Association.
American Psychiatric Association. (2022). *Diagnostic and statistical manual of mental disorders*, 5th edn. Text revision. American Psychiatric Association.
Beaudoin, C. (2023). Peut-on être trop sportif? Les enjeux de légitimation de l'addiction au sport à l'époque contemporaine. [Master's Thesis, University of Ottawa]. https://doi.org/10.20381/ruor-29567
Braun, V., & Clarke, V. (2006). Using thematic analysis in psychology. *Qualitative Research in Psychology, 3*(2), 77–101.

Brossard, B. (2019). Why mental disorders flourish and wither: Extending the theory of ecological niches. *Social Science & Medicine, 237*, 112445. https://doi.org/10.1016/j.socscimed.2019.112445

Brossard, B., & Chandler, A. (2022). *Explaining mental illness: Sociological perspectives*. Bristol University Press.

Brossard, B., Roy, M., Brown, J., Hemmings, B., & Larocque, E. (2023). On the social existence of mental health categories: The case of sex addiction. *Social Problems, 72*, spad024. https://doi.org/10.1093/socpro/spad024

Carnes, P. (2001). *Out of the shadows: Understanding sexual addiction*. Hazelden Publishing.

Carney, J., McGannon, K. R., & Atkinson, M. (2018). Exercise is medicine: Critical considerations in the qualitative research landscape. *Qualitative Research in Sport, Exercise and Health, 10*(4), 391–399. https://doi.org/10.1080/2159676X.2018.1476010

Ciciolla, L., & Luthar, S. S. (2019). Invisible household labor and ramifications for adjustment: Mothers as captains of households. *Sex Roles, 81*(7), 467–486.

Clark, M. A., Michel, J. S., Stevens, G. W., Howell, J. W., & Scruggs, R. S. (2014). Workaholism, work engagement and work-home outcomes: Exploring the mediating role of positive and negative emotions. *Stress and Health, 30*(4), 287–300. https://doi.org/10.1002/smi.2511

Cohen, B. M. Z. (2016). *Psychiatric hegemony: A marxist theory of mental illness*. Palgrave Macmillan.

Conrad, P. (2005). The shifting engines of medicalization. *Journal of Health and Social Behavior, 46*(1), 3–14. https://doi.org/10.1177/002214650504600102

Cook, B., Hausenblas, H., & Freimuth, M. (2014). Exercise addiction and compulsive exercising: Relationship to eating disorders, substance use disorders, and addictive disorders. In T. D. Brewerton & A. M. Dennis (Eds.), *Eating disorders, addictions and substance use disorders: Research, clinical and treatment perspectives* (pp. 127–144). Springer.

Dew, B. J., & Chaney, M. P. (2004). Sexual addiction and the internet: Implications for gay men. *Journal of Addictions & Offender Counseling, 24*(2), 101–104. https://doi.org/10.1002/j.2161-1874.2004.tb00186.x

Di Stefano, G., & Gaudiino, M. (2019). Workaholism and work engagement: How are they similar? How are they different? A systematic review and meta-analysis. *European Journal of Work and Organizational Psychology, 28*(3), 329–347. https://doi.org/10.1080/1359432X.2019.1590337

Eyal, G. (2010). *The autism matrix*. Polity.

Fraser, S., Moore, D., & Keane, H. (2014). *Habits: Remaking addiction*. Palgrave.

Glasser, W. (1976). *Positive addiction*. Harper and Row.
González-Hernández, J., Nogueira, A., Zangeneh, M., & López-Mora, C. (2021). Exercise addiction and perfectionism: A systematic review of the literature. *International Journal of Mental Health and Addiction, 8*, 144–155.
Gorgievski, M. J., Bakker, A. B., & Schaufeli, W. B. (2010). Work engagement and workaholism: Comparing the self-employed and salaried employees. *The Journal of Positive Psychology, 5*(1), 83–96. https://doi.org/10.1080/17439760903509606
Hacking, I. (1996). The looping effect of human kinds. In D. Sperber, D. Premack, & A. J. Premack (Eds.), *Causal cognition: A multi-disciplinary debate* (pp. 351–383). Oxford University Press.
Hacking, I. (1998). *Mad travelers: Reflections on the reality of transient mental illnesses*. University of Virginia Press.
Hacking, I. (1999). *The social construction of what?* Harvard University Press.
Hacking, I. (2002). *Historical ontology*. Harvard University Press.
Hacking, I. (2004). Between Michel Foucault and Erving Goffman: Between discourse in the abstract and face-to-face interaction. *Economy and Society, 33*(3), 277–302. https://doi.org/10.1080/0308514042000225671
Hacking, I. (2007). Kinds of people: Moving targets. *Proceedings-British Academy, 151*, 285–318.
Harbusch, M. (Ed.). (2022). *Troubled persons industries: The expansion of psychiatric categories beyond psychiatry*. Palgrave Macmillan.
Holland, G., & Tiggemann, M. (2017). "Strong beats skinny every time": Disordered eating and compulsive exercise in women who post fitspiration on Instagram. *International Journal of Eating Disorders, 50*(1), 76–79. https://doi.org/10.1002/eat.22559
Hughes, B. (2010). Understanding 'sexual addiction' in clinical practice. *Procedia-Social and Behavioral Sciences, 5*, 915–919. https://doi.org/10.1016/j.sbspro.2010.07.210
Irvine, J. M. (1995). Reinventing perversion: Sex addiction and cultural anxieties. *Journal of the History of Sexuality, 5*(3), 429–450.
Larocque, E., Brossard, B., & Namian, D. (2022). Unpacking the labelling process: Framing responsibility in sex addiction. In M. Harbusch (Ed.), *Troubled persons industries: The expansion of psychiatric categories beyond psychiatry* (pp. 193–219). Palgrave.
Larocque, E., & Moreau, N. (2023). When sport is taken to extremes: A socio-historical analysis of sport addiction. *International Review for the Sociology of Sport, 58*(2), 368–391. https://doi.org/10.1177/10126902221104956

Moreau, N. (2009). *État dépressif et temporalité. Contribution à une sociologie de la santé mentale*. Liber.

Moreau, N., Larocque, E., Jaimes, A., Vinit, F., Quidu, M., & Favier-Ambrosini, B. (2023). Embodying or resisting social normativity? A carnal inquiry into exercise addiction experiences. *Social Science & Medicine, 327*, 115948. https://doi.org/10.1016/j.socscimed.2023.115948

Moreau, N., Larocque, E., & Quidu, M. (2024). On becoming an "exercise addict": Analyzing exercise addiction processes through the sociology of dispositional and contextual plurality. *Staps, 143*(5), 99–121.

Morgan, W. P. (1979). Negative addiction in runners. *The Physician and Sportsmedicine, 7*(2), 55–77. https://doi.org/10.1080/00913847.1979.11948436

Namian, D., Kirouac, L., Binet, J., & Lambert, S. (2022). «À mon travail c'est valorisé, trop travailler»: La construction du trouble de dépendance au travail: Entre capitalisme émotionnel et méritocratie. *Service Social, 68*(1), 27–53. https://doi.org/10.7202/1089868ar

Negura, L., Plante, N., & Namian, D. (2023). The social construction of workaholism as a representational naturalization. *Heliyon, 9*(6), e17447.

Oates, W. E. (1968). On being a "workaholic": A serious jest. *Pastoral Psychology, 19*(8), 16–20.

Otero, M. (2012). *L'ombre portée: L'individualité à l'épreuve de la dépression*. Boréal.

Pearlin, L. I. (1989). The sociological study of stress. *Journal of Health and Social Behavior, 30*, 241–256. https://doi.org/10.2307/2136956

Pestaña, J. L. M. (2006). Un cas de déviance dans les classes populaires: Les seuils d'entrée dans les troubles alimentaires. *Cahiers d'Economie et de Sociologie Rurales, 79*, 67–95.

Reay, B., Attwood, N., & Gooder, C. (2013). Inventing sex: The short history of sex addiction. *Sexuality & Culture, 17*, 1–19. https://doi.org/10.1007/s12119-012-9136-3

Reid, R., & Kafka, M. (2014). Controversies about hypersexual disorder and the DSM-5. *Current Sexual Health Reports, 6*(4), 259–264.

Rose, N. (1998). *Inventing our selves: Psychology, power, and personhood*. Cambridge University Press.

Scheff, T. (1966). *Being mentally ill: A sociological study*. Aldine.

Shimazu, A., Schaufeli, W., Kamiyama, K., & Kawakami, N. (2015). Workaholism vs. work engagement: The two different predictors of future well-being and performance. *International Journal of Behavioral Medicine, 22*(1), 18–23.

Spence, J. T., & Robbins, A. S. (1992). Workaholism: Definition, measurement, and preliminary results. *Journal of Personality Assessment, 58*(1), 160–178. https://doi.org/10.1207/s15327752jpa5801_15

Sussman, S. (2012). Workaholism: A review. *Journal of Addiction Research & Therapy, 6*(1), 1–18.

World Health Organization. (2019). *International classification of diseases-11*. World Health Organization.

3

The Triangle of Medicalisation: Pathways for Interactive Negotiation of Diseases, Disorders and Addictions

Martin Harbusch

The Increasing Medicalisation of Society: A Paradoxical Phenomenon

Civilisation has always been understood as a process of increasing individualisation (see Elias, 2020). With social, historical and political developments and achievements and the differentiation of social structures, over the course of history more and more institutions and organisations are emerging, leading to an ever-greater diversity of social positions. The related specialisation and complexity of educational pathways leads to a growing demand for individuals to adapt, which in the face of multi-layered institutional knowledge systems and the associated more complex behavioural expectations also leads to more comprehensive forms of self-control. In contrast to Foucault (2024), who, from a power-oriented perspective, particularly emphasised the historical development of increasing

M. Harbusch (✉)
University of Siegen, Siegen, Germany
e-mail: martin.harbusch@uni-siegen.de

B. M. Z. Cohen et al. (eds.), *Addiction and the Medicalisation of Conspicuous Behaviour*, The Politics of Mental Health and Illness,
https://doi.org/10.1007/978-3-032-06313-7_2

disciplinary and surveillance apparatuses, Elias (2020) focused on the transformative interplay of social and personality structures in 'the civilisation process'. The metaphor of the 'inwardness' of the human being, the necessity of the dichotomisation of the inside and outside and increased forms of necessary (self-)control in Elias' work, can be seen to be consequences of the civilisation process and not—as in the case of Foucault—powerfully advanced forms of human training.

Nevertheless, both authors refer to a development that has not yet reached its end point but, even today, continues to progress, especially with the further differentiation of medicalisation processes: namely, the process of the increasing individualisation of society, which goes hand in hand with the increasing individualisation of social problems.

The development of the medical and psychiatric knowledge systems for describing and treating social problems also plays a central role in this process (see Foucault, 2016). In today's ever-expanding concept of health, ever more physical and mental relationships are being elevated to the status of medical problems. In the context of 'addiction', it can be noted that not only do addiction attributions occupy ever more 'niches' (see Brossard et al., 2023, and this volume) of social life, but also that the concept has increasingly evolved from a previously substance-dependent, physically assumed phenomenon to a description of problematic everyday behaviours.

On the one hand, there are interested professions and institutions (media, pharmaceutical industries, educational institutions, psychology, medicine, and so on) that professionally bring the ideas of endangered health and new possibilities of illness, disorder, and addiction to people. On the other hand, it is the individuals, particularly in Western societies, who experience themselves in an individualised manner, and contribute to the reproduction and maintenance of medical and psychiatric interpretations in everyday life through their efforts at prevention, problem recognition and self-optimisation. In this way, social problems are shifted to the 'interior' of the human being, so to speak, especially in the orientation of the concept of health toward human bodies and behaviours. The dependence on societal expectations of normality, against which many phenomena and behaviours can only be discussed as problems, fades from view in this perspective. In particular, the debates about the medicalisation, pathologisation and now 'addictification' of society (see for example, Loose, 2015) adopt these sociological concepts of internalisation and individualisation of social problems, and thus criticise the expansion of medical and psychiatric interpretative power. Instead of lamenting the increase in the number of sick, disturbed, and addicted people, sociology recognises the powerful processes of institutional attribution and, with increasing patient numbers, addresses the problem of narrowing social normality.

Since its emergence in the 1960s, the debate on medicalisation has criticised the fact that many human problems are discussed individually as 'medical problems', without legitimately being a condition of 'health' in need of medical intervention. On the one hand, these are physical conditions that are not really diseases, but which are perceived and treated as medical problems in the context of current societal discourses and the expansion of medical possibilities. Misshapen noses, protruding ears, or crooked teeth are today framed as avoidable and 'medically treatable' body characteristics. Putatively problematic pregnancies, postmenopausal symptoms or pubertal mood swings are examples of conditions that are depicted in (psychiatric) diagnostic catalogues. In addition to these issues, complex human emotions and behaviours have moved into the spectrum of medical categorisations using medical, psychiatric, psychological and therapeutic terminology. For example, restlessness or a lack of concentration at school or in the workplace, poor spelling or difficulty with arithmetic, abnormal eating behaviour, difficulties in dealing with one's own emotions or those of others, and many other difficult or confusing behaviours that are interpreted as 'too noticeable', 'too intense', or 'too uncontrolled' have fallen under the purview of medical and psy-based professionals. These are examples of situational constructions of deviant behaviour which, premised on social evaluations—mostly on the basis psychiatric categories or ideas of addiction—are now entering the domain of medicine.

Rather than framing the above examples of physical and action-oriented disturbances as simply existing abstractly in the social sphere and to be treated in isolation, these and other 'problems' can be argued to be based on situational assessments of modes of being and behaviour (see Frances, 2013). It is only in a social situation that they can be recognised as problems and interpreted as such by interested actors involved in the process of defining them. The same applies to the concept of addiction. What behaviour can be interpreted as 'problematic' or 'uncontrolled' is not determined by the treatment itself, but by the definitions of both professional and private actors, who have to make these interpretations in any given situation.

Medically discussed interpretations have experienced an enormous history of success on the coattails of societal developments: medicine has gained cultural and social authority in recent decades (Ballard & Elston, 2005, p. 229), and with this development the American Psychiatric Association (APA) has steadily expanded the number of diagnoses in their *Diagnostic and statistical manual of mental disorders* (DSM), thus shifting more and more behaviours into the realm of psychiatric control (see Blashfield et al., 2014; Cohen, 2016; Dellwing & Harbusch, 2013, 2019). As a consequence, in everyday life an increasing number of professionals are working in social spheres (including those outside medicine and psychiatry) with naturalistic interpretations of social processes. Social workers, educators, caregivers, teachers, employees of health insurance companies or private and public counselling services can all be considered here. Interestingly, people in these or similar professions use medical/psychiatric/addictifying knowledge systems in a field that is not their own, thereby becoming laypeople of the content they use and thus also making themselves servants of medicine and psychiatry (Harbusch, 2023). They become 'troubled persons industries' (Harbusch, 2022), which, in their low-threshold services, institutionally control and manage deviant behaviours, and thus at the same time counteract the revolutionary forces of populations living in disease and poverty under the guise of constituting 'caring' professions and services (see also Illich, 2007, p. 156); a development that was more or less covertly recognised as the goal of state interventions at the beginning of the social work profession (see for example, Sachse & Tennstedt, 1991). Furthermore, as a consequence of these developments, the interpretations and self-presentations of people in the echo chambers of everyday communication (for example, Youtube, TikTok, Instagram, and so on; see chapters from Arnsten and Campell; Hammersley, in this volume) are increasingly organised along psychiatric, medical and/or therapeutic lines (see for example, Dellwing, 2019).

Increasing processes of medicalisation thus lead to widespread feedback effects (see also Hacking, 1995) in general, since such labelled behaviours are increasingly perceived and communicated in public perception and discourse as 'real' diseases, disorders and addictions (Ballard & Elston, 2005, p. 229), and in this way also have consequences for the (self-) conceptualisation of all individuals in a society. After all, interpretations of deviant behaviour change with the process of medicalisation not only for the 'sick' themselves, but also for people who come into contact with disruptive phenomena and behaviours in everyday life, for professionals involved in the education or care of others, or for concerned healthy individuals (Frances, 2013) who strive to monitor and correct their own behaviour in the interests of health and self-optimisation. Medicalisation is a process that permeates social discourse on multiple levels in a multidimensional manner (see Ballard & Elston, 2005; Meyer, 2012); this can be seen in the discussion on the increasing addictification of society where the complexities of the phenomenon and the multitude of actors involved become a key focus for our analysis (see Taylor, 2019). Thus, the sociological examination of the concept of addiction is not only part of an increasingly differentiated debate on medicalisation, but also benefits from decades of sociological engagement with the fields of medicine and psychiatry.

That medicalising interpretations of behaviours can now occupy and defend such a prominent position in public discourse appears as paradoxical to sociologists: on the one hand, the complexity-reducing, problem-naturalising perspective of medicine and psychiatry is played out every day and may seem like common sense to us (for example, we usually discuss and experience our own and others' behaviour also in dichotomies of normal and deviant, appropriate and disrupting, and healthy and sick). On the other hand, however, this discourse often contradicts the established perceptions and interpretations of those in society, who are well aware of the contextual dependencies of their interpretations. We experience and describe ourselves every day as socially, highly complex beings, who align our behaviour and our emotions with the circumstances of the respective situation, who cannot determine the meanings of actions or things abstractly without a surrounding social context, whose view of the world reveals itself every day anew, and whose reactions to situations depend on moods, fellow human beings, or places where the communication takes place. In short, we experience ourselves in contact with the world as beings with a highly complex inner life, who in every situation (must) enter into an interaction with an equally complex external world and its people. Social deviation is also a socially negotiated and contextually differently produced interpretation, that performs specific functions in a situation and depends not only on social constellations and their people, but also that which cannot be formulated as a deviation without a social context; this is particularly the case in the medical and psychiatric sector (see Hunter, 1991; Jutel, 2011).

Furthermore, medicalisation contradicts publicly established images of human beings in a society characterised by diversity. Especially in Western societies, the acceptance of human diversity occupies a central place in current political as well as everyday debates and seems to us today as important as it is self-evident in many areas of social life. Against the backdrop of these complexity-conscious self-understandings, the fact that unifying concepts of medicine and psychiatry are breaking into the social sphere may be a cause for some concern. Because they strive for naturalisation and unification, they openly contradict widely accepted perspectives of diversity and self-determination.

The Critique of Medicalisation: A Classic Field in Sociology

Since the 1970s (Pitts, 1968; Schübel & Friele, 2023), the term medicalisation has been used to describe the social development of the increasing transfer of social contexts into the knowledge systems of medicine. According to the sociological argument, social problems are detached from their structural and social contexts in processes of medicalisation and are related to somatic functionalities. The dichotomous medical representations of 'healthy' and 'sick' or 'normal' and 'deviant' encode everyday phenomena and associated human perceptions, sensations and behaviours (see Schübel & Friele, 2023, p. 2), replacing context-specific explanations in an individual-centred manner and placing the social world in a purely dichotomous order in terms of the functionality and dysfunctionality of bodies; a perspective that is understood sociologically as a reduction in complexity. In contrast to socio-scientific theories that understand structural or social determinants as the cause of everyday problems, medicalising interpretations are thus interpreted as 'de-socialising' (Schübel & Friele, 2023). Likewise, they distinguish themselves from ideas of the importance of individual responsibilities for everyday problems and the choices of people in their everyday actions, and are thus also to be understood as a form of 'de-subjectivation' (Schübel & Friele, 2023).

The critique of the increasing medicalisation of society is a field of sociology that is both vast and classic, first in the US—which can be regarded as an intellectual home for the emergence and course of the debate (see Peter & Neubert, 2016, p. 282)—and later also in Europe. When Schübel and Friele (2023, p. 5) understand 'medicalisation' as an umbrella term for the processes of medicalisation (Illich, 2007), pathologization (Dellwing & Harbusch, 2019), and therapeutisation (Anhorn & Balzereit, 2016), they aim with this differentiation to draw attention to the importance of medicalising interpretations in the multi-faceted and multi-perspective private and public interpretations of social problems, which today are no longer confined to the field of medicine. Firstly, medicalisation is read as an increasing medicalisation of bodily diversity, for example when it comes to deviations in standardised pregnancy courses (Ballard & Elston, 2005, p. 232; Oakley, 1984), different processes of aging and dying, and dealing with the diversity of bodies. Secondly, it can be understood as pathologising behaviours, for example when deviant attention spans in class are perceived as problematic (Dellwing & Harbusch, 2013, 2019), shyness as social anxiety is included in the diagnostic catalogues of psychiatry (Lane, 2007), or when female emotional expressions before, during and after menstruation are framed as mental problems (Caplan, 1995). Thirdly, medicalisation can be interpreted as a form of therapy, for example when the difficulties of employees with their superiors are reinterpreted as a childhood-related psychological problems caused by hierarchy-abusing parents (Flick, 2025). From the current debates regarding the contemporary extension of the concept of addiction (see for example, Brossard et al., 2023; Castellani, 2000; Clarkson & Kopaczewski, 2013; Courtwright, 2019; Park, 2024), this medicalisation schema of Schübel and Friele (2023) could be expanded to include the aspect of addictification; in other words, the problematisation of pleasurable behaviours, which come under suspicion using the concept of addiction and are shifted into the contexts of psychiatric or medical control.

In the view of sociology, illnesses do not appear as problems requiring treatment per se, but rather as the result of a negotiation between social actors and in which they are made into medical facts (see Hunter, 1991; Jutel, 2011; Peter & Neubert, 2016, p. 274). This also brings into focus constellations of professional and private actors who marry certain interests with a diagnosis. Against the backdrop of medical knowledge, these actors not only reproduce and create the knowledge itself and the social places where it can be placed into a situational contexts and codified into diagnoses, but create themselves simultaneously as actors in the respective field.

These processes and practices of creating social reality are the subject of sociological analysis, which can analytically accompany the emergence, changes and expansions of diagnoses embedded in social, political and historical developments in a process-oriented and power-oriented manner. In the sociological concept of medicalisation, social events and activities that are highly diverse in terms of content and form are reflected and appear as a single social trend which, in sum, means an expansion of medical responsibilities to ever broader contexts of social life (Ballard & Elston, 2005, p. 230).

Such a conflation of diverse social processes and practices into a single term can be seen as an opportunity both sociologically and medically, but at the same time it opens up possibilities for criticism. Thus, in the idea of a social 'trend' of medicalisation, diverse contexts come into focus together, which would otherwise initially stand isolated next to each other. The expansion of psychiatric diagnostic catalogues, interactions between doctors and patients, the development of new drugs in the pharmaceutical industry, everyday interpretations of social problems in everyday life, evaluations of uncontrolled behaviours, and so on, can all be seen as examples of the diversity of empirical phenomena that sociologists refer to when they discuss 'medicalisation'. All of these and many other contexts emerge in the concept as a phenomenon that appears to be more than the sum of its individual parts and that indicates directions, trends, shifts in the social construction of meaning, which could be less clearly addressed without the idea of a cross-practice logic of 'medicalisation'.

In the concept of medicalisation, not only does the current social development become apparent, but also that medical, psychiatric, therapeutic, addictifying interpretations gain influence in the public discourse regarding the interpretation of social deviations. But the category also performs the function of enabling other social phenomena to be related to this shift in public and private interpretative habits. For example, it could be noted across phenomena and in terms of social diagnosis that with an ever-expanding concept of illness, not only the idea of 'health' (formerly the absence of disease) is idealized and socially narrowed, and in this context, more and more people are becoming 'clients' of the psychosocial and medical systems. At the same time, a process of alienation can be observed, in which people, in their constant pursuit of health through medical and psychiatric self-reflection, are putting themselves under continuous observation and constantly imagining the possibility that they or others may fall victim to a potential 'disease'. They become critical observers of (their own) behaviours and emotions, and simultaneously laypersons of their problems. Due to interpreting and addressing their problems as individual problems, they consequently promote individualizing interpretations in everyday life. At the same time, they learn to understand the difficulties of people in the social sphere as naturalistic problems, to turn to institutions for solutions and, in this context, may no longer consider themselves as experts at interpreting their own problems in their own everyday lives (see Harbusch, 2019).

However, this advantage of the concept of medicalisation in unifying socially different phenomena can also be understood as a disadvantage, especially when it simply assumes a common connection of diverse events and actions. As Peter and Neubert (2016) fear, we run the risk of attributing unilateral partialities to the involved professional and private actors, and thus negate reflection on our own motivations for actions and the consequences of those actions. This criticism also applies to sociology.

Interested in medicalisation, the social sciences may miss other, central aspects of the respective context that are equally, if not more, important to its design. Sociology, which in the field of medicine is itself only a layperson, ultimately runs the risk in these or similar societal diagnostic statements of adopting precisely the paternalistic position that it attributes to medicine (Conrad & Schneider, 1980, p. 76; Peter & Neubert, 2016, p. 277). Medicalisation can be discussed as a social trend in contemporary diagnostics and performs a social function at this point; however, it is also important sociologically to note that medicalisation itself is also a social and communicative construction (for further discussion, see chapters from Cohen et al.; Möll; Reichertz, in this volume)

Early Criticism: Medicalisation as a One-Way Street

In the course of early critiques of psychiatry, which emerged in the 1960s (Szasz, 1961) and critically examined the moral and socio-political dependence of psychiatric diagnoses (see also Szasz, 1977), disease categories increasingly came under suspicion from a sociological perspective which suggested the medical capture of the social world (see Ballard & Elston, 2005). With ideas of 'medical dominance' (Freidson, 1970), 'medical imperialism' (Conrad & Schneider, 1980; Taylor, 1979), or a "medical takeover of everyday life" (Ballard & Elston, 2005, p. 231), authors used belligerent metaphors to criticise the codes and approaches through which the medical apparatus were taking over additional areas of social life and bringing them under their control. With increasing diagnoses of illnesses, medicine changed our understanding of illness and health (Illich, 2007, p. 32) by framing more and more physical conditions as medical issues, by changing public discourse about tolerable suffering (thereby lowering associated individual tolerance thresholds for discomfort and pain), and by concealing the rights to (self-)healing beyond the medical system as a legitimate possibility (see also Barker, 2014, p. 169). As a radical monopoly (Illich, 2007), medicine not only shifted the ways in which people were perceived, turning them into dependent clients of the medical system, but it also fundamentally impaired individual freedom, independence and self-determination, and thus became a powerful normative authority in society.

These early critiques of the dominance of medicine were taken up and elaborated in various critical contexts of the 1970s and 1980s. They received special attention in feminist literature (see for example, Ballard & Elston, 2005, p. 232; Oakley, 1984), with authors noting that not only had female emotional expressions always been considered particularly pathological to psychiatry, but that medicine also placed the female body (especially the female reproductive system) under critical scrutiny. Marxist-oriented discussions (see for example, Navarro, 1976; Waitzkin, 1978) spoke of a power-oriented creation of social roles in hierarchical terms which were legitimised with the help of the medical system, as well as the growing pharmaceutical industry that maximized its profits on the backs of patients, based on the increasing rates of diagnosis. Especially in recent debates about psychiatry, Marxist arguments are once again playing a role (see Cohen, this volume), reaching beyond socially constructionist, interactionist, and action-theoretical approaches in a structure-oriented manner. In doing so, however, such theorisations of medicalisation and power have become less important since the 1980s.

Expanding the Debate: Medicalization as Action

In his later and more moderate critique of medicine, Peter Conrad (2007) emphasised that understanding medicalisation processes cannot solely focus on medical doctors as key figures, nor on a unilateral medical-driven hegemonisation of public discourse (Schübel & Friele, 2023, p. 3). Conrad finds the assumption of an active subjugation of social reality and its people by supposedly cunning, strategically acting doctors just as implausible as the notion of an irreversibility of the medicalisation process (Ballard & Elston, 2005, p. 229). The hypothesis of the one-sidedness of its driving forces is empirically just as untenable as the abstract denunciation of an entire profession in light of its (sometimes very respectable) results.

Since the 1980s, the debate about the medicalisation of society has become increasingly diversified (Conrad & Schneider, 1980). This is in part due to the recognition that other profession groups within the extended medical and psychosocial systems also appear as important actors today, and are actively involved in the creation of medicalising interpretations with their own interests, content and action strategies. Already in early critiques, actors in the everyday use of medical categories were mentioned (see Illich, 2007, p. 84). At this point, however, they appeared as secondary instances of social action with a supporting role but no decision-making function. The interplay of disciplines in the public sphere was unilaterally resolved in early critiques in favour of the hegemonic position of medicine; a perspective that does not adequately reflect the active role of secondary, strategically operating user disciplines (see Conrad & Schneider, 1980, p. 76; Harbusch, 2022). Additionally, a changed perception of patients in the diagnostic process was also an important argument for advancing the diversification of the debate. This is because the early critiques overlooked the diverse forms of contextual involvement of patients (Peter & Neubert, 2016, p. 274) which they showed when seeking out doctors as well as in the negotiation of symptoms and (mental) illnesses (see Hunter, 1991).

Especially online, people who are not experts now play an important role in the reproduction of medical categories. Their views and practices can certainly also be understood as an act of reproducing medical knowledge—a kind of feedback effect (Peter & Neubert, 2016). Or it could be noted that the echo chambers of social media have always followed their own logic, and that current trends towards the use of medicalising interpretations align more with the approaches and forms of logic presentation used by online platforms rather than with the logic of medicine. Increasing medicalisation at this point does not necessarily imply a positivistic approach to diagnoses, although identity formations with reference to or in demarcation from disease categories are widespread on social networks in particular (Dellwing, 2019). However, it was not only important for a newer, increasingly differentiated medicalisation discourse over the years to take the constructions of medical and psychiatric interpretations seriously beyond expert cultures. Rather, it seemed particularly important for those affected by medical interpretations to simultaneously have access to their own voice in public discourse with the latter. Taking an active role in the negotiation of (psychiatric) disease and addiction categories may offer those affected a way out of the position of pure victimisation. Peter and Neubert (2016) point out that important medicalisation movements do not occur at hospitals or in general practitioner (GP) offices, but rather in the social arenas of support groups, subcultures, and/or in online communities. This is where increasingly recognised themes of physical and psychological suffering ignite and spread, which only translates into medical and psychiatric disease patterns as a secondary step. For example, the Alcoholics Anonymous (AA) movement was of central importance to the discussion and development of alcoholism as an official, medical category of addiction (see Ballard & Elston, 2005). Paradoxically, medicalisation discourse appears within affected populations—contrary to early power-oriented and Marxist perspectives—as a type of empowerment and liberation (see Ballard & Elston, 2005, p. 233).

In addition to a focus on clinically relevant groups, Conrad also emphasised the mobility of medical discourse, which eludes purely power-orientated critiques. If today, for example, almost all sexual preferences in Western societies are no longer considered pathological, or births are framed again as a natural process rather than as a medical event, or, in the context of disability, there a central constructivist discussion of types of social production of disability which avoid focusing on the supposedly deviant functionality of the body in a proto-normalistic manner (Link, 1998), then these can be considered as 'de-medicalising' developments that contradict the image of an irreversibility of the medicalisation process (see Conrad, 1992, p. 225). Furthermore, in this way contemporary political discourse appears in processes of de-medicalisation as central instances in the construction of everyday meanings in the first step and also in the second step, they also enlist medicine in their service. Conrad and Schneider (1980) note that increasingly more types of social deviance are being transferred into the realm of medical control and that the medicalisation of society can be read as a medical appropriation of social problems.

Thus, medicalisation—which cannot be formulated without contemporary interpretive horizons, transinstitutional negotiations and accounting logics, and/or political framings of deviant behaviour—itself remains a dependent variable. If one wants to say something about processes of medicalisation today, the question of the underlying paradigmatic interpretation of a society and especially the construction of social deviance always arises (see also Reichertz, this volume). Processes of demedicalisation in this context reveal another paradox of the medicalisation movement. For a medical system of knowledge that strives for naturalisation and rationalisation, it must become apparent in the confrontation with everyday interpretations as well as with the postmodern (social) scientific self-reflections of contemporary society, that their perspectives are to be understood as more political than medical and also more normative than rational in many contexts. Increasing rationalisation in the medical sense thus goes hand in hand with an understanding of one's own irrationality. In psychiatry—and especially in the area of addiction—this paradox is arguably coming into full bloom.

The Triangle of Medicalisation: Disease, Disorder and Addiction as Interaction

Medicalisation is a debate that addresses the handling of medical knowledge in various stages of disciplinary, institutional, cultural and social life and, over the course of its development, has identified more and more actors as not only involved, but also, in terms of action theory, actively participating. In this context, I argue that medicalisation today can no longer be understood as a unilateral power structure, but rather as a multi-perspective, interpretative framework. With regard to the reproduction of medical knowledge in various everyday contexts, both the content being conveyed and the structure-creating situational practices of the actors involved are up for debate, as they apply medical knowledge based on different motivations and strategies.

The debate on the addictification of society greatly benefits from the above discussion. Taylor (2019) can, for example, reconstruct the concept of pornography addiction, identifying the paradigmatic prerequisites, historical developments, and institutional and individual interests needed to pinpoint this problematic concept today. Likewise, Hacking (1995, 1998)—who moves between constructivism and realism with his concept of the 'ecological niche' (see also Brossard, 2019)—sees the emergence of mental disorders and addiction as an interplay of medical concepts, cultural perceptions, and everyday reproductions. The struggles and achievements of the medicalisation debate are directly or indirectly also reflected in the perspectives of some of the chapters in the present volume (see for example, Arntsen and Campbell on extreme sports and addiction attributes; Brossard et al. on exercise, work, and sex addiction; Lacey et al. on social media addiction), and it becomes evident that the comparatively young debate about the addictification of society can already take place in a very complex manner.

In the proposed 'triangle' of medicalisation (see Fig. 3.1 below), existing lines of discussion can be newly ordered and related so as to redefine the field in a unified manner and to indicate pathways along which theoretical ideas and empirical research can advance in the future. Even though the focus here is on the debate about medicalisation, the paths and negotiating positions outlined in the triangle are equally relevant for

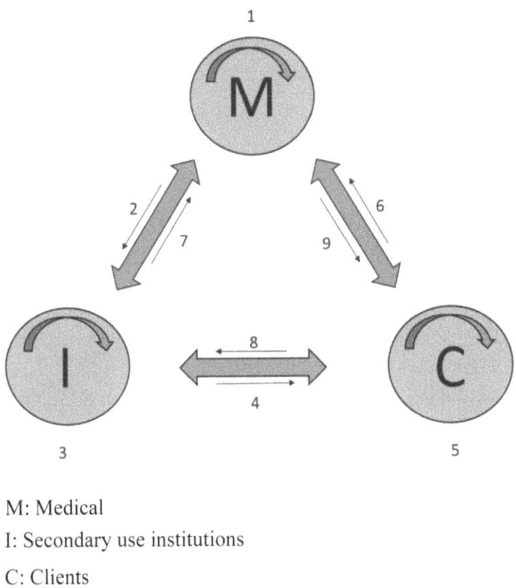

Fig. 3.1 The triangle of medicalisation. M: Medical, I: Secondary use institutions, C: Clients

the debates on pathologisation and the addictification of society. Other contributions have also attempted, with the help of a pictorial structure (or at least a pictorial language) to imagine a comprehensive context of medicalisation and to thereby give it direction (Conrad & Schneider, 1980; Hacking, 1995; Illich, 2007; Schübel & Friele, 2023; Zola, 1979). However, these representations so far have mostly remained within the logic of a typical cause-and-effect relationship, which—as with the debate over recent decades—has indeed become more differentiated over the years, but which cannot adequately and uniformly represent the multidimensionality and interwoven nature of the phenomenon.

While Illich (2007) and other proponents of early critiques (see also Zola, 1979) base their arguments on the dichotomous logic of 'top and bottom', and juxtapose everyday life with a world of experts, the more moderate types of critique use images that are more differentiated in terms of content, but very similar in terms of structure. In relation to the importance of medicalisation processes for social work, Schübel and Friele (2023) for example maintain a dichotomous logic of 'top and bottom', but also concede that the actors 'at the bottom' have their own interests and scope of actions. Thus, they speak of different directions of movement in medicalisation, which can either start 'at the top' or 'at the bottom' and then each one follows a different path. While "top down" (Schübel & Friele, 2023, p. 3) takes up the direction of movement of early critiques and discusses the power-oriented relationship between doctors on the one hand and their clients on the other, a "bottom up" approach (Schübel & Friele, 2023, p. 3) has also emerged from this relationship. By this, Schübel und Friele (2023) mean that the (self-)demands of a population that has been trained in medical vocabulary now also adopt these interpretations independently from medical actors, making it a guiding principle in their lives. Specific dietary habits, fitness orientations, or health-oriented work-life balances are examples of 'bottom-up' medicalisation movements, which are brought forward by laypeople in the form of expectations towards institutions of the medical and psychosocial systems as well as towards themselves and their social environment. A similar reciprocal relationship is assumed in the strategic interaction between various professions and disciplines. Referring to the dissemination of medical knowledge into the social sphere from medical institutions, 'push' strategies can be seen as contrasting with 'pull' strategies which arise from explicitly non-medical professions and institutions (Schübel & Friele, 2023). With the help of medicalising interpretations, application disciplines pursue strategies of legitimisation or professionalisation of their own content by actively adopting knowledge from other fields.

Conrad and Schneider (1980) discuss at least three different levels through which medicalisation processes can take place—these are figuratively to be understood as a kind of 'chain' since they also imply a hierarchical and temporal order of medicalisation. The 'conceptual level' refers to the active production and dissemination of medical categories in specialist discourses, and is followed by an 'institutional level' that marks the adoption of these concepts into everyday life (Conrad & Schneider, 1980, p. 75). As gatekeepers, medical researchers are introducing new categories into everyday practice before they are used by other professionals from medical and non-medical institutions to interpret social problems in a more routine way. Finally, at a 'doctor-patient-level', the results of conceptual and institutional work are available for the communication between doctors and patients as interpretations for non-medical contexts as well (Conrad & Schneider, 1980, p. 75). In this way, medicalisation eventually finds its way through the social and cultural interpretative patterns of society.

In a kind of circular movement, Ian Hacking (1995) contrasts the interaction between people and institutional knowledge systems as a 'looping effect'. Through categorisations, institutions create constructions of people that centrally determine both their own perspectives and approaches, and their own self-perceptions. However, these categorisations do not arise in a vacuum and do not function abstractly, but rather they arise while closely interacting with everyday life. Medical examinations and their results are aimed at 'moving targets' and thus are made flexible in their application. For Hacking (1995), science and humans are in an interdependent relationship with each other, which is best characterised by a circular or looping motion. In this way, dependencies and fluidities become visible in the definition process, whose directions—the possible starting and end points of medicalisation practices—become blurred in the figure of the loop.

The triangle of medicalisation, on the other hand, is a proposal to take up these and other aspects of the medicalisation debate and the related constructions of social roles and relationships associated with them and to re-systematise them with a common image. In this way, not only diverse conceptual understandings of past and new critiques come into play together. In addition, the different arenas for negotiating medical interpretations in professional and private worlds of participating actors can be seen at and between the levels. Similarly, the interrelationships between the levels of actors are evident. The numbering in Fig. 3.1 indicates the various levels and directions that may play a role in the negotiation of diseases/disorders/addictions. While levels one, three and five refer to intradisciplinary negotiation processes which have been hinted at but not spelled out in the sociological discussion on medicalisation/pathologisation/addictification (Frances, 2013), the other levels of negotiation are each devoted to the possibility of interdisciplinary negotiation. The complex dynamics of the medicalisation process outlined in Fig. 3.1 are discussed in greater detail below.

M: Medical

The classic sociological view of medicalisation—that is, the hegemony of medical and psychiatric discourses (see also Cohen, 2016)—is symbolised by the position at the apex of the triangle. According to the physicians (which refers both to medical doctors and psychiatrists themselves as well as to the researching and producing medical industries and interest groups), the movement of medical knowledge produced here runs from 'top' to 'bottom' (2 and 9). In his contribution to this volume, for example, Bruce Cohen follows this classical perspective of a 'top-down' movement based on Marxist theory. Also in this collection, the discussions from both Thaddeus Müller and Tehseen Noorani begin with historical considerations of the intradisciplinary negotiation and differentiation of medical knowledge (1), which then in the second step has consequences for disciplinary categories and the thematization of patients (9). At the same time, however, 'bottom-up' movements (Schübel & Friele, 2023) are also conceivable (6 and 7), which can be initiated either from the position of other (psycho)social, economically oriented, media and cultural or political institutions, or by clients themselves. A one-sided view of medicalisation as a 'top-down' movement overlooks the dependence of medical and psychiatric categories on cultural, political, and historical conditions. The processes of de-medicalisation and the adaptive performance of physicians have not been given sufficient consideration in the current debate.

Negotiations with actors in the 'outside world' have consequences for additional encounters between doctors and patients in day-to-day interactions (Hunter, 1991; Jutel, 2011), for intradisciplinary negotiations of doctors' roles as well as for conceptual readjustments of both medical and psychiatric diagnostic categories. In this sense, the medical profession can also to be understood as a group dependent on processes of medicalisation. This point seems to have been conceptually and empirically overlooked in the entire debate on medicalisation so far, perhaps because consideration of a more nuanced process appears counterintuitive at first glance and challenges the classic sociological critique.

I: Secondary Use Institutions

Recent research on secondary use institutions (see for example, Harbusch, 2022) has also shown that medicalisation/ pathologisation/addictification is a fluid discourse driven by a variety of motivations. In various arenas of everyday application in political, cultural and educational institutions or in contexts of care and counselling, medical and psychiatric interpretations as well as attributions of addiction are expressed in field-specific usage (Harbusch, 2023). These do not necessarily align with the medical logic of their production. Developed in the respective field, medical and psychiatric categories are intradisciplinary negotiated (3) and also in contact with the medical profession, neighbouring disciplines, and clientele (2, 7, 4 and 8), and are always interpreted with regard to the respective situation. Professionals involved in politics, economics, and institutional (self-)interest are also oriented towards their clientele and their interests. Thus, these groups act as important and powerful agents in the dissemination of medical vocabulary. In this volume for example,

Matilda Hellman examines the relationship between online reporting and public discourse (4), Gerd Möll investigates the powerful enforcement of political agendas using addiction concepts (4), Jo Reichertz discovers political motives for the oppression of less privileged populations in institutional constructions of gambling addiction (4), Baptiste Brossard and Benjamin Hemmings analyse the varieties of representations of sex addiction in cinema (4), and Mark Elam notes that technological innovations precede official, psychiatric conceptions of nicotine and gambling addictions (7).

Institutions are often closer to the clientele than doctors and can act as 'grey eminences' between the spheres of influence of various institutions and their terminologies, deciding which problematic constructions they want to take on and which not and, consequently, which solution pathways they want/can/must pursue. Sometimes they use medical arguments to legitimise their own actions and decisions in their daily work in front of their colleagues, representatives of other institutions, and/or their clients. In their analysis also in this collection, Cherie Lacey, Ian Goodwin and Antonia Lyons show how constructions of addiction arise as a result of negotiations between the interests of different economic and political institutions, and subsequently enter political discourse. In doing so, they not only refer to the influence of institutional actors on the topics in medicine and everyday life (4 and 7), but they also recognise the connection between different non-medical institutions as a central field of negotiation for addiction categories (3).

Sometimes, however, institutions also choose other discursive paths, especially in the interests of their clients. Under the guise of medical interpretations, for example, they may refer people seeking help to the medical or psychiatric field when they do not necessarily need to. In this context, too, a medical discipline that is dependent on only supposedly 'subordinate' areas of the psychosocial system is emerging. Instead, however, it is usually professionals from secondary use institutions who recognise and (can/must) express suspicions of a possible disease/disorder/addiction in the interpretation of broader social problems, so as to then transfer people into the diagnostic and accounting logics of the medical system (7). Recent research shows that many professionals in these fields are often aware of their crucial role (see for example, von Kardorff et al.,

2025), strategically use medicalising concepts situationally (or do not do so at all), and thereby place both their clientele and the medical profession under their control.

C: Clients

In the everyday (self-)interpretations of clients (on and offline), there are also various ways of addressing medicalising interpretations, which on the one hand arise in cooperation with other institutions or with the medical system (2, 6, 8 and 9), but on the other hand also develop in exchange with other laypeople (5). The contemporary success of medicalising interpretations is particularly evident from the fact that, although medical vocabulary is also reproduced in professional contexts, it is precisely in the micro-situations of everyday life that actors actively promote medicalising interpretations in their private lives as well (see Harbusch, 2022). For example, Richard Hammersley demonstrates in this volume how the public (de)medicalization of addictive behaviour also depends on the willingness of people to recognise these attributions (8 and 6). Similarly, the chapter in this collection from Lars Arntsen and Nancy D. Campbell uses extreme sports as an example of how people actively create addictive descriptions of their own behaviour (8, 6 and 5).

In conversations over garden fences, at school events, coffee gatherings, supermarkets or sports clubs, the problems of people and their interpretations are discussed and negotiated today in everyday life with the help of medical and psychiatric categories. Psychiatric diagnoses make this possible in particular because the logic of diagnostic catalogues interprets behaviours from people as symptoms of an 'underlying' disease; a logic that is consistent with everyday observations and assessments of actions. People thus become agents towards putatively abnormal behaviours of themselves and others. Kris Taylor demonstrates this, for example, in his chapter in the volume which profiles the self-descriptions of people 'addicted' to pornography (5). The success of medicalising/pathologising/addicting discourses leads to a situation of constant (self-)observation of actions and emotions, internalises related social conflicts, the relationship between normality and deviation, as well as the mechanisms of social control, and forces people into the 'tyranny of the public' (Harbusch, 2019) requiring constant readiness for self-opposition (5).

In contrast, the reproduction of medical and psychiatric vocabularies in everyday life can also fulfil important functions for those affected and, in this sense, can also be used strategically. This is because diagnoses can be seen as helpful and relieving, since they professionally address personal tensions and uncertainties with the outside world, thus providing a conceptual place with well-developed solution strategies (8). At the same time, the questions about social as well as individual causes and responsibilities for the development of the respective problems are also resolved against the backdrop of the idea of medicalisation. This is of interest both to those affected and their immediate social environment.

Conclusion: The Addictification of Society

The debate about the medicalisation of society has been going on for half a century now. It has not lost its contemporary relevance. On the contrary, sociological discussion in this area have expanded, and the struggle for adequate theories to describe everyday problems in an individualised society is still raging. In the process, the focus of the debate has shifted from the medicalisation of society to the pathologisation of society and—especially since the release of the fifth edition of the DSM (American Psychiatric Association, 2013)—the addictification of society. This article has argued that all three forms are basically the same phenomenon and that pathologisation and addictification are ultimately to be understood as further differentiations of the classical medicalisation discourse. After all, everyone shares the common logic of creating naturalising explanations for highly complex social phenomena and behaviours. In this context, the medicalised behaviours do not just emerge in a complex sociological context of family, work, education, care, and counselling; even the medicalising interpretations themselves conceal the moral, political, religious, institutional, monetary, and cultural backgrounds and interests, without which they would not recognise deviant behaviour as such and be able to define it in medical terms. Medicalisation is a discursive network that has experienced tremendous success in recent decades, especially in the areas of pathologisation and addictification, which currently permeates large parts of social and individual (self-)interpretation and involves various actors in different ways.

Sociology has responded comprehensively in the associated debates and has continued to differentiate itself in recent decades. The present chapter (and indeed, the present volume as whole) are parts of this process. Nevertheless, sociology has only had an outsider position in public discourse. Although previously unexplored counter-positions are emerging in the echo chambers of social networks, and people online are no longer willing to accept standard of medical interpretations without question, this is probably to be interpreted more as a marginal phenomenon.

The debate on the addictification of society has benefited enormously from sociological work over the past decades. What began in the medicalisation discourse with respect to putative physical abnormalities and continued in the pathologisation discourse with respect to unwanted, socially disrupting behaviour, now emerges as a starting point for the discussion of addictification, which concerns the problematisation of pleasurable behaviours. Recent research in the addiction field (see for example, Brossard et al., 2023; Taylor, 2019) demonstrates a theoretical and empirical complexity of analysis that has only recently recognised the medicalisation and the pathologisation of society (Hacking, 1995, 1998). The triangle of medicalisation proposed in this chapter has aimed not only to merely represent and organise the complexity of the entire debate—and this includes the debates on medicalisation, pathologisation, and addictification—but also to clarify the ways in which topics can advance theoretically as well as empirically in this context in the future.

References

American Psychiatric Association. (2013). *Diagnostic and statistical manual of mental disorders*, 5th edn. American Psychiatric Association.

Anhorn, R., & Balzereit, M. (Eds.). (2016). *Handbuch Therapeutisierung und Soziale Arbeit* [Handbook of therapy and social work]. Springer VS.

Ballard, K., & Elston, M. A. (2005). Medicalisation: A multi-dimensional concept. *Social Theory and Health, 3*, 228–241. https://doi.org/10.1057/palgrave.sth.8700053

Barker, K. K. (2014). Mindfulness meditation: Do-it-yourself medicalization of every moment. *Social Science & Medicine, 106*, 168–176. https://doi.org/10.1016/j.socscimed.2014.01.024

Blashfield, R. K., Keeley, J. W., Flanagan, E. H., & Miles, S. R. (2014). The cycle of classification: DSM-I through DSM-5. *The Annual Review of Clinical Psychology., 10*(1), 25–51. https://doi.org/10.1146/annurev-clinpsy-032813-153639

Brossard, B. (2019). Why mental disorders flourish and wither: Extending the theory of ecological niches. *Social Science & Medicine, 237*, 112445. https://doi.org/10.1016/j.socscimed.2019.112445

Brossard, B., Roy, M., Brown, J., Hemmings, B., & Larocque, E. (2023). On the social existence of mental health categories: The case of sex addiction. *Social Problems, 72*, spad024. https://doi.org/10.1093/socpro/spad024

Caplan, P. J. (1995). *They say you're crazy: How the world's most powerful psychiatrists decide who's normal.* De Capo Press.

Castellani, B. (2000). *Pathological gambling: The making of a medical problem.* State University of New York Press.

Clarkson, J., & Kopaczewski, S. (2013). Pornography addiction and the medicalization of free speech. *Journal of Communication Inquiry, 37*(2), 128–148. https://doi.org/10.1177/01968599134823

Cohen, B. M. Z. (2016). *Psychiatric hegemony: A marxist theory of mental illness.* Palgrave Macmillan.

Conrad, P. (1992). Medicalization and social control. *Annual Review of Sociology, 18*(1), 209–232. https://doi.org/10.1146/annurev.so.18.080192.001233

Conrad, P. (2007). *The medicalization of society: On the transformation of human conditions into treatable disorders.* John Hopkins University Press.

Conrad, P., & Schneider, J. (1980). *Deviance and medicalization: From badness to sickness.* Temple University Press.

Courtwright, D. T. (2019). *The age of addiction: How bad habits became big business.* Harvard University Press.

Dellwing, M. (2019). Half a liberation: Using parallel narratives of psychiatry in social networks and the success of psychiatric discourses in digital cultures. In M. Dellwing & M. Harbusch (Eds.), *Pathologisierte Gesellschaft? 12. Beiheft des Kriminologisches Journal* (pp. 172–196). Beltz-Juventa.

Dellwing, M., & Harbusch, M. (Eds.). (2013). *Krankheitskonstruktionen und Krankheitstreiberei: Die Renaissance der soziologischen Psychiatriekritik*. Springer VS.

Dellwing, M., & Harbusch, M. (Eds.). (2019). *Pathologisierte Gesellschaft?: 12. Beiheft Kriminologisches Journal*. Beltz-Juventa.

Elias, N. (2020). *Über den Prozess der Zivilisation. Soziogenetische und psychogenetische Untersuchungen. Erster Band: Wandlungen des Verhaltens in den weltlichen Oberschichten des Abendlandes* (32nd ed.). Suhrkamp.

Flick, S. (2025). Arbeitsleiden in psychosomatischen Settings: Zur (Un) Möglichkeit gesellschaftliche Strukturen zu behandeln. In E. von Kardorff, M. Harbusch & D. Robin (Eds.), *Zur Gesellschaft der verletzten Seelen: Neue soziologische Perspektiven auf Psychiatrie, Gesellschaft und Subjekt* [On the society of injured souls: New sociological perspectives on psychiatry, society and the subject]. Springer VS.

Foucault, M. (2016). *Wahnsinn und Gesellschaft* [Madness and civilization]. Suhrkamp.

Foucault, M. (2024). *Überwachen und Strafen: Die Geburt des Gefängnisses* [Discipline and punish: The birth of the prison]. Suhrkamp.

Frances, A. (2013). *Saving normal: An insider's revolt against out-of-control psychiatric diagnosis, DSM-5, big pharma, and the medicalization of ordinary life*. Harper Collins.

Freidson, E. (1970). *Profession of medicine: A study of the sociology of applied knowledge*. University of Chicago Press.

Hacking, I. (1995). The looping effect of human kinds. In D. Sperber, D. Premack, & A. J. Premack (Eds.), *Causal cognition: A multi-disciplinary debate* (pp. 351–383). Oxford University Press.

Hacking, I. (1998). *Mad travelers: Reflections on the reality of transient mental illnesses*. University of Virginia Press.

Harbusch, M. (2019). Eine Tyrannei der Öffentlichkeit: Drei Schritte der subjektiven Aneignung therapeutischer Narrative. *Kriminologisches Journal, 51*(2), 107–125. https://doi.org/10.3262/kj1902107

Harbusch, M. (Ed.). (2022). *Troubled persons industries: The expansion of psychiatric categories beyond psychiatry*. Palgrave Macmillan.

Harbusch, M. (2023). Reiserouten der Medikalisierung: Über Traveling Concepts und die verschlungenen Pfade zwischen Akademie und Lebenswelt. In T. Schübel & B. Friele (Eds.), *Medikalisierung und Soziale Arbeit [Medicalisation and social work]* (pp. 139–155). Springer VS. https://doi.org/10.1007/978-3-658-40507-6_9

Hunter, K. M. (1991). *Doctors' stories: The narrative structure of medical knowledge*. Princeton University Press.
Illich, I (2007). *Die Nemesis der Medizin: Die Kritik der Medikalisierung des Lebens* [Medical nemesis: A critique of the medicalisation of life], 6th edn. C.H. Beck.
Jutel, A. G. (2011). *Putting a name to it: Diagnosis in contemporary society*. John Hopkins University Press.
Lane, C. (2007). *Shyness: How normal behavior became a sickness*. Yale University Press.
Link, J. (1998). *Versuch über den Normalismus: Wie Normalität produziert wird*. Westdeutscher Verlag.
Loose, R. (2015). The hijacking of the symptom and the addictification of society. *Subjectivity, 8*, 165–179. https://doi.org/10.1057/sub.2015.2
Meyer, P. C. (2012). Gesellschaftliche Hintergründe der Medikalisierung. *Bioethica Forum, 5*(2), 52–58.
Navarro, V. (1976). Social class, political power, and the state: Their implications in medicine—Parts I and II. *Journal of Health Politics Policy and Law, 1*(3), 256–284. https://doi.org/10.1215/03616878-1-3-256
Oakley, A. (1984). *The captured womb: A history of the medical care of pregnant women*. Basil Blackwell Publisher Ltd..
Park, J. (2024). *Addiction becomes normal: On the late-modern American subject*. University of Chicago Press.
Peter, C., & Neubert, C. (2016). Medikalisierung sozialer Prozesse. In M. Richter, & K. Hurrelmann (Eds.), *Soziologie von Gesundheit und Krankheit* [Sociology of health and illness] (pp. 273–285). Springer VS.
Pitts, J. R. (1968). Social control: The concept. *International Encyclopedia of Social Sciences, 14*, 381–396.
Sachse, C., & Tennstedt, F. (1991). Armenfürsorge, soziale Fürsorge, Sozialarbeit. In *Handbuch der deutschen Bildungsgeschichte. Band IV. 1870–1918*. C.H. Beck.
Schübel, T., & Friele, B. (Eds.). (2023). *Medikalisierung und Soziale Arbeit* [Medicalisation and social work]. Springer VS.
Szasz, T. (1961). *The myth of mental illness: Foundations of a theory of personal conduct*. Harper & Row.
Szasz, T. (1977). *The manufacture of madness: A comparative study of the inquisition and the mental health movement*. Syracuse University Press.

Taylor, K. (2019). Pornography addiction: The fabrication of a transient sexual disease. *History of the Human Sciences, 32*(5), 56–83. https://doi.org/10.1177/0952695119854624

Taylor, R. (1979). *Medicine out of control: The anatomy of a malignant technology*. Sun Books.

von Kardorff, E., Harbusch, M., & Robin, D. (Eds.) (2025). *Zur Gesellschaft der verletzten Seelen: Neue soziologische Perspektiven auf Psychiatrie, Gesellschaft und Subjekt* [On the society of injured souls: New sociological perspectives on psychiatry, society and the subject]. Springer VS.

Waitzkin, H. (1978). A Marxist view of medical care. *Annals of Internal Medicine, 89*(2), 264–278. https://doi.org/10.7326/0003-4819-89-2-264

Zola, I. K. (1979). Gesundheitsmanie und entmündigende Medikalisierung. In I. Illich, J. MacKnight, & K. Zola (Eds.), *Entmündigung durch Experten: Zur Kritik der Dienstleistungsberufe* (pp. 57–80). Rowohlt.

4

The Communicative Construction of Addiction

Jo Reichertz

It comes to this, that a disease is what the medical profession recognizes as such.
Jellinek (1972, p. 12)
The concept of the normal is properly a variant of the concept of the good.
Benedict (1934, p. 82)
Is social construction itself not a social construction?
Gergen (2019, p. 261)

In his study on the emergence of the psychiatric profession, Robert Castel (1979) argues that when we cannot explain the actions of other people, we begin to wonder (as individuals and as groups) whether these people are possibly different from us. If we cannot find the reasons for the strange behaviour of the other person, then we often might label that person as 'mentally ill'. In this case, social behaviour takes place in a space that is

J. Reichertz (✉)
Institute for Advanced Study in the Humanities, Essen, Germany

B. M. Z. Cohen et al. (eds.), *Addiction and the Medicalisation of Conspicuous Behaviour*, The Politics of Mental Health and Illness,
https://doi.org/10.1007/978-3-032-06313-7_3

outside of what is *normal* and *expected*, and consequently, the concept of illness is used by a group of people to label certain behaviours of others not as different, but rather as 'sick'. Illness is therefore a social or communicative construction of reality; the statement that a certain person is sick is a social attribution or, in other words, a communicative construction of a person's identity.

The position that what people in a society believe to be 'real' is a social or communicative construction has been highly influential in the humanities and the social and psychological sciences since the 1960s. This theoretical perspective has repeatedly shown how deviant forms of behaviour, such as passionate gambling at electronic gaming machines, the intensive consumption of alcoholic beverages or the willing taking of risks, were regarded as *addictions* and as *illnesses* for which medical personnel were made primarily responsible. The gradual expansion of medical professionals' responsibility for such deviant behaviour over the course of the twentieth century has been referred to as the process of *medicalisation.*

In debating the concepts of addiction as well as medicalisation, many social scientists have taken the position that both are *social* or *societal* constructions. Yet in recent years, myself and some other scholars have suggested that we should instead understand them as *communicative* constructions. Therefore, in this chapter, I will take a communicative constructivist approach to understanding 'addiction', using passionate gambling as my example. In doing so, I will draw on my own empirical research findings to look at some relevant concepts from Erving Goffman and Stephen Lyng, and then make some innovations in my analysis, drawing on Foucault and his concept of the 'technologies of the self'.

Background

The Communicative Constructivism of Reality

In recent years, the concept of *communicative constructivism* has been developed in German-speaking countries in dialogue with the social constructivism of Berger and Luckmann (1967), the social constructionism of Kenneth Gergen (1991), the discourse theory of Foucault and the actor-network theory of Latour (Couldry & Hepp, 2016; Hepp, 2020; Keller, 2024; Keller et al., 2013, 2018; Knoblauch, 2020; Knoblauch & Steets, 2022; Reichertz, 2015, 2017, 2019, 2024). This theoretical direction, which is primarily based on empirical work in the spirit of the sociology of knowledge, does not see language and knowledge as the most important components for the construction of reality, but rather in power-structured *communication* (that is, concrete speech) from person to person (Reichertz, 2021, 2024) and the *power-structured public media debate* (Keller, 2024) regarding the content and practices of a culture. If, above all, we give primacy to public discourse and its significance for the communicative construction of reality, then we can also speak of the *discursive construction of reality* (Keller, 2024; Keller et al., 2018) or the *mediated construction of reality* (Couldry & Hepp, 2016; Hepp, 2020).

In this view, the communicatively constructed reality always and necessarily transcends the perspective of the individual actors, whose actions primarily represent the expression and result of either their conscious or embodied knowledge. However, these knowledge components themselves are also the result of communicative and media processes that systematically transcend the individual perspective. In this respect, communicative action serves to construct or rebuild the world, one's own identity and the identity of others. In this sense, communication 'creates' identity, relationships and the world (in other words, reality), because communication is social action with consequences. To be less precise, we could also say that communication *constitutes* the world, our own identity and that of others. Or that *communication constitutes identity, relation and reality*.

Construction Does Not Mean Arbitrariness

When communicative constructivism speaks of 'construction', it primarily addresses 'production'—meaning the creation of a reality that everyone (at least for a certain time) considers to be real (and without alternative). The term 'construction' therefore does not emphasise the arbitrary, but rather focuses much more on the concept of the construction of architects; here 'construction' means formation, the creation of a particular reality. Beyond the communicatively created possibility, there is no other more 'real' reality; there is only one reality, and that is the one that is communicatively created. In this respect, communicative constructivism is entirely compatible with realist concepts, as it does not denounce the communicatively created possibility as an illusion, as ideological or even as false, but says that there is only one reality for the respective society, namely the communicatively created one.

Objective statements are certainly possible about this communicatively created reality, if 'objective' is translated as 'socially shared'. Communicative constructivism is therefore not 'radically' constructivist or relativist, but clearly differentiates itself from both. What is communicatively created is 'real' because it is real for the respective society and also has real consequences. Socially shared statements are possible about this reality and its consequences—statements that can be substantiated on the basis of empirical research. It is very easy to distinguish between 'fake news' and communicative constructions with *good reason*, because whoever can explain more of social reality with their constructions, whoever can give more good reasons, is also more right; or, in short, *whoever sees more is more right* (see for example, Reichertz, 2021).

Passion: A Kind of Self-Destruction or Self-Punishment?

One might argue that, while there is a tendency in the psychological sciences (and perhaps the pharmaceutical industry) to pathologise various human behaviours that were once considered 'normal' (see for example, Cohen, 2016; Schivelbusch, 1992; Wiesemann, 2000), gambling with money also has a *destructive* side. For it could ruin the lives of gamblers and the lives of those close to them. Gambling on slot machines or 'pokies' is therefore a self-destructive strategy (regardless of what the players themselves think of it). Such an interpretation is essentially based on the psychoanalytic understanding of gambling addiction brought into the world by Sigmund Freud.

Partly coinciding with this view, Freud theorised that gamblers do not gamble for money, but for excitement. Thus, in his perceptive 1928 article on Dostoevsky's passion for gambling, Freud (1969, p. 283) writes that "Dostoevsky was perceptive enough to recognize it [his gambling as a problem], and honest enough to confess it. He knew the main thing was play in and of itself, *le jeu pour le jeu*." At this point, Freud (1969, p. 283) quotes (without citing a source) a letter by Dostoevsky in which he writes about his motivation for gambling: "I swear to you, it [his gambling] is not a matter of greed, although I certainly needed money above all else." But behind this fun of playing the game, according to Freud, there was something else (and here we no longer agree with his argument): namely, the desire for self-punishment deeply rooted in the gambler's personality and biography. "All the details of his libidinously nonsensical behaviour prove this and something else", argued Freud (1969, p. 283) of the gambler, "[h]e never rested, he had not lost everything. Play was for him also a way of self-punishment."

This psychoanalytic reading of passionate gambling with money was later expanded by Bergler (1958) into a theory that passionate gamblers would rebel against the authority of their parents. I don't think this statement is true. However, I can only note here that this theory is again a way of explaining unusual behaviour in medical terms and then certifying passionate gamblers as having problems with their mental health.

The Communicative Construction of Medicalisation

A sociology that deals with the communicative construction of knowledge must always be aware that its own constructions, no matter how plausible they may seem to a society or a group of people, are also constructions. In other words, there is nothing in the culture of a society that is beyond the social perspective; one always remains in the discourse of one's society, and thus also expresses it, no matter how much one may try to resist it. This also applies to the concept of medicalisation—it too is a communicative construction, albeit a construction of psychotherapists and sociologists, but without doubt a construction, albeit a construction with good reasons.

In periods when passionate gambling was considered as a moral problem someone was understood as either possessed by 'the gambling devil' (as it was during the Middle Ages; see Quassowski, 1921; Reith, 1999) or of bad character. This meant that either religion and the priests or education and the teachers were in charge of managing this social problem (Möll, 2021). When it was considered as a legal problem, gambling was forbidden—and law and the police were in charge (Quassowski, 1921).

According to Peter Adams (2023, pp. 90–113), the 'discovery of mental illness' by the psychiatrists Emil Kraepelin (1856–1926) and Robert Spitzer (1932–2015) played a major role in the process of medicalisation. Kraepelin and Spitzer succeeded in establishing physical illness as a metaphor for mental illness: in this view, just as the body can become ill due to certain substances or due to certain stresses, the mind is also said to become ill due to certain substances or overloads. This 'discovery' of mental illness was accompanied by the relabelling of addiction as a special form of mental disorder. This view has largely prevailed in recent decades (Möll, 2021), and it has become normal to speak of *mental* illness and to build a healthcare system around mental pathologies that correspond to the nosology for physical illnesses (for a socio-historical overview of addiction, see the Introduction chapter in this volume).

As I have outlined in my previous research (Möll, 2021; Reichertz, 2012, 2018; Reichertz et al., 2010, 2011), in the gambling halls people play with great passion and great willingness to suffer—and they will do this over and over again. The latter probably accounts for the fact that, in the past few decades, the somatising term of addiction has established itself for the passion to play at slot machines. In this way, an attempt is made to recode the passion for repeatedly getting involved in dangerous situations in a medical and scientific discourse, and to grasp the temptation of adventure as an addiction or pathology.

Therefore the cause of passionate gambling is today seen as an expression of physical or psychological dysfunctionality (see also Cohen, 2016; Rose, 1999, 2007). This 'problematic' behaviour is now understood as a disorder/disease that should or must be treated medically. Doctors and therapists are now responsible. There is no doubt that this view of passionate gambling is also a communicative construction, albeit a communicative construction *with good reasons.* In my opinion, such an explanation can explain the behaviour of players much better than the labels of addiction and illness. The creation of the 'pathological gambler' is an expression of the process of *medicalisation* society is currently undergoing (Campbell, 2008, 2012; Castellani, 2000;). In view of the resulting opportunities and the expansion of the range of therapies on offer, the German magazine *Der Spiegel* speaks of a 'jackpot for therapists' (Schmidt, 2012, p. 47) and social scientists speak of 'medicalisation' (Conrad, 1992).

Informed by the *sociology of knowledge*, we can take a closer look at the circumstances that have led to the prevailing communicative construction that passionate gambling is an addiction (see also the field of critical addiction studies, for example Fraser et al., 2014; Keane, 2002; Palm, 2023; Sedgwick, 1993; Valverde, 1998). The term 'medicalisation' addresses the "process by which nonmedical problems become defined and treated as medical problems, usually in terms of illness and disorder" (Conrad, 1992, p. 209; Conrad & Schneider, 1980). For Conrad (2009, p. 480), medicalisation goes "far beyond psychiatry and was not always the product of medical imperialism, but of more complex social forces". By medicalising the passion to prove oneself in risk and call it an addiction one has indeed explained why people do something that is economically absurd.

The thesis of medicalisation, mainly brought into play by Thomas Szasz (1961, 1970), Ronald D. Laing (1971, 1985) and Laing and Cooper (1964), Irving Zola (1972), and Ivan Illich (1976), and then elaborated on by Peter Conrad and Joseph Schneider (1980, see also Conrad, 1992, 2007) as well as Michel Foucault (2003), assumes that what is considered medical knowledge owes much to historical and social processes. 'Medicalisation' is the term for the social process that began at the end of the nineteenth century and continues to this day, which conceptualises and attempts to understand and treat certain human behaviours that society considers harmful (such as alcohol and tobacco consumption, but also the use of drugs and medications, and increasingly, the use of media, gambling and much more) as *medical* rather than religious or criminal problems.

This process is largely driven by the changes in scientific knowledge about the human body and the human soul in the eighteenth and nineteenth centuries, but certainly also by the increased importance and influence of medical professionals and a health complex made up of doctors and pharmaceutical companies, as well as various providers of therapies and therapy facilities. In the course of this process, more and more expressions of life are declared to be the area of responsibility of medicine, and then understood as a disease or disorder, which are not only medically and therapeutically treatable, but *should* or *must* be treated. It is therefore also an expression of a historical tendency (Foucault 2003) to summarise human action, but above all social problems, in medical terms and also to treat them medically (see also Rose, 1999, 2007). Assessing a problematic activity as an addiction worthy of treatment is one form of medicalisation that sees the cause of a person's impaired or disturbed behaviour as a mental health issue (Dellwing & Harbusch, 2019; Schetsche, 2013; Schmidt-Semisch, 2016). Another form of medicalisation, however, is to label *substances* that produce intoxication as poison that ultimately harms or destroys the user (see for example, Schivelbusch, 1992). Whichever meaning one chooses, medical professionals are always called upon to 'treat' and 'cure' this problem.

What is special about this process is that responsibility for social problems is attributed to the problematic behaviour of *individuals* and they are held responsible for it. The individual is thus certified as having a pathological abnormality that, especially here, can be cured by experts using their expert knowledge, practices and pharmacological means (Anhorn & Balzereit, 2016; Harbusch, 2022). In recent decades, this view has become widespread, which has also led to the emergence of new therapies, hospitals and clinics for the treatment of addiction. As Wiesemann (2000, p. 11) has summarised this process of the medical capture of social problems,

> By naming the causes of diseases, medicine always exerts a direct influence on their social management and control. Once a medical cause has been identified, both those responsible and those to blame are named, competences are defined and areas of responsibility assigned.

The concept of medicalisation was popularised in the writings of Thomas Szasz (1961), who argued that illness was invented by doctors in the interests of medical professionals and the state in order to better contain and control undesirable behaviour in society. For him, psychiatry, as the historical successor to the Inquisition (Szasz, 1970, 1979a, 1979b), clearly adopts the position of the rulers. He claims that the manual of the witch hunters (the *Malleus Maleficarum*) is comparable to the American Psychiatric Association's *Diagnostic and Statistical Manual of Mental Disorders* (the DSM) (Szasz, 1970). For Szasz (1970, p. 63), there is a fundamental separation and conflict between those "who hold power and use it to oppress others, and those who are oppressed by power and seek to free themselves of it." 'Health' and 'illness' in this view are the result of communicative and discursive constructions (Anhorn & Balzereit, 2016; Feustel et al., 2019; Herwig-Lempp, 1987; Netherland, 2012; Reichertz, 2018; Reichertz et al., 2010; Schmidt, 1999, 2012; Wiesemann, 2000), which, in a power-structured process, also result from medicine extending its jurisdiction to social behaviour that was previously considered either a moral or legal problem.

Of course, the discovery and rise of the concept of medicalisation is a result of a historically situated process that did not emerge by chance in the 1960s with the anti-psychiatry movement. Just as the term 'communicative construction' is a communicative construction, the concept of medicalisation is also a communicative construction that can certainly be explained sociologically. It is also a resistance to the prevailing social culture of adaptation, incorporation and governance of the seemingly objective criteria of a neutral medical culture. Because this is the case, leading authors in this discourse have expressed criticism of the concept of medicalisation (Kaye, 2012; Keane, 2004, 2009; Palm, 2023; Valverde, 1998). But, as already explained, acknowledging that a sociological explanation is historically situated does not necessarily make it a 'bad' explanation, rather the decisive point is what one can explain through this account—that is, whether one understands more with this approach compared to others. And here, in my view, the concept of medicalisation is very helpful.

Addiction as a Specific Form of Being Different

Currently, the altered *brain* is very much held responsible for addiction and, in particular, the genes associated with the dopamine system (Cohen, this volume; Heather et al., 2022; Lawrence et al., 2003; Molina et al., 2000; Wise, 1994). Computer-generated images of altered neuro-structures are often shown to prove that the brain and the production of neurotransmitters have changed as a result of human behaviour, and that the brain ultimately incites people to repeat a certain action (for instance, sex, gambling, or drug taking) again and again.

The bottom line is that, if you are prepared to call it a disease, addiction is a very *special* disease. Firstly, this is because medical science has yet to determine the specific biological mechanism that causes the disease, describe what effect this mechanism has, and explain how this disease-causing mechanism can be cured by a specific therapy. None of this seems to be the case with much of what is currently categorised as 'addiction' (see also Wiesemann, 2000, p. 47). Secondly, addiction is special because this term is used to describe all those behaviours of people which are outside the norm and which are regarded by society as inappropriate or morally reprehensible because they disrupt the moral order of a society, impair a person's ability to work, and/or are a bad example to others (Illich, 1976; Möll, this volume; Schivelbusch, 1992; Szasz, 1979a, 1979b). Additionally, addiction is a special case because it shakes up the cultural norms of a society. As Wiesemann argues, the disease of addiction calls into question,

> what people in the western world today consider to be their highest values: Freedom, individuality and rationality. … It deceives reason and replaces individuality with the mechanism of an external compulsion. It is a secret illness, perhaps the secret illness of modernity par excellence, because it leaves the subject's self-certainty unimpaired and yet it is precisely the

> subject's most important characteristics that are called into question.... It is not a disease of manifest symptoms or of disturbed well-being. An addict can perhaps be someone who subjectively still feels well. Everyone is called upon to constantly check whether their consumption of alcohol and nicotine, as well as their relationship to work and sport, does not already show signs of addiction. (Wiesemann, 2000, p. 7; see also Valverde, 1998).

If we take the idea of the social or communicative construction of social reality seriously, then from the perspective of the sociology of knowledge, the behaviour that doctors have been calling addiction for the last two centuries is a special form of being different, of being outside normality, which, in order to be able to deal with it better, is now called an illness for which a certain professional group—namely doctors—are responsible.

In my view, this does not do justice to the actions of gamblers. Addiction is not the answer to the question as to the reasons for gambling at slot machines, but addiction is the current social discourse of medicalisation imposed on events in gambling halls. This discourse restricts the freedom of the individual to do risky things of their own volition by doctors and therapists working to 'free' the addicts from their illness (Dellwing & Tietz, 2019; Schetsche, 2013).

The addiction discourse offers *one* pattern to explain why gambling is played in arcades. This pattern is contemporary because it attributes an unusual kind of devotion to physical processes in the brain, labels it as sick and disturbing, and thus removes it from the actors' sphere of knowledge and freedom. However, the 'addiction' explanation only fits the time, but not the observed gambling behaviour in arcades. There, 'addiction' is not the issue, but the constant need to prove oneself. Yet the discourse on addiction does not make something clear, but rather buries the underlying problem. You need more than a simple reductionist biological or medical understanding to explain such behaviour. As Palm (2023, p. 492) confirms, these understandings "must be supplemented with more complex and social explanations".

Here is my suggestion for such an explanation: arcades are not really about winning money, nor are they about addiction. Instead the automaton game can be understood, in general terms, as a means of the 'technology of the self' that enables individuals,

> to perform, by their own means, certain operations with their bodies, with their own souls, with their own conduct of life, in such a way that they transform themselves, modify themselves, and attain a certain state of perfection, happiness, purity and supernatural power. (Foucault, 2005, p. 968; see also Foucault, 2008)

In this sense, slot machine play is an exercise, a competition, a challenge that demands and gives one identity. Arcades, like gambling houses, turn their users into subjects in two ways. They subject players to a series of regulations and disciplines. But they also open up the possibility for players to form themselves as sovereign and self-regulating subjects who seek out and face their own challenges (however small they may be), as well as offering the possibility of going against the spirit and reason of the times.

In the next section, I will use the example of passionate gambling on slot machines to show that such an otherness could also be called something else, and that social power and social differences always play a role in this labelling process. This is because passionate gambling on gaming machines can also be understood as a special form of *edgework*. This explanation is also supported by my own empirical field studies and discourse analyses on gambling addiction conducted over several years.

The aim of my scientific research was always to answer some general questions, such as: why do people do what they do (even when their actions are strange to me and I do not understand at first sight what they do)? When I think their behaviour is strange, who is really 'strange' here? Me or the people? Maybe I do not understand because I am the stranger in this field of actions? If so, I have to come into closer contact with such actors to try and understand them better; in other words, I have to do fieldwork (see Möll, 2021, and this volume; Reichertz, 2012, 2018; Reichertz et al., 2010, 2011). In the research work, myself and my team made extensive use of participant observation and document analysis. We also conducted interviews with 43 male players, four female players, four gambling hall managers and two service assistants, one team leader, two technicians (these are the people who perform background programming and machine maintenance tasks), and the head of the market research department of a large gaming arcade chain.

Passionate Gambling: Addiction or Edgework? A (Re-)Construction

In contemporary society, there appears to be a popular consensus that excessive gambling can be considered an *addiction* (Adams, 2008; Dennis, 2021; Heinz et al., 2019; Ladouceur, 2004; Livingstone, 2005; Meyer, 1983; Orford, 2005; Schüll, 2012). According to the *recent* prevailing view, people who gamble too much—which often only means losing more money than they can afford—are *addicted*. Is passionate gambling also a *disease*? I do not think so. Nowadays, everyone seems to know that the phenomenon called 'gambling addiction' is real and that those who are diagnosed as gambling addicted need medical help. The fact that there are so many institutions that deal with the problems of gambling addicts reinforce this view. However, myself and other scholars disagree (see for example, Granfield & Reinarman, 2015; Livingstone et al., 2018; Möll, 2021; Reith, 2007, 2018; Venuleo & Marinaci, 2017). Instead, gambling addiction can be considered as a communicative construction and, at other times and under other circumstances, the behaviours involved would not be called a 'disease' but rather a *risky behaviour* (Goffman, 1970), an *excessive appetite* (Orford, 2001), *sensation seeking* (Zuckerman, 1994), *edgework* (Arntsen and Campbell, this volume; Lyng, 1990, 2005) or simply a *deviant consumption practice* (Cohen, this volume).

To strengthen this thesis, we can begin by considering the passionate use of slot machines and the view of the gamblers: in the fieldwork on slot machines (see Möll, 2021; Reichertz, 2018; Reichertz et al., 2010, 2011; see also Reith, 1999, 2004, 2007, 2018), one quickly observes that the difference between playing *with* money and playing *for* money is constitutive. While in the first case it is a matter of receiving an appropriate compensation, in the second case the focus is on the chance for a profit. In the arcade, (almost) nobody assumes that one can live from playing at the machines. Money is not invested to achieve long-term financial success. (Almost) everyone knows that in the long run the player will only lose. That is why the gamblers play *with* money, not *for* money (see also Möll, this volume). In the gambling hall you bring your money as a sacrifice, so to speak, to bring about what is important to you in this place: namely, the joy of playing.

So the attraction of the game is the game itself, or more precisely, knowing about the danger of the game. You can forfeit the game if you lose control. But keeping control is fun. For a good player, the game is about the attraction of exposing themself to danger, not to succumb to the game and the danger, but to use the proximity of the danger to enjoy it. The risk brings the attraction, and competent play is thus the controlled taking and enjoying of risks. If you like, it is an adventure with a return ticket, which also results in the de-banalizing of your own everyday life. The constant and strong desire of many people to repeatedly make their everyday life more colourful, to give it meaning, can be understood as a passion. Gambling halls represent an offer that enables you to live out this passion.

So much for the players' view, but how does science, especially *sociology* see it? First of all, from an economic point of view, gambling is unproductive, since no value is being created, it is merely a redistribution between the players, or the players and the establishment. Gambling does not contribute to the success of a society either. On the contrary, it questions fundamental social-cultural basics, "because they [the players] logically oppose a society based on the work ethic. … The certain element of emotional excitement that occurs when money is being bet or gambled for undermines values of self-discipline, prudence and sober rationality" (Lutter, 2010, p. 29). In western societies, avoiding risks is viewed as rational, whereas taking risks is either viewed as irrational or as an expression of being poorly informed or having poor perception.

Outlined in the following section, a significantly differing point of view is provided by Erving Goffman, one of the very few well-known sociologists who dealt with gambling early and often, and attests that gamblers serve an important function in society. As one of the American founding fathers of qualitative research, Goffman was employed as a card-dealer in different casinos in Las Vegas for an extended period in the 1960s. He was also a passionate blackjack-player.

Erving Goffman: Action—A Question of Character

Goffman's (1970) essay *Where the Action Is* describes not only the culture of legalised gambling, but in a further sense is also about the phenomenon of the voluntary taking of serious risks. For his analysis, Goffman uses the term 'action', which he uses to name actions that are rich in consequences and uncertainty (Goffman, 1970, p. 203). These are believed to be engaged in for their own sake. Goffman does not trace the motivation to participate in 'action' back to individual traits of the actors, such as impulsiveness, irrationality or other idiosyncratic traits of personality. In contrast, the relation of 'action' and morally important qualities which make up the 'character' of a person is much more important to him. "Taking serious risks voluntarily", states Goffman (1970, p. 258), "is a medium to acquire and maintain character; it is a goal in itself only in relation to other causes." For this reason, the voluntarily taking of risks is about demonstrating and building a (strong) character.

Actors oriented towards action develop qualities that, to a certain degree, all members of a society need to possess, in order to secure the continuance of society and its order. So Goffman's thesis (and mine) is that the voluntarily taking of risks in general—and thus also in gambling—is not only about money and excitement, it is also about identity and image. And it is about society and its grounding.

Lyng: 'Edgework' and Reflexivity

Goffman's concept of 'action' is nowadays in competition with other sociological attempts to explain the voluntary taking of risks. In his work on general economics, George Battailles (2021) points out that the *unproductive expenditure* of goods and money is important in every society—which would also make the actions of passionate gamblers (both the rich and the less rich) understandable. Another explanation could be based on Foucault's work: in *The Order of Discourse* (Foucault, 1970; see also Foucault, 2003), for example, he conceptualised the 'drawing of boundaries' and 'rejection' as elementary components of the procedures and experiences of exclusion. Stephen Lyng (1990, 2005) took a different approach with his concept of *edgework*. The term 'edgework' has its roots in the writings of American author and journalist Hunter S. Thompson, who made a name for himself by dealing with experiences of excessive drug use. Lyng borrows this term in his research investigating the reasons why more and more people prefer risky activities during their free time; among others are those engaged in skydiving, paragliding and extreme climbing. The searching and experiencing of physical or psychological boundary crossing behaviour is central to 'edgework'.

In its original form, edgework means consciously entering a situation that intentionally risks physical and psychological well-being and the imaginations of a well-ordered mind. All edgework activities have one central feature in common:

> they all involve a clearly observable threat to one's physical or mental well-being or one's sense of an ordered existence. The archetypical edgework experience is one in which the individual's failure to meet the challenge at hand will result in death or, at the very least, debilitating injury. (Lyng, 1990, p. 857)

Eruptions of good feelings grow out of deliberately caused self-endangerment (Lyng, 1990, p. 861). The boundaries that the 'edge-worker' tests are not only between life and death. They also run between order and chaos, sanity and madness, or between conscience and abeyance. It is, however, always about getting as close to the boundary as possible, without crossing it. An example of this is the skydiver, who aims to pull the trigger of his or her parachute as late as possible and still land safely, or the mountain climber, who tries to master greater and greater heights without using an oxygen mask (see also Arntsen and Campbell, this volume).

Emotions like fear and excitement may count as central elements of edgework, but it is not only the wish for intense feelings that is the main reason for taking risks voluntarily. Edgeworkers are not looking for the adrenaline kick they get in highly risky situations that cannot be controlled or influenced anymore. This is why, for Lyng (1990), gambling does not count as edgework. Situations with uncertain endings are engaged in by edgeworkers, according to Lyng (1990), because they want to master them in a smart, clever manner. Therefore Lyng sees a major difference between his edgework-concept and Goffman's action-concept: edgework is committed for its own sake and not for other and 'higher' aims.

In line with my own argument, however, Gerda Reith claims that gambling very much can be understood as edgework, since it is totally sufficient when the gambler believes that he or she is in control of what is going on. "Lyng (1990) is critical of the inclusion of gambling as edgework due to the lack of control it involves, and to the presence of 'fate'", states Reith (1999, p. 243),

> However, it has been found that gamblers believe they are in control of their destiny and can influence fate. Their very feelings of omnipotence, transcendence, hyperreality, and the alteration of perceptions of time and space … derive from this, and this is what gives gamblers the 'thrill' they pursue … Therefore it is appropriate to classify gambling as edgework here.

With the action and edgework concepts, we have two sociological perspectives of the phenomenon of voluntary risk-taking. In this perspective the users of slot machines are not hell-bent on destroying their lives or those of their family and friends (and the vast majority of them don't). But their voluntary risk-taking means proving themselves, and so it makes sense to them—it gives not only a thrill in their lives, but identity and self-respect as well. To gamble passionately means taking risks voluntarily. And that means to live more intensely. At least for a limited time. And once you lose, your strength is to get back up again and keep playing—again and again.

Conclusion: Gambling as Resistance Against the Demands of the Meritocracy

To place the interpretation of my data in a different theoretical horizon, I have followed Foucault (2008) in arguing that the slot machine game can be meaningfully understood as a 'technology of the self' that enables individuals to shape themselves and their subjectivities too, even if they are not completely aware of it. Arcades turn their users into subjects in two ways: they subject players to a series of regulations and disciplines, but they also open up the possibility for players to form themselves as sovereign and self-regulating subjects who seek out and face their own challenges (however small these might be). Users do not bow to the economic rationality that dominates their everyday lives, but rather in the arcade they find a place where economic rationality is suspended (at least for the players). In other words, at the slot machines they resist the rationalisation of their lives, where everything has to make economic sense; they give money with great perseverance and what they get in return is worth the money they spend. Because what they get in return is the voluntary assumption of real risks and the proof that they can stand it.

Furthermore, slot machine gambling can be understood as a means of the less well-off to transform themselves in order to attain a certain state of happiness, because gambling is experienced as the (re)acquisition of individual freedom and self-determination. Without a doubt, slot machine gambling is a kind of risky competition, a challenge that challenges you. The machine gamblers are always looking for their individual self-assertion in risk, seeking to experience temptations. Their real enjoyment only arises when they surrender to the charms of slot machines without completely falling for them. Players do not want to be deterred from this behaviour by well-intentioned, yet paternalistic, admonitions to refrain from dangerous, 'addictive' activities in the interests of family and society. Rather, they want to prove themselves and they are always looking for the challenge (see also Keane, 2002; Reith, 2007, 2018). Such passionate gamblers do not want to fail even though they know about the danger. But only this knowledge makes the difference: it turns a child's game into a competition. And one demonstrates strength by continuing to play the machines despite the losses. That is the hidden message of using slot machines.

Society sanctions some costly forms of voluntary risk-taking (carried out chiefly by the middle classes), labelling them as forms of edgework, yet those practiced by the working classes are labelled as pathological and grounds for medical intervention. In this way, passionate gambling at slot machines can also be seen as a resistance by the less well-off to the capitalistic principle of meritocracy (even if it is only a symbolic resistance). It is resistance to the demands of the meritocracy, and the dominant norm that we should value money rather than spending it on nothing. To label the passionate slot machine gambling as an addiction and a disease can therefore also be understood as an attempt by the ruling groups to stop such resistant activity.

The bitter irony of this issue is that this message applies not only to losers, but above all to winners, since it is the central message of every capitalist meritocracy to lose repeatedly and yet to keep playing. That is not only the hidden message of using slot machines but the heart of this society as well. Therefore using slot machines passionately is not a complete and direct form of political resistance against meritocracy, but rather only a symbolic one. The question is: is it worth fighting for? Apparently at least for the gamblers.

References

Adams, P. J. (2008). *Gambling, freedom and democracy*. Routledge.

Adams, P. J. (2023). *Monster metaphors: When rhetoric runs amok*. Routledge.

Anhorn, R., & Balzereit, M. (Eds.). (2016). *Handbuch Therapeutisierung und Soziale Arbeit* [Handbook of therapy and social work]. Springer VS.

Battailles, G. (2021). *Der verfemte Teil*. Matthes & Seitz.

Benedict, R. (1934). Anthropology and the abnormal. *The Journal of General Psychology, 10*(1), 59–82. https://doi.org/10.1080/00221309.1934.9917714

Berger, P., & Luckmann, T. (1967). *The social construction of reality: A treatise in the sociology of knowledge*. Bantam.

Bergler, E. (1958). *The psychology of gambling*. International Universities Press.

Campbell, N. D. (2008). *Discovering addiction: The science and politics of substance abuse research*. University of Michigan Press.

Campbell, N. D. (2012). Medicalization and biomedicalization: Does the diseasing of addiction fit the frame? In J. Netherland (Ed.), *Critical perspectives on addiction* (pp. 3–25). Emerald Group Publishing.

Castel, R. (1979). *Die psychiatrische Ordnung: Das goldene Zeitalter des Irrewerdens*. Suhrkamp.

Castellani, B. (2000). *Pathological gambling: The making of a medical problem*. State University of New York Press.

Cohen, B. M. Z. (2016). *Psychiatric hegemony: A Marxist theory of mental illness*. Palgrave Macmillan.

Conrad, P. (1992). Medicalization and social control. *Annual Review of Sociology, 18*(1), 209–232. https://doi.org/10.1146/annurev.so.18.080192.001233
Conrad, P. (2007). *The medicalization of society: On the transformation of human conditions into treatable disorders*. John Hopkins University Press.
Conrad, P. (2009). The shifting engines of medicalization. In P. Conrad (Ed.), *The sociology of health and illness* (pp. 480–492). Worth Publisher.
Conrad, P., & Schneider, J. (1980). *Deviance and medicalization: From badness to sickness*. Temple University Press.
Couldry, N., & Hepp, A. (2016). *The mediated construction of reality*. Polity Press.
Dellwing, M., & Harbusch, M. (Eds.). (2019). *Pathologisierte Gesellschaft?: 12. Beiheft Kriminologisches Journal*. Beltz-Juventa.
Dellwing, M., & Tietz, A. (2019). Pathologisierte Sozialität: 'Spielsucht' als institutionelle Verteidigung. *Kriminologisches Journal, 51*, 50–73.
Dennis, K. (2021). *Gambling: The hidden addiction—Overcoming gambling addiction* (2nd ed.). Independently published.
Feustel, R., Schmidt-Semisch, H., & Bröckling, U. (Eds.) (2019). *Handbuch Drogen in sozial- und kulturwissenschaftlicher Perspektive* [Handbook of social and cultural science perspectives on drugs]. Springer VS.
Foucault, M. (1970). *Die Ordnung des Diskurses*. Ullstein.
Foucault, M. (2003). Die Geburt der Sozialmedizin. In M. Foucault (Ed.), *Dits et Ecrits, Tome III: 1976–1979* (pp. 272–298). Suhrkamp.
Foucault, M. (2005). Technologie des Selbst. In M. Foucault (Ed.), *Dits et Ecrits, Tome IV: 1980–1988* (pp. 966–1015). Suhrkamp.
Foucault, M. (2008). *The birth of biopolitics*. Palgrave Macmillan.
Fraser, S., Moore, D., & Keane, H. (2014). *Habits: Remaking addiction*. Palgrave Macmillan.
Freud, S. (1969). Dostojewski und die Vatertötung. In S. Freud, *Bildende Kunst und Literatur* (Studienausgabe Band X) (pp. 267–286). Fischer Verlag.
Gergen, K. G. (1991). *The saturated self: Dilemmas of identity in contemporary life*. Basic Books.
Gergen, K. G. (2019). The social construction of reality. In M. Pfadenhauer & K. Knoblauch (Eds.), *Social constructivism as paradigm* (pp. 259–272). Routledge.
Goffman, E. (1970). *Interaktionsrituale*. Suhrkamp.
Granfield, R., & Reinarman, C. (2015). *Expanding addiction: Critical essays*. Routledge.
Harbusch, M. (Ed.). (2022). *Troubled persons industries: The expansion of psychiatric categories beyond psychiatry*. Palgrave Macmillan.

Heather, N., Field, M., Moss, A. C., & Satel, S. (2022). *Evaluating the brain disease model of addiction*. Routledge.
Heinz, A., Romanczuk-Seiferth, N., & Potenza, M. N. (Eds.). (2019). *Gambling disorder*. Springer.
Hepp, A. (2020). *Deep mediatization*. Routledge.
Herwig-Lempp, J. (1987). Das Phänomen der sogenannten neuen Süchte. *Neue Praxis, 17*, 54–64.
Illich, I. (1976). *Limits to medicine: Medical nemesis—The expropriation of health*. Marion Boyars Publishers Ltd..
Jellinek, E. M. (1972). *The disease concept of alcoholism*. Hillhouse Press.
Kaye, K. (2012). De-medicalizing addiction: Toward biocultural understandings. In J. Netherland (Ed.), *Critical perspectives on addiction* (pp. 27–52). Emerald Group Publishing.
Keane, H. (2002). *What's wrong with addiction?* New York University Press.
Keane, H. (2004). Disorders of desire: Addiction and problems of intimacy. *Journal of Medical Humanities, 25*(3), 189–204. https://doi.org/10.1023/B:JOMH.0000036637.03254.38
Keane, H. (2009). Foucault on methadone: Beyond biopower. *International Journal of Drug Policy, 20*(5), 450–452. https://doi.org/10.1016/j.drugpo.2008.10.005
Keller, R. (2024). *The sociology of knowledge approach to discourse*. Springer.
Keller, R., Hornridge, A. K., & Schünemann, W. J. (2018). *The sociology of knowledge approach to discourse: Investigating the politics of knowledge and meaning-making*. Routledge.
Keller, R., Knoblauch, H., & Reichertz, J. (Eds.). (2013). *Kommunikativer Konstruktivismus: Theoretische und empirische Arbeiten zu einem neuen wissenssoziologischen Ansatz*. Springer VS.
Knoblauch, H. (2020). *The communicative construction of reality*. Routledge.
Knoblauch, H., & Steets, S. (2022). From the constitution to the communicative construction of space. In G. B. Christmann, H. Knoblauch, & M. Löw (Eds.), *Communicative constructions and the refiguration of spaces* (pp. 19–35). Routledge.
Ladouceur, R. (2004). Gambling: The hidden addiction. *The Canadian Journal of Psychiatry, 49*(8), 501–503. https://doi.org/10.1177/070674370404900080
Laing, R. D. (1971). *The politics of the family*. Tavistock.
Laing, R. D. (1985). *Wisdom, madness, and folly: The making of a psychiatrist 1927–57*. Macmillan.
Laing, R. D., & Cooper, D. (1964). *Reason and violence*. Tavistock.

Lawrence, A. D., Evans, A. H., & Lees, A. J. (2003). Compulsive use of dopamine replacement therapy in Parkinson's disease: Reward systems gone awry? *The Lancet Neurology, 2*(10), 595–604.

Livingstone, C. (2005). Desire and the consumption of danger: Electronic gaming machines and the commodification of interiority. *Addiction Research & Theory, 13*(6), 523–534. https://doi.org/10.1080/16066350500338161

Livingstone, C., Adams, R., Cassidy, R., Markham, F., Reith, G., Rintoul, A., Dow Schüll, N., Woolley, R., & Young, M. (2018). On gambling research, social science and the consequences of commercial gambling. *International Gambling Studies, 18*(1), 56–68. https://doi.org/10.1080/14459795.2017.1377748

Lutter, M. (2010). *Märkte für Träume: Die Soziologie des Lottospiels*. Campus.

Lyng, S. H. (1990). Edgework: A social psychological analysis of voluntary risk taking. *American Journal of Sociology, 95*(4), 851–886.

Lyng, S. H. (Ed.). (2005). *Edgework: The sociology of risk taking*. Routledge.

Meyer, G. (1983). *Geldspielautomaten mit Gewinnmöglichkeit—Objekte pathologischen Glücksspiels*. Brockmeyer.

Molina, J. A., Sáinz-Artiga, M. J., Fraile, A., Jiménez-Jiménez, F. J., Villanueva, C., Ortí-Pareja, M., & Bermejo-P, F. (2000). Pathologic gambling in Parkinson's disease: A behavioral manifestation of pharmacologic treatment? *Movement Disorders, 15*(5), 869–872. https://doi.org/10.1002/1531-8257(200009)15:5<869::AID-MDS1016>3.0.CO;2-I

Möll, G. (2021). *Mit Geld spielt man nicht! Glücksspiel und »Glücksspielsucht« im parlamentarischen Diskurs* [You don't gamble with money! Gambling and 'gambling addiction' in parliamentary discourse]. Transcript. https://doi.org/10.14361/9783839460719

Netherland, J. (Ed.). (2012). *Critical perspectives on addiction*. Emerald Publishing Limited.

Orford, J. (2001). Addiction as excessive appetite. *Addiction, 96*(1), 15–31. https://doi.org/10.1046/j.1360-0443.2001.961152.x

Orford, J. (2005). *Problem gambling and other behavioural addictions*. University of Birmingham.

Palm, F. (2023). Addiction phobia: Foucault, abstract governance, and the fascination with materiality in contemporary critical studies of addiction. *Distinktion: Journal of Social Theory, 24*(3), 488–507. https://doi.org/10.1080/1600910X.2023.2235907

Quassowski, B. (1921). Obrigkeitliche Wohlfahrtspflege in den Hansestädten des Deutschordenslandes bis 1525. *Zeitschrift des Westpreußischen Geschichtsverein, 61*, 103–148.
Reichertz, J. (2012). Vom verführerischen Gesang der Spielautomaten. In N. Schröer, V. Hinnenkamp, S. Kreher, & A. Poferl (Eds.), *Lebenswelt und Ethnographie* (pp. 217–231). Oldib.
Reichertz, J. (2015). Communication, identity, and power. In P. Meusberger, D. Gregory, & L. Suarsana (Eds.), *Geographies of knowledge and power* (pp. 315–333). Springer.
Reichertz, J. (2017). Die Bedeutung des kommunikativen Handelns und der Medien im Kommunikativen Konstruktivismus. *Medien & Kommunikationswissenschaft, 65*(2), 252–274.
Reichertz, J. (2018). Die kleinen Freuden am Automaten. In C. Lövenich & J. Richardt (Eds.), *Geniessen verboten* (pp. 131–141). Novo Argumente.
Reichertz, J. (2019). From understanding to impact: Communicative power. In M. Pfadenhauer & K. Knoblauch (Eds.), *Social constructivism as paradigm* (pp. 292–310). Routledge.
Reichertz, J. (2021). "Wer mehr sieht, hat mehr Recht": Über die Notwendigkeit und die Grenzen der Säkularisierung von Forschung. In G. Betz, M. Halatcheva-Trapp, & R. Keller (Eds.), *Soziologische Experimentalität* (pp. 274–290). Juventa.
Reichertz, J. (2024). *Kommunikationsmacht: Wirkungen und Potentiale kommunikativen Handelns* (2nd ed.). Springer VS.
Reichertz, J., Niederbacher, A., Möll, G., Gothe, M., & Hitzler, R. (2010). *Jackpot: Erkundungen zur Kultur der Spielhallen* (2nd ed.). VS Verlag.
Reichertz, J., Niederbacher, A., Möll, G., & Hitzler, R. (2011). *Erwartungsräume: Spielkultur in großen und kleinen Spielhallen*. Oldib.
Reith, G. (1999). *The age of chance: Gambling in Western culture*. Routledge.
Reith, G. (2004). Consumption and its discontents: Addiction, identity and the problems of freedom. *The British Journal of Sociology, 55*(2), 283–300. https://doi.org/10.1111/j.1468-4446.2004.00019.x
Reith, G. (2007). Gambling and the contradictions of consumption: A genealogy of the "pathological" subject. *American Behavioural Scientist, 51*(1), 33–55. https://doi.org/10.1177/0002764207304856
Reith, G. (2018). *Addictive consumption: Capitalism, modernity and excess*. Routledge. https://doi.org/10.4324/9780429464447
Rose, N. (1999). *Governing the soul: The shaping of the private self* (2nd ed.). Free Association Books.

Rose, N. (2007). *The politics of life itself: Biomedicine, power, and subjectivity in the twenty-first century.* Princeton University Press.

Schetsche, M. (2013). Pathologization as strategy for securing the Wirklichkeit: The example of paranormal experiences. In M. Dellwing & M. Harbusch (Eds.), *Krankheitskonstruktionen und Krankheitstreiberei: Die Renaissance der soziologischen Psychiatriekritik* (pp. 271–286). Springer VS. https://doi.org/10.1007/978-3-531-18784-6_11

Schivelbusch, W. (1992). *Tastes of paradise: A social history of spices, stimulants, and intoxicants.* Vintage.

Schmidt, L. (1999). *Psychische Krankheit als soziales problem: Die Konstruktion des "Pathologischen Glücksspiels".* Leske+Budrich. https://doi.org/10.1007/978-3-322-97456-3

Schmidt, L. (2012). Glücksspielsucht: Aufkommen der Problemdefinition und anhaltende Kontroversen. *Soziale Probleme, 23*(1), 40–66.

Schmidt-Semisch, H. (2016). "Sucht" als leerer Signifikant: Zur Pathologisierung und Medikalisierung von Alltagsverhalten. In R. Anhorn, & M. Balzereit (Eds.), *Handbuch Therapeutisierung und soziale Arbeit* [Handbook of therapy and social work] (pp. 837–852). Springer VS. https://doi.org/10.1007/978-3-658-10870-0_31

Schüll, N. D. (2012). *Addiction by design: Machine gambling in Las Vegas.* Princeton University Press. https://doi.org/10.1515/9781400834655

Sedgwick, E. K. (1993). *Tendencies.* Duke University Press.

Szasz, T. S. (1961). *The myth of mental illness.* Hoeber/Harper.

Szasz, T. S. (1970). *The manufacture of madness: A comparative study of the inquisition and the mental health movement.* Harper & Row.

Szasz, T. S. (1979a). *The myth of psychotherapy: Mental healing as religion, rhetoric and repression.* Oxford University Press.

Szasz, T. S. (1979b). *The theology of medicine: The political-philosophical foundations medical ethics.* Oxford University Press.

Valverde, M. (1998). *Diseases of the will: Alcohol and the dilemmas of freedom.* Cambridge University Press.

Venuleo, C., & Marinaci, T. (2017). The social construction of the pathological gambler's identity and its relationship with social adaptation: Narratives from members of Italian gambling anonymous and gam-anon gamily groups. *Journal of Gambling Issues, 36,* 138–163. https://doi.org/10.4309/jgi.2017.36.7

Wiesemann, C. (2000). *Die heimliche Krankheit: Eine Geschichte des Suchtbegriffs.* Frommann-Holzboog Verlag.

Wise, R. A. (1994). A brief history of the anhedonia hypothesis. In C. R. Legg & D. Booth (Eds.), *Appetite: Neural and behavioural bases* (pp. 243–263). Oxford University Press.

Zola, I. K. (1972). Medicine as an institution of social control. *The Sociological Review, 20*(4), 487–504. https://doi.org/10.1111/j.1467-954X.1972.tb00220.x

Zuckerman, M. (1994). *Behavioral expressions and biosocial bases of sensation seeking*. Cambridge University Press.

5

A Marxist Theory of Addiction

Bruce M. Z. Cohen

The status of addiction as a common malady in Western society is hard to refute. Park (2024, p. 1) speaks of a current milieu in which the confluence of media, legal and medical discourse has successfully produced the idea that addiction is normal, "simply human nature", and that we are all addicts in waiting. As will be profiled in this chapter, however, there is a paradox at the heart of this normalisation process when considering the highly contested nature of addiction as an established medical disease; for 'addiction' has never been adequately defined, the claims to aetiology remain shaky, and the treatments continue to lack efficacy.

Following Marxist theory, I will argue in this chapter that we can better understand such a paradox if we consider how addiction discourse can serve the needs of capitalist society. In brief, behaviour commonly labelled as 'addiction' will be more accurately referred to

B. M. Z. Cohen (✉)
Waipapa Taumata Rau/University of Auckland, Auckland, New Zealand
e-mail: b.cohen@auckland.ac.nz

B. M. Z. Cohen et al. (eds.), *Addiction and the Medicalisation of Conspicuous Behaviour*, The Politics of Mental Health and Illness,
https://doi.org/10.1007/978-3-032-06313-7_4

here as *deviant consumption practices*. Consumption is a vital activity for the continuance of capitalism (Marx, 1887), so it is actively encouraged among the workers through various means. There is, however, a point where these consumer and leisure activities can cause problems for capital and the generation of surplus value; where passionate consumption leads to a negation of people's responsibilities as producers in their various roles which contribute to the survival of the current economic system. These so-called 'pathological' levels of consumption are what psy-professionals and associated institutions have labelled as addictions. As issues of productivity have become a greater anxiety for twenty-first century capitalism (Davies, 2015), so the addiction discourse has proliferated. Thus, I will argue here that addiction discourse serves an increasingly important ideological role in labelling 'irrational' consumers as 'addicts'. At the same time, this analysis does not ignore the great potential for surplus value to also be generated by servicing deviant consumers through the expanding addiction wing of what Harbusch (2022) calls the 'troubled persons industries' (in this case, including psy-professionals and health practitioners, detox clinics, pharmaceutical corporations, insurance companies, biotech enterprises, and online media firms engaged in the addiction area). As Marx & Engels (1965, p. 37) argued, capitalism "must nestle everywhere, settle everywhere, establish connections everywhere", and these addiction experts and organisations can also be understood as spaces for increasing capital accumulation.

Focusing on definitions, theories of aetiology, and the efficacy of treatments, the following background section will perform a deconstruction of addiction science, highlighting some of the major problems with considering addiction as a valid medical disease. This is followed by two analysis sections: the first focusing on the political economy of addiction and the accumulation of surplus value by addiction experts, institutions, and corporations; and the second, analysing the precise ideological role played by addiction discourse in neoliberal society. The chapter ends with some brief recommendations for future directions of analysis for critical addiction researchers.

Background: The Magic and Mystery of Addiction Science

Contested Definitions

Survey research in the US has suggested that two percent of the population are currently addicted to alcohol, one and half percent addicted to other drugs, and the same proportion addicted to gambling (Adams, 2008, p. 3). The text-revised version of the fifth edition of the American Psychiatric Association's (APA) *Diagnostic and Statistical Manual of Mental Disorders* (DSM-5-TR) estimates the lifetime rate for alcohol use disorder to be 29 percent, with 14 percent of the US population classed as 'severe' cases (American Psychiatric Association, 2022, p. 557). Current rates for opioid use disorder are estimated to be somewhere between 0.6 and 0.9 percent (American Psychiatric Association, 2022, p. 612) and, for gambling disorder, 0.2 to 0.3 percent (American Psychiatric Association, 2022, p. 663). From a single page in the first edition of the DSM in 1952 (American Psychiatric Association, 1952, p. 39), the official nosology on 'substance-related and addictive disorders' has expanded to a bulky section of 123 pages in the latest DSM-5-TR (American Psychiatric Association, 2022, pp. 543–665). Representing the APA's official position, Petry (2016, p. 4) suggests this may only be the tip of the addiction iceberg; just because disorders related to sex, shopping, tanning, exercise and other behaviours do not currently feature in the DSM, "does not mean they are not psychiatric disorders", but only that there is a lack of available research evidence at this time.

Yet despite claims that the disease is pervasive and continually growing (see Courtwright, 2019), the definition of addiction remains highly contested. This has been admitted as much in the DSM-5-TR where the APA note the "uncertain definition" of addiction (American Psychiatric Association, 2022, p. 543); a sentiment echoed by Petry (2016, p. 1) who describes addiction as "a loaded term", which "has different meanings to different people." Adams (2008, p. 4) points out that this ambivalence has been informed by a historical conceptualisation of addiction as a 'loss of control'; of people as unable to avoid repeated inebriation and increasing their 'dependency' on certain substances (for a historical overview, see Cohen et al., this volume). Considering the problematic interplay between choice and compulsion in defining such behaviour, it may be a case that using the term addiction in such contexts reveals "more about the speaker's background than about a common meaning" (Adams, 2008, p. 4). Following Shaffer (1985), Keane (2002, p. 9) has noted that the ongoing debates over the nature of addiction within the medical and psychological fields means that the area is in a permanent state of 'conceptual chaos' and a 'crisis of categories'. In Room's (1998, p. 316) view, the changing diagnostic classifications of addiction witnessed in the DSM over time can be seen as much "like a shifting kaleidoscope—beautiful, mysterious, but not of much practical use."

Contested Aetiology

Since the DSM-III in 1980, scholars have noted the rise of neurological theories of addiction, to a point where, by the end of the twentieth century, it had become (and remains) the hegemonic view within and beyond medicine (Campbell, 2012; Park, 2024; Reith, 2019). Following earlier beliefs of physicians that addiction was hereditary, Robert Dupont, director of the National Institute on Drug Abuse (NIDA), theorised in 1978 that addiction was genetic and "a brain disease that affects behavior" (cited in Anderson et al., 2010, p. 489). By 1996, researchers also claimed to have found a specific gene for pathological gambling (Castellani, 2000, p. 49). The current DSM-5-TR (American Psychiatric Association, 2022, p. 557) claims that 40–60 percent of the causation variance in alcohol use disorder (the current medical label for alcoholism) can be explained by genetic influences, with one to two percent of cases being the result of a single gene. Behavioural disorders such as sex and pornography addiction are now typically theorised in line with this biomedical view, in which extended exposure can disrupt normal neurochemical pathways in the brain (Clarkson & Kopaczewski, 2013). This mirrors NIDA's current understanding of drug addiction, as they note that researchers "have also found that chronic drug abuse alters the brain's anatomy and chemistry and that these changes can last for months or years after the individual has stopped using drugs" (cited in Anderson et al., 2010, p. 489; see also Leshner, 1997). Campbell (2012) has outlined how this 'biomedicalisation' of addiction as brain disease has captured the public imagination over the past few decades, seemingly destigmatising addiction through more acceptance that it is something beyond one's control, encouraging more people to accept they have a 'problem' and to engage with treatments which are assumed to be efficacious (see discussion below).

Yet despite the current dominance of the brain disease model of addiction (BDMA), there remains a surprising lack of consensus on aetiology from researchers, and indeed the validity of the diagnostic category of addiction also continues to be questioned (Campbell 2007, 2012; Clarkson & Kopaczewski 2013; Hammersley & Reid, 2002). As Campbell (2007, p. 4) has remarked of substance abuse researchers, for instance, "[w]hile no science speaks with a unified voice, [they] comprise a remarkably disunified chorus." Evidence for the BDMA, argues Peele (1985, pp. 7–8), has never been effectively established, though contradictory evidence has often been ignored. Clarkson & Kopaczewski (2013, p. 130) summate some the key issues with the research when they state that,

> There is no threshold of consumption that one reaches before one is considered an addict that does not rely on the emergence of social problems tied to the behavior itself. Knowledge of addict behavior comes mainly from those who cannot control their behavior and not from functional participants for whom the behavior lacks serious social consequence. The disease model of addiction does not adequately address nonbiological factors that influence behavior, including cultural, social, situational, ritualistic, developmental, personality, and cognitive elements.

As with other areas of mental illness, rather than producing scientifically credible evidence, psychiatry's faith in the diagnostic category of addiction has come from technological interventions which appear to demonstrate a positive correlation with biological theory. For researchers of opiate use, this was the belief that the substitution of one drug (heroin) with another (methadone)—through the health intervention of methadone maintenance treatment (MMT), more recently re-named as opioid substitution treatment (OST)—reduced the reliance on illegal substances and stabilised user behaviour, meaning that a successful pharmacological intervention appeared to confirm biological causation. In Dupont's words, addiction

> has to do with the brain. And that the [replacement] drugs really work. And they work better for some people than others. The vulnerability is not equal in the population. There are many factors, including genetic factors, which influence that vulnerability. (cited in Anderson et al., 2010, p. 485).

Yet positive evaluations of such programmes in 1970s and 1980s did not last, and by 2009 Dupont (cited in Anderson et al., 2010, p. 490) was bemoaning that "the search for a silver bullet for drug abuse, the drug that stops—or better yet prevents—drug abuse has been disappointing" (see also Hall et al., 2015, p. 107). In considering smoking as addictive, Elam (2012, and this volume) has noted the same pattern, with the medical community only theorising smoking as a biologically determined addiction following the successful introduction of another drug replacement technology (in this case, Nicorette gum), which appeared to show that smokers' cravings and compulsions for cigarettes mirrored the same behaviours as cocaine and heroin users. As Hall et al. (2015, p. 107, emphasis added) confirm, "[t]he most widely used drugs in addiction", such as methadone and nicotine replacement therapy, "*preceded* the BDMA by more than 30 years." The perceived successes of pharmaceutical interventions have led to a false belief that addiction has a biological aetiology, which in turn has aided medicine's claims to expertise and authority in understanding addiction and treating addicts.

The hegemony of the BDMA is being constantly reinforced by the popular reporting of addiction research from neuroscience (see Hellman, this volume; Hellman et al., 2022) which reproduces the narrative of progress and new discoveries aided by more precise technological interventions. Perhaps most symbolic among these has been the relatively recent introduction of the positron emission tomography (PET) and functional magnetic resonance imaging (fMRI) brain imaging technologies to addiction science. As Keane (cited in Clarkson & Kopaczewski, 2013, p. 133) notes, these machines have been used as strategies by scientists to produce "the universal truth of addiction", through—to use Reith's (2019, p. 110) caustic phrase—"the magic tunnel of the fMRI scanner" which has only in fact revealed binaries of normal and abnormal based on pre-assessments (and self-reports) of social conduct, rather than actually identifying chemical or biological indicators of dependence. Reporting on the modest results of brain imaging for understanding addiction, Hall et al. (2015, p. 107) have confirmed that "[t]he fact that decreased activity in frontal brain regions is modestly correlated with self-reported drug craving does not show that drug use is driven by irresistible impulses." This finding was part of a more general review conducted by Hall et al. (2015, p. 105) of the BDMA in which they argue that there is no consensus among neuroscientists regarding the validity of the model, and that it is "not supported by animal and neuroimaging evidence to the extent its advocates suggest; it has not helped to deliver more effective treatments for addiction; and its effect on public policies toward drugs and people with addiction has been modest." As Park (2024, p. 2) summates of the neuroscientific paradigm, while it has facilitated the production of a large amount of recent research in the area,

> has had a huge effect on the scientific literature, and on what is cited as the science of addiction in public media, legal arguments, and state policy … it has not yet yielded a novel and widely useful technique for treatment; hence, its power to change how institutions treat and respond to addiction has been weak.

The efficacy of treatments for behaviour which have been labelled as 'addictive' is the issue to which I now turn.

Contested Efficacy

As has been discussed so far, the definitions of addiction are vague and imprecise, while theories for aetiology have proved to be inaccurate and weak in assessing such problematic behaviours. Peele (1985, p. 1) concludes from this that the common-sense view of addiction that currently dominates understanding of such behaviour "derives more from magic than from science." That said, what of the treatments—such as medications and therapy—which are often said to aid recovery from such dependency? To what extent does the available research suggest they are effective? This sub-section considers the evidence and the implications towards the Marxist analysis I perform in the latter half of this chapter.

Despite high estimates of the amount of people who will suffer from alcohol use disorder in their lifetime (see above), there is no effective treatment currently available. Alcoholism differs from traditional medical issues, states Peele (1989, p. 119, emphasis original), in that "[t]he disease of alcoholism is *defined* by people's behavior, and the treatment is to get people to stop drinking." Doctors can do little more for the patient than encourage detoxification, note Conrad & Schneider (1992, p. 74), and then refer users on to a support group, usually Alcoholics Anonymous (AA). Previous research has, however, questioned the effectiveness of such programmes, finding that some former alcoholics subsequently return to 'social' or moderate levels of drinking (Armor et al., 1978; Davies et al., 1969; Pattison et al., 1977). For Peele (1989), the great irony of the continued ineffectiveness of groups like AA and the growing number of therapeutic interventions for alcoholism is that their many failures are then used as evidence for the 'deep seated' nature of the disease. "Relapse is so common" in such services, he notes, "that it is used to justify the disease idea. Failures are not evidence of the futility of treatment; they simply indicate that, as the treatment personnel assert, people can never fully recover from the disease" (Peele, 1989, pp. 116–117).

For opioid addiction (most commonly meaning heroin use), both therapy and MMT/OST are argued to be effective as treatment modalities (Leshner, 1997). Initial evaluations of MMT services in the 1960s appeared to demonstrate improvements in life chances for clients, along with a reduction in social problems (such as levels of criminality related to the procurement of illegal substances). On this basis, governments have continued to show enthusiasm for the funding of such health initiatives, and MMT/OST remain the most widely used opioid replacement therapy in many Western countries (Bennett, 2011, pp. 130–131). Biomedicine's assertion of drug replacement technologies as a 'magic bullet' for addiction have, however, clashed with the available evidence (Bourgois, 2000, p. 165). Conrad & Schneider (1992, pp. 139–140) have commented that relapse rates following the intervention of MMT/OST remain high, with various evaluations in the 1970s and 1980s suggesting the creation of a black market for methadone, the continuation of heroin use for some clients while still in the programmes, and little noticeable effect on subsequent crime rates. Bennett (2011, p. 131) puts the figure of relapse to heroin following MMT/OST detox at 90 percent within the first twelve months; more recently, Klein et al. (2022, p. 97) have reported that 75 percent of those "who misuse opiates or psychostimulants, particularly crack, relapse within 3–6 months of exiting treatment." As Campbell (2012, p. 22) notes, no precise medication has been yet developed which effectively treats *any* addiction. This includes smoking replacement technologies, where the introduction of Nicorette gum had little to no effect on smoking cessation (Elam, 2012). As Hall et al. (2015, p. 107) have plainly stated "[t]he promised treatment benefits associated with the BDMA have not materialised."

Peele (1985, p. 6) suggests that addiction professionals' belief in the BDMA may be a result of confirmation bias in which they regularly encounter clients who effectively mimic and self-report the behaviours of being 'out of the control', 'unable to stop', and suspecting that they may have 'a brain disease'. Despite doctors and counsellors witnessing "a context-limited sample of addictive behavior", it reinforces their beliefs in the 'realness' of the BDMA (Peele, 1985, p. 6). In contrast, evidence suggests that changes in the socio-economic context of the user can have a much greater effect on potentially changing the behaviours perceived as addictive. As Heyman (2009, p. 21) reports, "[m]ost people [around 95 percent] who use addictive drugs do not become addicted to them" (see also Hari, 2015). Additionally, most addicts quit drugs without professional assistance (Hall et al., 2015; Heyman, 2009, p. 167; Kincaid &

Sullivan, 2010; Satel & Lilienfeld, 2013), with typical social and economic obligations experienced after the age of 30 meaning drug usage tends to dissipate (Heyman, 2009, pp. 154–156); addiction is therefore theorised by Heyman (2009) as a voluntary rather than a biological condition. Evidence for these claims includes the famous study of Vietnam veterans by Robins et al. (cited in Peele, 1985, p. 8) in 1975, in which only 14 percent of narcotic addicts became re-addicted after their return to the US.

Typically, MMT/OST clinics will also provide psychosocial support to their clients through on-site counsellors and social workers. Following a review of 35 randomised control trials of such MMT/OST provision, Amato et al. (cited in Epstein, 2019, p. 73) reported that "[p]resent evidence suggests that adding psychosocial support does not change the effectiveness of retention and opiate use during treatment". In a more general survey of the efficacy of such interventions, Epstein (2019, p. 68) states bluntly that "[p]sychotherapy offers no apparent cure for drug addiction." While meta-analyses of therapeutic interventions will usually contradict this finding, he notes a plethora of issues with such research, including: the reliance on self-reporting with no independent verification; publication bias (that is, the reporting of positive results only, while ignoring or under-reporting negative findings); non-blind studies; a lack of objective testing (for example, no urine or blood analysis); a lack of non-treatment controls (such as waitlists or placebos); and a lack of consideration as to whether the treatment was actually harmful to clients (Epstein, 2019, p. 68). "[T]he problems of assessing the prevalence, incidence, and social effects of addiction as well as the pervasive methodological pitfalls of the studies", concludes Epstein (2019, p. 68), "undercut any claim of abstinence, remission, or harm reduction that is systematically related to psychotherapeutic treatment of any kind."

To summarise this section, addiction science has successfully promoted the BDMA to hegemonic status despite a lack of adequate definitions, measures, and treatment interventions. Variations in patterns of nonaddictive use among the population have been systematically ignored by the research community (Clarkson & Kopaczewski, 2013, p. 130), as have the lives of the vast majority of supposed 'addicts' who recover without any need for treatment. Agreeing with Hammersley & Reid (2002), I argue here that addiction is a convenient myth constructed by medicine to avoid more complex investigations of behaviours that have been labelled as such. In line with other critical scholars, addiction can be better understood as a socially constructed and increasingly medicalised form of social deviance (Campbell, 2012; Keane, 2002; Suissa, 2006); specifically, I refer to these in the discussion which follows as *deviant consumption practices* (that is, specific consumption practices which have been variously labelled as 'dark', 'passionate', 'dangerous', 'risky,' or 'excessive').

As I demonstrate below, addiction discourse, and the medical and therapeutic troubled persons industries that have grown up around it, operate as institutions of social control on those in danger of crossing certain dominant moral boundaries of acceptable behaviour in Western society. It should be noted here however that, in line with cultural Marxist theory, this analysis is not ignorant of the contradictions inherent in capitalism's desire for us to consume more but then label some as consuming too much; there are always points of resistance where the working classes challenge ruling ideas, whether symbolically, socially, or politically, and that includes through their consumption practices sometimes labelled as 'addictive' (see Reichertz, this volume). But it is my contention that capitalism gains from the establishment and expansion of the addiction discourse in two distinct ways: firstly, it facilitates the expansion of capital and surplus value through the promotion of an industry of addiction experts, institutions, and organisations; and secondly, it increasingly serves an ideological role in reinforcing the primacy of productivity in neoliberal society. I will take these issues in turn in the two sections which follow.

A Political Economy of Addiction: The Tiger Woods Effect

While some scholars have taken aim at the dynamics of capitalism which encourage addictive behaviours (see for example, Courtwright, 2019), I argue in this section that a Marxist analysis should focus much more on the addiction wing of the troubled persons industries which have been established with the increasing medicalisation of deviant consumption practices over time; this includes groups of psy-professionals and health practitioners, pharmaceutical corporations, wellness and detox clinics, insurance companies, biotech enterprises, new media businesses, NGO and government organisations, and research institutions who have all benefited extensively from the expansion of the addiction discourse. Capitalism needs workers to keep consuming for the survival of the system (Marx, 1887). For Courtwright (2019), the growth in the number of addicts and varieties of addiction witnessed over the past few decades follows an increase in levels of consumerism; as capitalism has "engineered excess" (Courtwright, 2019, p. 224) in leisure activities such as gambling, eating and videogaming, addictions have become more common place. In Reith's (2019, p. 71) words, "we can see the globalisation of consumer capitalism matched by the global march of addictions." Focusing on the gambling industry as a case study, Courtwright (2014, p. 6) argues that "[s]ince the late nineteenth century [the industry] has become increasingly mechanized, digitized, and rationalized to minimize costs and maximize profits, but at the price of increasing the risk of addiction." The profits to made from gambling in the US alone are indeed eye-watering, with a gross gaming revenue of $67 billion in 2023 (Statista, 2024). For Reith (2019, p. 125, p. 129), gambling is "almost [the] perfect [vehicle] for capital accumulation", with electronic gaming machines (EGM)—which account for 70–85 percent of the industry's profits—often conceptualised as 'reverse cash machines'.

The establishment of such consumption practices in capitalist society may then appear as a contradiction, for we are being increasingly encouraged to engage in such consumer behaviour at the same time as we are also in danger of being subject to the medicalised label of an addict (Reith, 2019). In the section which follows I will give an answer to this seeming contradiction, but for now it is enough to say that while I recognise the accumulation of surplus value from such consumption activities (and that it can lead to problems for some), this can distract our attention from the profits to be made by the parallel creation and expansion of the troubled persons industries who are supposedly responsible for supporting those who have been labelled as addicts.

While they may claim to be in operation to care for and treat addicts, Peele (1989, p. 145) argues that the addiction movement succeeds "principally at expanding their industry by finding more addicts and new types of addictions to treat." For example, Conrad & Schneider (1992, p. 87) note that the identification by medicine of 'chronic drunkenness' as a disease in the twentieth century brought about a "virtual 'industry' of professional and lay persons charged with the identification, treatment, counselling, and study of such persons." These groups were "clearly interested parties in perpetuating and expanding [the] growing number of organizations, both public and private, dedicated to the diagnosis and treatment of alcoholism" (Conrad & Schneider, 1992, p. 87). The number of estimated alcoholics in the US expanded rapidly in the post-war period, with a shift from government funding of public facilities to support for third-party financing, leading to a significant expansion of private inpatient treatment in the 1970s and early 1980s, and resulting in most therapy being paid by insurers (Peele, 1989, p. 49). These actors have obvious vested interests in increasing their business, which they do through exaggerating the numbers of people going untreated, and falsely promoting addiction as a treatable disease (see also Midanik, 2006).

While AA claimed that as many as 22 million Americans could be considered as alcoholics in the 1980s, Room (cited in Peele, 1989, p. 47) suggested there was in fact little evidence that large numbers were going untreated, with 1.7 million people already in treatment, while less (1.5 million) actually reached the DSM criteria for 'alcohol dependence'. Peele (1989, p. 49) theorises that many of the people in for-profit facilities are high functioning individuals who do not appear as alcoholics and must be persuaded by the professionals that they *really do* have a problem. Ideas of the progressiveness of addiction to alcohol (that is, that consuming one or two drinks can quickly lead to levels of problem drinking) have been increasingly used by organisations like AA and private inpatient services to convince more and more people that they are alcoholics 'in denial'; indeed, Peele (1989, p. 51) notes that private treatment centres state that their biggest issue is the denial of a drinking problem among many of their clients. The main source of referrals to such facilities are via the criminal justice system where those found guilty of drunk driving face a stark choice between incarceration or treatment (Peele,

1989, p. 50). In a similar threatening manner, Employee Assistance Programs will often force workers into treatment programmes as an alternative to losing their jobs (Peele, 1989, p. 50). Young people and 'early stage' problem drinkers are also targeted by such organisations to further expand their client base, claiming that alcohol is a potential 'gateway drug' for which the population requires closer surveillance and capture (Peele, 1989, p. 50).

Noting the increase in MMT programmes in the US in the early 1970s, Conrad & Schneider (1992, p. 139) acknowledge that, at the time, "[e]ntrepreneurship and profitability undoubtedly contributed to methadone maintenance's rapid spread." Often operated by private physicians, hospitals, and mental health facilities, by 1974 there were 80,000 addicts involved in such services, suggesting to the authors "a virtual counterepidemic of methadone programs" (Conrad & Schneider, 1992, p. 139). The growth in the global market for nicotine replacement therapies between 1978 and 1985 also aided an expansion in both the selling of pharmaceutical products as well as an uptake in interest from private research companies (Elam, 2012); thus, smoking and cessation became "too lucrative … to be overlooked as a medical problem" (Peele, 1989, p. 118). By the late 1980s, the total expenditure on drug and alcohol treatment in the US was estimated to be around $2 billion, with private hospitals generating half, and federal and state government spending the other half (Peele, 1989, p. 126). In 2018, figures showed that the US medical expenditure on alcohol-related disorders was $10 billion, while a further $7 billion was spent on opioid-related disorders (Li et al., 2023).

The introduction of pathological gambling to the DSM-III in 1980 and the subsequent diagnostic creep of other behavioural addictions has only served to further produce surplus value. While, ironically, the DSM has remained silent on the issue of money itself, the psychiatric classification has led to a further proliferation in interest from a range of professionals (from medical to legal), with Reith (2019, p. 137) noting that the label's reliance on "one's own subjective feelings about wins and losses" meaning that potentially any gambler can be labelled as such. By the end of the twentieth century, insurance companies had recognised pathological gambling as a treatable condition for which they would provide payment (Castellani, 2000, p. 105). Despite the problematic criteria, obesity discourse and eating addictions in the twenty-first century have also been hyped in Western society as another epidemic of excess and, more than coincidentally, very profitable areas for further disease-mongering (Reith, 2019, pp. 103–124). Often suggested by the addiction industry as an incurable and lifetime illness (Peele, 1989, p. 118), the obesity discourse has facilitated yet more lucrative industries including in publishing (for example, popular books on diet and nutrition), medical and therapeutic treatments (for instance, diet pills, bariatric surgery, private wellness clinics, and weight-watcher programmes), and the fitness industry (Peele, 1989, p. 119). Given the fact that everyone must eat, and with more than half the US population qualifying as 'over-weight', Peele (1989, p. 134) suggests that the potential for these troubled persons industries to make money through the construction of eating disorders is substantial (see also Fixsen, 2024).

In their research on sex addiction, Brossard et al. (2023) offer a salient case study to illustrate how the expanding addiction discourse provides a range of increasing marketable products and services, even in the absence of an officially recognised disorder. In fact, sex addiction's exclusion from the DSM in 1994, note the authors, led to a dramatic increase in the use of the term by actors outside medicine, including counsellors and therapists, the media, religious groups, and the legal profession. The media, for instance, increasingly use sex addiction as a buzzword to profile celebrity lives; lawyers can utilise the label in offering mitigating circumstances in custody cases; religious organisations establish counselling groups (and even start-up apps) aimed at clients questioning sexual abstinence, their sexual identity, or general sexual acts considered a 'sin' by their church; and therapists advertise their services as experts on working with sex addicts. Questioned about their use of the term, the researchers found the latter group to be contradictory; there was a preference not to use the label in sessions unless their clients did, yet they still promoted their services as including work with 'sex addicts'—"I want people to find me", states one therapist, "so I do it for them [the clients], right?" (cited in Brossard et al., 2023). The need for more customers is, of course, at the forefront of sex therapists' operations. This is bluntly stated by another therapist who proclaimed of the world-famous golfer who declared himself to be suffering from sex addiction, "[w]e want more of the Tiger

Woods of the world." Another explained, "[w]ithin about 48 hours after Tiger Woods told the world [of his many infidelities] … I got something like a 300 percent increase in cases of people who were calling me saying 'Do you treat sex addiction?'" (cited in Brossard et al., 2023).

As Brossard et al.'s (2023) research illustrates, the lack of a formal psychiatric diagnosis—along with ineffective treatment regimens—is no barrier to expanding addiction discourse and its utilisation to increase surplus value; selling deviant consumption practices as 'addiction' produces markets for numerous treatments and services. Yet, as will be explored in the following section, just as important to a Marxist analysis of addiction discourse is an understanding of the increasing ideological role it plays in neoliberal society.

The Ideological Role of Addiction: (Still) Losing Control

Up until the 1970s, the history of addiction can be considered as the history of policing marginalised populations (including the working classes, the poor, young black men, and immigrants) considered a threat to respectable society and thus marked as social deviants (see Cohen et al., this volume). While these groups remain a key focus of addiction discourse, due to the increased emphasis on (and anxiety towards) *worker productivity* in neoliberal society (see Davies, 2015), the medicalisation of deviant consumption practices has expanded to also encompass members of the middle classes. As Davies (2017) notes, the DSM-III was the first edition of the manual to introduce 'occupational functioning' as a symptom of mental disorder (it appeared over a hundred times in the manual; see Cohen, 2022). For example, one of the three criteria that distinguished substance abuse from nonpathological use in the DSM-III (and the one discussed in most detail in the manual) was "*[i]mpairment in social or occupational functioning* caused by the pattern of pathological use" (American Psychiatric Association, 1980, p. 164, emphasis added). The current section on substance-related and addictive disorders in the DSM-5-TR (American Psychiatric Association, 2022) witnesses how much the symptomologies related to the failure to fulfil major 'role obligations' at work, in school, and at home have become almost ubiquitous in addiction discourse. In agreement with Reith (2019), the pathologisation of consumption practices takes place in the DSM when such behaviour is seen to effect productivity. For Keane (2002, p. 4), "[t]he addict is someone who has lost control over their desires and thereby over their life, as evidenced in their failure to meet work, family and social expectations." As an increasing threat to capitalism, these uncontrolled forms of consumption require closer monitoring and intervention by the psy-professionals. Keane (2002) suggests there remains here strong parallels with the original addiction discourse regarding the loss of control and a need for medicine to closely surveil and discipline the body.

Critical scholars have also drawn on the example of MMT/OST to argue that, rather than aiming to 'cure' opioid users, the central purpose of such interventions is to morally discipline addicts; therefore, MMT/OST can be better understood as a form of social control. MMT/OST has been claimed to lead to improvements for addicts "in employment, education, and family reconciliation" (Conrad & Schneider, 1992, p. 135), but the system has also been criticised as a form of 'chemical parole' in which clients can often only access methadone through regular attendance at clinics and being subject to evasive urine and blood tests. Reflecting on the efficacy issues of MMT/OST (see discussion above), professionals have responded in turn by pointing out that the regime also forces the client to make contact with counselling and medical staff attached to the service; in Conrad & Schneider's (1992, p. 140) view this confirms that the use of methadone is not a drug treatment but "a social control mechanism". "The techniques, technologies, and procedures utilised in methadone programs", agrees Bennett (2011, p. 130), "aim to produce a more compliant, conforming, and self-regulating subject."

Such medical regimes serve to discipline clients through technologies which 'responsibilise' and normalise the user as 'sick' rather than as an 'addict' (see also Müller, this volume). In the words of Bourgois (2000, p. 165, emphasis added), "[t]reatment in this context becomes a hostile exercise in disciplining the unruly misuses of pleasure and in *controlling economically unproductive bodies.*" Heavy drug use and other forms of deviant consumption are seen to undermine productive activities

(Heyman, 2009, p. 167) and are thus at odds with the neoliberal values of individualism, hard work and self-sufficiency as the only way to true happiness and success (Greenberg, 2008, p. 30). "Addiction and its vilification", reflects Epstein (2019, p. 78), "reinforce cherished social values of individualism and sin in the United States."

I have previously argued that psychiatric discourse has significantly expanded in neoliberal society as a nuanced and highly effective form of social control which regulates our everyday lives in the service of capital (see Cohen, 2016). Psy-professional activities and the claims they make, enshrined in official documents like the DSM, reflects the dominant norms and values of capitalism. We should therefore understand addiction discourse in the same way. As Reith (2019, p. 68) has also clarified, the assumptions made in the language of the addiction criteria represents "a mirror image of the neoliberal ideal." For example, she notes that the oft-repeated DSM-5-TR (American Psychiatric Association, 2022, p. 609) symptom of addiction as "[r]ecurrent … use resulting in a failure to fulfill major role obligations at work, school, or home", should be understood as "essentially relat[ing] to the impacts of spending what is judged to be too much time or money on particular forms of consumption and from spoiled relationships, unsatisfactory jobs and general existential ennui" (Reith, 2019, p. 69). Neoliberalism requires "controlled consumption" (Reith, 2019, p. 142) and has increasingly medicalised what is seen as 'irrational' forms of such behaviour—for instance, too much gaming, shopping, drinking, drug taking, gambling, sex and pornography use at the expense of labouring 'productively' for the ruling classes. It is, suggests Reith (2019, p. 142), a continuation of the dominant puritanical morality on consumption from the eighteenth and nineteenth centuries, yet given increased emphasis in neoliberal capitalism "as a means of affirming the self and demonstrating responsible citizenship."

Conclusion

Despite ongoing claims from professionals and researchers that addiction is a brain disease for which effective treatments exist, this chapter has demonstrated that the area remains poorly defined, with strong internal disagreements over aetiology, and 'treatments' which continue to lack efficacy. As Szasz (1974) previously argued of mental illness, we can also understand addiction as a metaphor rather than a medical disease; in this case, a metaphor for socially deviant consumption practices. This chapter has used a Marxist framework to demonstrate that the recent growth in the numbers and varieties of addictions can be explained through an understanding of the political economic and ideological roles addiction discourse plays in serving capitalism: firstly, more addictions mean the further expansion of the troubled persons industries through which actors such as insurance companies, pharmaceutical corporations, new media and biotech businesses, research organisations, and private doctors, therapists and clinics produce surplus value for capitalism; and secondly, addiction discourse works as a form of social control through which capitalism asserts the need for citizens to be more productive, while labelling those considered to be engaged in irrational consumption practices as addicts and, thus, socially deviant.

The sad fact of the establishment and growth of the troubled persons industries related to 'addictions' and 'addicts' is that the treatments and services offered have been of little help to those who have sought solutions to their consuming problems. As we have seen in this chapter, while changes in behaviours described as 'addictions' may be difficult, many do change their behaviour, and do so voluntarily as their circumstances alter. Keane (2002, p. 3) makes this point clearly when she states that

> It may be extremely difficult for people to change behaviours defined as addictive, but many do, often without any formal treatment. Other habitual and routine patterns of behaviour regarded as benign or positive may well be just as resilient to change; the strength of their hold generally escapes notice because attempts are not made to give them up.

As addiction appears to become more 'normalised' and commonplace in our world (Park, 2024), critical scholars of addiction need to recognise the troubled persons industries for the snake oil entrepreneurs that they really are. We need to further analyse and understand the structural dynamics through which capitalism allows psy-professionals and associated institutions to claim expertise and expand in an area which is so obviously flawed. It is worth reminding ourselves how a fellow sociologist researching in the area of social deviance and drug-taking conceived such 'rule enforcers' in Western society over 60 years ago:

> First, they say that by reason of their efforts the problem they deal with is approaching solution. But, in the same breath, they say the problem is perhaps worse than ever (though through no fault of their own) and requires renewed and increased effort to keep it under control. Enforcement officials can be more vehement than anyone else in their insistence that the problem they are supposed to deal with is still with us, in fact is more with us than ever before. In making these claims, enforcement officials provide good reason for continuing the existence of the position they occupy. (Becker, 1963, p. 157)

References

Adams, P. J. (2008). *Fragmented intimacy: Addiction in a social world.* Springer.

American Psychiatric Association. (1952). *Diagnostic and statistical manual: Mental disorders.* American Psychiatric Association.

American Psychiatric Association. (1980). *Diagnostic and statistical manual of mental disorders* (3rd ed.). American Psychiatric Association.

American Psychiatric Association. (2022). *Diagnostic and statistical manual of mental disorders* (5th ed.), text rev. American Psychiatric Association.

Anderson, T., Swan, H., & Lane, D. C. (2010). Institutional fads and the medicalization of drug addiction. *Sociology Compass, 4*(7), 476–494. https://doi.org/10.1111/j.1751-9020.2010.00292.x

Armor, D. J., Polich, J. M., & Stambul, H. B. (1978). *Alcoholism and treatment.* Wiley.

Becker, H. S. (1963). *Outsiders: Studies in the sociology of deviance.* The Free Press.

Bennett, C. (2011). Methadone maintenance treatment: Disciplining the 'addict'. *Health and History, 13*(2), 130–157. https://doi.org/10.1353/hah.2011.0019

Bourgois, P. (2000). Disciplining addictions: The bio-politics of methadone and heroin in the United States. *Culture, Medicine and Psychiatry, 24*(2), 165–195. https://doi.org/10.1023/A:1005574918294

Brossard, B., Roy, M., Brown, J., Hemmings, B., & Larocque, E. (2023). On the social existence of mental health categories: The case of sex addiction. *Social Problems, 72*, spad024. https://doi.org/10.1093/socpro/spad024

Campbell, N. D. (2007). *Discovering addiction: The science and politics of substance abuse research*. University of Michigan Press.

Campbell, N. D. (2012). Medicalization and biomedicalization: Does the diseasing of addiction fit the frame? In J. Netherland (Ed.), *Critical perspectives on addiction* (pp. 3–25). Emerald Group Publishing.

Castellani, B. (2000). *Pathological gambling: The making of a medical problem*. State University of New York Press.

Clarkson, J., & Kopaczewski, S. (2013). Pornography addiction and the medicalization of free speech. *Journal of Communication Inquiry, 37*(2), 128–148. https://doi.org/10.1177/0196859913482З

Cohen, B. M. Z. (2016). *Psychiatric hegemony: A Marxist theory of mental illness*. Palgrave Macmillan.

Cohen, B. M. Z. (2022). Psychiatric expansion and the rise of workplace mental health initiatives. In M. Harbusch (Ed.), *Troubled persons industries: The expansion of psychiatric categories beyond psychiatry* (pp. 129–145). Palgrave Macmillan.

Conrad, P., & Schneider, J. (1992). *Deviance and medicalization: From badness to sickness* (2nd ed.). Temple University Press.

Courtwright, D. T. (2014). Learning from Las Vegas: Gambling, technology, capitalism, and addiction. *University of Nevada Las Vegas center for gaming research occasional paper series, 26*. University Libraries.

Courtwright, D. T. (2019). *The age of addiction: How bad habits became big business*. Harvard University Press.

Davies, D. L., Scott, D. F., & Malherbe, M. E. L. (1969). Resumed normal drinking in recovered psychotic alcoholics. *International Journal of the Addictions, 4*(2), 187–194. https://doi.org/10.3109/10826086909062013

Davies, J. (2017). Political pills: Psychopharmaceuticals and neoliberalism as mutually supporting. In J. Davies (Ed.), *The sedated society: The causes and harms of our psychiatric drug epidemic* (pp. 189–225). Palgrave Macmillan.

Davies, W. (2015). *The happiness industry: How the government and big business sold us well-being*. Verso.

Elam, M. (2012). Pharmaceutical incursion on cigarette smoking at the birth of the brain disease model of addiction. In J. Netherland (Ed.), *Critical perspectives on addiction* (pp. 53–75). Emerald Group Publishing.

Epstein, W. M. (2019). *Psychotherapy and the social clinic in the United States: Soothing fictions*. Springer Nature.
Fixsen, A. (2024). *The construction of eating disorders: Psychiatry, politics and cultural representations of disordered eating*. Palgrave Macmillan.
Greenberg, G. (2008). *The noble lie: When scientists give the right answers for the wrong reasons*. Wiley.
Hall, W., Carter, A., & Forlini, C. (2015). The brain disease model of addiction: Is it supported by the evidence and has it delivered on its promises? *The Lancet Psychiatry, 2*(1), 105–110.
Hammersley, R., & Reid, M. (2002). Why the pervasive addiction myth is still believed. *Addiction Research & Therapy, 10*(1), 7–30. https://doi.org/10.1080/16066350290001687
Harbusch, M. (Ed.). (2022). *Troubled persons industries: The expansion of psychiatric categories beyond psychiatry*. Palgrave Macmillan.
Hari, J. (2015). *Chasing the scream: The first and last days of the war on drugs*. Bloomsbury.
Hellman, M., Egerer, M., Stoneham, J., Forberger, S., Männistö-Inkinen, V., Ochterbeck, D., & Rundle, S. (2022). *Addiction and the brain: Knowledge, beliefs and ethical considerations from a social perspective*. Palgrave Macmillan.
Heyman, G. M. (2009). *Addiction: A disorder of choice*. Harvard University Press.
Keane, H. (2002). *What's wrong with addiction?* Melbourne University Press.
Kincaid, H., & Sullivan, J. A. (2010). Medical models of addiction. In D. Ross, H. Kincaid, D. Spurrett, & P. Collins (Eds.), *What is addiction?* (pp. 353–376). MIT Press. https://doi.org/10.7551/mitpress/8439.003.0014
Klein, M., Dixon, J., & Butler, C. (2022). Multiple relapses into opiate and crack misuse among people in recovery: An interpretative phenomenological analysis. *Journal of Addictions & Offender Counseling, 43*(2), 97–110. https://doi.org/10.1002/jaoc.12106
Leshner, A. I. (1997). Addiction is a brain disease, and it matters. *Science, 278*(5335), 45–47. https://doi.org/10.1126/science.278.5335.45
Li, M., Peterson, C., Xu, L., Mikosz, C. A., & Luo, F. (2023). Medical costs of substance use disorders in the US employer-sponsored insurance population. *JAMA Network Open, 6*(1), e2252378. https://doi.org/10.1001/jamanetworkopen.2022.52378
Marx, K. (1887). *Capital: A critique of political economy: Volume I*. Progress Publishers.
Marx, K., & Engels, F. (1965). *Manifesto of the Communist Party*. Foreign Languages Press.

Midanik, L. (2006). *Biomedicalization of alcohol studies: Ideological shifts and institutional challenges*. Routledge.

Park, J. (2024). *Addiction becomes normal: On the late-modern American subject*. University of Chicago Press.

Pattison, E. M., Sobell, M. B., & Sobell, L. C. (1977). *Emerging concepts of alcohol dependence*. Springer.

Peele, S. (1985). *The meaning of addiction: An unconventional view* (Rev. edn.) Jossey-Bass Publishers.

Peele, S. (1989). *Diseasing of America: How we allowed recovery zealots and the treatment industry to convince us we are out of control* (Rev. edn.) Jossey-Bass Publishers.

Petry, N. M. (2016). Introduction to behavioral addictions. In N. M. Petry (Ed.), *Behavioral addictions: DSM-5® and beyond* (pp. 1–5). Oxford University Press.

Reith, G. (2019). *Addictive consumption: Capitalism, modernity and excess*. Routledge.

Room, R. (1998). Alcohol and drug disorders in the international classification of diseases: A shifting kaleidoscope. *Drug and Alcohol Review, 17*(3), 305–317. https://doi.org/10.1080/09595239800187141

Satel, S., & Lilienfeld, S. (2013). *Brainwashed: The seductive appeal of mindless neuroscience*. Perseus Books Group.

Shaffer, H. J. (1985). The disease controversy: Of metaphors, maps and menus. *Journal of Psychoactive Drugs, 17*(2), 65–76. https://doi.org/10.1080/02791072.1985.10472325

Statista. (2024). Commercial gross gaming revenue (GGR) of the gambling industry in the United States from 2020 to 2023. *Statista Research Department*. https://www.statista.com/statistics/1332999/gross-gaming-revenue-us/#:~:text=The%20gross%20gaming%20revenue%20of,compared%20to%20the%20previous%20year

Suissa, A. J. (2006). Gambling addiction as an individual pathology: A commentary. *International Journal of Mental Health and Addiction, 4*, 195–199. https://doi.org/10.1007/s11469-006-9029-5

Szasz, T. S. (1974). *The myth of mental illness: Foundations of a theory of personal conduct* (Rev. edn). Harper & Row.

Part II

Negotiating 'Addiction'

6

The Social Construction of 'Good' and 'Bad' Addicts: How Relabelling Addiction Shaped the Opioid Epidemic

Thaddeus Müller

In a period of 30 years, the US landscape of addiction has drastically changed. Where there were in the early and mid-1990s between 4000 and 8000 drug-related deaths, this has risen to over 100,000 since 2021. This is related to the introduction of strong opioid pain killers, with a similar addictive quality as heroin, in the second half of the 1990s. Pharmaceutical companies have been named as the main culprits causing the opioid epidemic. They created an aggressive marketing campaign in which they supplied false information about the addictive potential of opioid painkillers. Pain specialists have been described as their accomplices as they were supported by these companies financially. Pharmaceutical companies funded pain management-societies, opioid therapy publications, prescription opioid research, conferences and lectures on the benefits of opioid painkillers (Van Zee, 2009).

T. Müller (✉)
Lancaster University, Lancaster, UK
e-mail: t.muller@lancaster.ac.uk

B. M. Z. Cohen et al. (eds.), *Addiction and the Medicalisation of Conspicuous Behaviour*, The Politics of Mental Health and Illness,
https://doi.org/10.1007/978-3-032-06313-7_5

In public debate, the focus has been on the financial relationship between the pain specialists and the pharmaceutical industry, indicating that the former supported the use of opioid pain killers out of economic gain (see for example, Berg, 2023; Keefe, 2021; Macy, 2018; Meier, 2018; Poitras, 2022). But in fact, their pro-opioid narrative was already developed before OxyContin was available. As a result of the focus on financial motives, no systematic attention has been given to the social construction of the medicinal pro-opioid narrative (Müller, 2018). My argument here is that this narrative played a crucial role in the normalisation of strong opioid pain killers, together with the aggressive and incorrect marketing by pharmaceutical companies. This publication is the first to analyse medicinal publications on opioids, pain and addiction in a historical, critical and systematic way to unpack the development of the pro-opioid narrative. Within this narrative, medical specialists redefined addiction in order to remove the stigma of opioid drug use, which is related to the perceived 'moral weaknesses' of its users (Goffman, 1963). The redefinition of addiction was crucial in having opioid painkillers accepted as normal medication by family physicians, nurses, specialists and their patients. This chapter contributes to our understanding of the opioid public health crisis by describing and analysing the social construction of addiction by physicians in their academic publications, and thus creating one of the contributing circumstances which caused an unhampered prescribing of strong opioid pain killers for more than a decade, until 2010 when prescribing opioids became more regulated.

Removing the original label of 'addiction' and its stigma was crucial in the acceptance of opioid painkillers, and thus in the development of the opioid epidemic. Within this redefinition a differentiation was constructed between 'good' and 'bad' addicts. Those patients who showed symptoms of physical dependence and tolerance but stuck to the medical guidelines were 'good' addicts. Those who showed signs of aberrant behaviour were, by default, labelled as 'bad' patients (and 'bad' addicts) because they did not follow the medical guidelines. The core theme of the narrative was that the pill was not the problem; the patient was the problem.

Before I focus on how medical specialists redefined addiction, I will give a short description of the opioid epidemic and discuss the methods that I have used.

The Opioid Epidemic

In the beginning of the first phase of the opioid epidemic (1996–2010), prescription opioid analgesics—OxyContin by Purdue Pharma—were introduced for the treatment of non-malignant (cancer related) pain, such as lower back pain, migraine and post operative pain. At its peak in 2010 the annual opioid prescribing rate was 81.2 prescriptions per 100 persons (Guy et al., 2017). Where in 1999, 180 morphine milligram equivalents (MME are quantities that indicate the strength of opioid medication in relation to morphine) were prescribed per person in the US, this peaked in 2010 at 782 MME per person (Schuchat et al., 2017). In addition, through diversion, a substantial increase of recreational use of prescription opioid drugs took place. It turned out that the time release system of OxyContin (12 hours) could be bypassed by crushing the pill and getting immediate access to the active substance, oxycodone. In less than a decade, 25 million people initiated nonmedical use of prescription opioids (Center for Behavioral Health Statistics and Quality, 2012).

The second phase (2010–2015) was triggered by a tighter regulation of prescribing opioid pain killers and creating a tamper resistant pill. Those who had no access to prescription opioids anymore turned to heroin, which was at the time of high quality, easily available and cheaper. The third phase (2015–present) started with the introduction of fentanyl, which is 50 times stronger than heroin, and increased the number of overdoses dramatically.

Methods

The method I have used for this chapter is qualitative document analysis (QDA) (Altheide et al., 2008, p. 127). In QDA the emergence of conceptual insights while doing document analyses plays a crucial role. In the process of gathering, sampling and analysing documents, concepts are developed by constant comparison. Researchers submerge themselves in the data and interact in an ethnographic way with the documents, comparing them and grounding their developing insights in the developing data. Because its starting point is a sensitizing concept (Blumer, 1954), QDA is an excellent method to explore new fields and develop new angles.

Since 2017, I have been involved in researching the opioid epidemic. My research focuses on a wide range of publications, such as newspaper publications, online publications, medical publications, videos, documentaries, court documents and books (see Müller, 2018). Here I will mainly pay attention to medical publications in academic medical journals, which has not been done before in a systematic way. In my analysis of how pain specialists redefined the concept of addiction in the pro-opioid narrative, I will critically pay attention to how they support their claims with data and by referring to publications.

Redefining Addiction

The redefinition of addiction took place over a period of three decades. Two periods can be distinguished as outlined below.

In the first period (1970–1986) themes were developed by liberal and progressive physicians who identified with the hospice movement (palliative care) and the pain management movement. This narrative focussed predominantly on patients within a hospital setting and patients with malignant pain. In general, they were patients under close medical supervision. It is due to these humanitarian physicians that nowadays continuous opioid treatment is common for cancer patients and persons in palliative care in the Global North.

In the second phase (1986–2010) a pro-prescription opioid narrative developed which focussed on the treatment of *chronic non-malignant* pain. The themes from the first period, which were developed in relation to cancer patients and palliative care, were uncritically applied to outpatients with non-malignant pain. The aim was to destigmatise the use of opioid pain killers for these patients. One crucial difference from the first period is that a distinction was socially constructed between 'good' addicts (physically dependent) versus 'bad' addicts (psychologically dependent), which coincides respectively with patients following and patients not following the medical guidelines.

A Pro-Opioids Narrative Directed at Chronic Malignant Pain Patients (1970–1986)

In the normalisation narrative three themes played an essential role: undertreatment, opiophobia, and addiction (its definition and prevalence). Undertreatment is a legitimate theme that refers to situations in which patients do not get access to the accurate amount of pain killers to manage their pain. Already in the 1950s, Bonica, Houde and Rogers in the US and Saunders and Twycross in the UK focused on developing palliative care (Meldrum, 2005). They were the early pioneers in the pain management community and highlighted undertreatment of those who suffered severe and chronic pain, including terminal cancer patients.

The campaigners for the medicinal use of opioids had to deal with opposing medical, legal and cultural definitions that stigmatised the use of opioids to manage pain. The establishment of the US's 'war on drugs' policy in the 1970s created a scare among physicians in relation to opioid drugs; they could get arrested and prosecuted for prescribing opioid pain killers to patients over an extended duration. It also established a negative representation of drugs as leading to addiction and, subsequently, to crime and immorality, suggesting the weak moral fibre of opioid users. The resulting stigma dehumanised users, with addiction to opioids being defined as a moral problem (Blumberg, 1973; Himmelstein, 1978). In addition, religious beliefs, especially within the Christian tradition, defined pain and suffering as a constitutive part of life. Accepting pain was seen as a moral act. Those who did not complain and suffered in silence were seen as good persons and good patients. In addition, in the medical world, pain was not prioritised. The dominant perspective was that pain was irrelevant as it was seen as a symptom, not as a physical state to be treated (Meldrum, 2005).

Marks and Sachar's (1973) publication, 'Undertreatment of medical inpatients with narcotic analgesics', forms a landmark in researching undertreatment. They show that during hospitalisation most patients experience severe to moderate pain. Their research also indicates that physicians lack accurate information about the strong painkillers they prescribe, especially in relation to addiction. Morgan (1985) indicates in his foundational publication, 'American opiophobia: Customary underutilization of opioid analgesics', that many physicians in hospitals tend to give a lower dosage than is recommended. This is related to what he calls 'opiophobia', an illogical fear that the use of medical opioids will automatically lead to addiction. In his moral quest to destigmatise opioid painkillers, Morgan (1985, p. 172) differentiates between physical dependence and addiction, proposing that "[p]hysical dependence is something that happens to individuals who use or are given opioids appropriately."

Morgan (1985, p. 171, emphasis original) indicates that many physicians are not aware of the difference; they think physical dependency and addiction are similar, but he states that addiction is different:

> *Addiction* is a word which has only social determinants. It refers to a life in which drug use has become paramount. An addicted human sacrifices to his drug and its use a large measure of what the larger culture holds dear; e.g. resources, savings, family, respect, sexual activity, non-criminal status, joy of eating, health and even life itself. This commitment and ability to give over life to a drug is rare and unusual…

Morgan (1985, p. 172) argues for the destigmatisation of opioids by stating that, though they do lead to physical dependence, they do not automatically lead to what he understands as 'addiction': "[f]ew users of opioids, although physically dependent, proceed to addiction. It is a rare individual who will proceed from drug use as an incidental event in life to the cardinal event in life." In his groundbreaking publication, Morgan normalises legal drug use by normalising all drug use. He minimises the risk of getting addicted to illegal drugs and thus claims that addiction to legal opioids is also not as problematic as the conservative narrative claims it to be.

Robert Newman, a famous physician, scientist and methadone activist, counters the conservative opiophobic narrative in his 1983 publication, 'The need to redefine addiction', in the *New England Journal of Medicine*. He states that the idea that 'once an addict, always an addict' is based on a selective group of opioid users who seek treatment. To normalise drugs he refers to a wide range of studies on a more general group of users. For instance, he includes the well-known study of Vietnam veterans, that shows that a vast majority stopped using heroin when they returned to the U.S. (Robins et al., 1974). Referring to Graeven and Folmer (1977), Newman (1983, p. 1095) indicates that the prevalence of heroin "in the United States has been estimated to be as high as 4 million."

In line with the dominant conception of alcoholism, Newman states that many are able to use heroin, but are not addicted as they are able to stop and start whenever they choose to do so. He suggests formulating a more restricted definition, differentiating addicts from other narcotic users, which can counter the notion that addiction is the default result of frequent drug use. Newman redefines narcotic addiction as: "an *atypical* response to exposure to opiates, characterised by a tendency toward progressively greater consumption of the drug and a persistent disposition to relapse to drug use when abstinence has been achieved and physical dependence reversed" (1983, p. 1096, emphasis added). This definition destigmatises illegal and legal drugs. As I will show later, the notion that addiction is an atypical response to exposure to opiates would also be adopted in the pro-opioid narrative of pain specialists.

Kathleen Foley, the most prominent pro-opioid campaigner in the 1980s, includes the previous discussed references in her destigmatising narrative. She advocates opioid pain medication for cancer patients and patients in palliative care and resists the conservative notion that opioid use would enslave and demoralise its users. In the 1980s, she published many articles on cancer pain in which the three themes—undertreatment, opiophobia and a redefinition of addiction—are all an integral part of her pro-opioid narrative (see for example, Foley, 1985, 1986,

1988, 1989). In 1981, she and Ronald Kanner state that addiction is rare among cancer patients: "[o]ur experience with narcotic drug use in chronic pain is in sharp contrast to the anecdotal data suggesting that patients with chronic pain receiving narcotic analgesics are at high risk to become 'addicted'" (Kanner & Foley, 1981, p. 170). In their effort to normalise opioids analgesics they state that addiction does not lie in the drugs itself; psychological, social and economic circumstances cause addiction. This leads to the following reformulation of addiction: "[a]ddiction (now, preferably referred to as *psychological dependence*) is a behavioural pattern of compulsive drug use and preoccupation with securing its supply" (Kanner & Foley, 1981, p. 162, emphasis original).

In this narrative, tolerance and physical dependence do not automatically lead to addiction. In a later publication, Foley (1989, p. 2263) states that in order to fully understand the negative effect of opioids, the concept of addiction should be redefined as "a pattern of drug use characterised by a continued craving for an opiate manifested as compulsive drug seeking behaviour and overwhelming involvement in drug procurement and use." Referring to the famous study of Porter and Jick (1980), which I will discuss later in detail, Foley (1989, p. 2263) states that "the medical use of opioids is rarely associated with the development of addiction." In this context, she also refers to the aforementioned study of Vietnam veterans and their recovery from drugs; once they were home and stopped using heroin, only a small minority relapsed (Robins et al., 1974).

In sum, the first period of destigmatisation of opioids had a humanitarian character and was mainly concerned with those in palliative care and patients with cancer, mostly in a hospital setting. This pro-opioid narrative normalised the use of legal and illegal drugs. It promoted a more liberal approach to pain management to counter undertreatment. It labelled the resistance against prescription opioid analgesics as opiophobia, an illogical fear that these painkillers would lead by default to addiction. It emphasised that physical dependency and tolerance were common aspects of the use of opioids. The destigmatisation narrative indicated that these physical reactions were not problematic, in that they would not automatically lead to addiction. Opioids themselves were not the problem, the context—social, economic, and psychological—created the problem. But in the case of palliative care and malignant pain this did not matter, as it was rare that patients showed signs of addiction in the hospital setting due to their continued access to opioid pain medication. This narrative turned out to be highly successful, as the World Health Organization (WHO) included it in their policy advice on cancer treatment in 1990 (Meldrum, 2005).

A Pro-Opioids Narrative Directed at Chronic Non-Malignant Pain Patients (1986–2010)

In the late 1980s and early 1990s the pro-opioid narrative had reached its initial aim: a medical acceptance of the use of opioid medication for cancer patients and palliative care. In this period, pain specialists created a normalising narrative that made medicinal opioid use acceptable for patients without malignant pain. This narrative was supported by many publications, of which I will discuss the foundational ones here.

Portenoy and Foley's publication, 'Chronic use of opioid analgesics in non-malignant pain: Report of 38 cases' (1986), was a gamechanger as it deliberately changes the pro-opioid narrative to include chronic non-malignant pain patients. The authors' rationale for their research was triggered by a lack of studies on non-malignant pain treated with opioid analgesics. Their study has a retrospective character and is based on a mere 38 patients. Because it does not include a control group, this publication falls below the required standard for rigorous medical research. Still, they conclude "that opioid maintenance therapy can be a safe, salutary and more humane alternative to the options of surgery or no treatment" (Portenoy & Foley, 1986, p. 171). In the following decades, the research has been cited frequently as proof that addiction is rare among users of opioid analgesics for non-malignant pain (Tafreshi et al., 2022).

An innovative element in their narrative on addiction is that they constructed a new category of patients to explain that some did show signs of addiction: namely, the problematic patient with a history of drug use. This patient was contrasted with patients that stuck to the medical guidelines; patients who had no history of drug abuse. With the introduction of this differentiation, it created a divide between unproblematic and problematic users of prescription opioids, stigmatising the latter. This element was used to construct two new interrelated themes in the pro-opioid narrative: 1) a focus on problematic users and how to 'identify' them, and 2) that addiction with 'good' patients, as a rule, was exceptional.

In addition, Portenoy and Foley's article describes clinical guidance for prescribing opioids for chronic non-cancer pain. To reiterate, the development of these guidelines are not based on rigorous research. In the words of Tafreshi et al. (2022, p. 517), "[b]y contemporary standards of evidence-based medicine, this guidance can certainly be criticized regarding both the quality of the underlying evidence but also on the opaque and likely idiosyncratic process through which this guidance was developed." The article was the first of many publications to follow in which Portenoy further developed these themes. Before I focus on his work in more detail, I will describe two other publications that shaped the new pro-opioid narrative.

Three years after Portenoy and Foley's publication, Weissman and Haddox (1989) published a crucial article, 'Opioid pseudoaddiction—an iatrogenic syndrome', that solves a recurrent problem in pain-management: in contrast to the pro-opioid narrative, physicians do observe signs of addiction in the controlled setting of a hospital treating patients without a history of drug abuse. An example is given by Weissman and Haddox; they present the case of a young man (17 years old) who was diagnosed with acute leukaemia. He was hospitalized and given morphine, but within days his behaviour changed. He started to complain about pain to get more drugs. But the authors did not relate his behaviour to addiction but rather to undertreatment. In line with their observation, they developed a new concept, 'pseudoaddiction', described as "the iatrogenic syndrome of abnormal behavior developing as a direct consequence of inadequate pain management" (Weissman & Haddox, 1989, p. 363). The solution is obvious: to deal with this situation patients had to be given more analgesics until they calmed down.

This redefinition of addiction into pseudoaddiction has been one of the foundations of the pro-opioid narrative and has been used repeatedly by pain specialists (see for example, Elander et al., 2004; Portenoy, 1996; Sees & Clark, 1993; Weaver & Schnoll, 2002). Just as the article from Portenoy and Foley lacked a rigorous research plan, pseudoaddiction was not supported by valid research. In addition, Greene and Chambers

(2015, p. 313) state that "we find no empirical evidence yet exists to justify a clinical 'diagnosis' of pseudoaddiction".

Another common way to construct the pro-opioid narrative was by misrepresenting studies on opioid analgesics (see for example, Medina & Diamond, 1977; Perry & Heidrich, 1982; Porter & Jick, 1980). Pro-opioid campaigners tended to refer to these and other publications to prove that addiction among patients using opioids for their pain is rare, less than one percent. A famous example is the Porter and Jick study, which I mentioned previously above in relation to Foley's research. It has been described as reporting that opioid abuse only took place in four of 11,882 patients. Though this study is published in the *New England Journal of Medicine*, its scientific status is limited. It is published as a letter to the editor and contains just over 100 words. In addition, the letter is *not* about managing chronic non-malignant pain for out-patients but focusses on inpatients who received a low dose of opioid analgesics for acute pain. The journal has added on their website that the "letter has been 'heavily and uncritically' cited as evidence that addiction is rare with opioid therapy" (Zhang, 2017).

Since the mid-1980s, Portenoy has published many articles and gave many presentations redefining addiction in line with his predecessors (Chou et al., 2009; Fine & Portenoy, 2007; Portenoy, 1990, 1996; Portenoy et al., 1997, 2005; Rosenblum et al., 2008). As the leader of the pro-opioid movement his main goal was to re-educate physicians and nurses, and highlight misconceptions around addiction and the use of opioid medication. He acted, in line with Foley, as a campaigner, fighting for the rights of pain patents to have access to opioids, which he called a 'gift from nature' (Lurie, 2021).

Here we will focus on Portenoy's (1996) article, 'Opioid therapy for chronic nonmalignant pain: A review of the critical issues', which captures all the main themes of the new pro-opioid narrative. In this publication he states that an understanding of the positive contribution of opioid therapy is "hampered by a confusing nomenclature" (Portenoy, 1996, p. 208). Portenoy explains that addiction is a physiological phenomenon related to what he calls the "abstinence syndrome" (Portenoy, 1996, p. 208), which is related to the decrease of opioid use. He makes clear that anybody who uses opioids, even for a few days, should be seen as "physically dependent" (Portenoy, 1996, p. 208). Consequently, he states that physical dependence does not align with addiction:

> Although some definitions of addiction refer to physical dependence, the potential for abstinence is neither necessary nor sufficient for the diagnosis of addictions. Clinicians sometimes use the general term, 'dependent,' or the inaccurate label, 'addicted,' to describe patients who are presumed to be physically dependent. Given the stigma that may accompany the use of an incorrect term, this language should be avoided. Clinicians should use 'physically dependent' when referring to the potential for abstinence. Physical dependence is usually perceived to be clinically unimportant as long as abstinence is avoided. (Portenoy, 1996, p. 208)

Portenoy wants to avoid the term 'addiction' because this stigmatises prescription opioid users. In his eyes, the accurate term is 'physical dependence'. And as he states in the last sentence, addiction will not follow from physical dependence because opioid-treated patients will have ample access to prescribed opioids, meaning that in a medical setting abstinence as a rule does not take place. Following this tautological reasoning the difference between patients (physical dependence) and 'real' addicts is the legal access to opioid drugs.

In line with this statement, he disagrees with definitions accepted by the WHO and the American Psychiatric Association's fourth edition of the *Diagnostic and Statistical Manual of Mental Disorders* (DSM). He argues that, according to the criteria of the DSM-IV, most opioid-treated patients would indeed be labelled as 'addicted'. In order to distinguish 'bad' addicts from 'good' addicts, Portenoy introduces a new concept to diagnose addiction: 'representative aberrant drug-related behaviors' (1996, p. 209). It is unclear how 'representative' this is as he does not support this concept with data or references to any academic literature but his own. He also claims that some aberrant behaviour is more predictive than others, which is a quite bold move as there does not seem to be any rigorous research to support the predictive quality of these behavioural indicators. Some examples of "[p]robably less predictive" indicators are: the "[a]ggressive complaining about the need for more drug[s]"; "[d]rug-hoarding during periods of reduced symptoms"; and "[r] equesting specific drugs" (Portenoy, 1996, p. 209). Examples of "[p]robably more predictive" indicators are: "[s]elling prescription drugs"; forging prescriptions; and "[s]tealing or 'borrowing' drugs from others" (Portenoy, 1996, p. 209).

In addition to these differences of aberrant behaviour between patients and addicts, Portenoy also highlights another difference which has a physiological character. He states that "addicts who receive opioids in the absence of pain report euphoria, whereas patients and volunteers rarely report this effect, and indeed, more commonly described dysphoric feelings" (Portenoy, 1996, p. 210). This is related to the assumption that pain somehow cancels the blissful effect of opioids. In line with this way of reasoning, many within the pain management community thought that because of this inability to get high, pain patients could not become addicted.

Another difference between real addicts and patients with chronic pain, according to Portenoy, is that they do not share the same social psychological and physiological characteristics. Again, this is a bold statement not supported by rigorous medical research. Portenoy (1996, p. 210, emphasis added) states that,

> In sum, these data [Portenoy does not refer to data, only to references] suggest that the development of addiction results from an interaction between the inherent reinforcing properties of opioid drugs and predisposing psychological, social and physiological factors that are presumably *uncommon in the heterogenous population of patients with chronic pain.*

What we see here is a rhetoric strategy that Portenoy commonly applies in his publications. In the first part of a sentence, he relates something that most of his readers will agree to be true, and is supported by references. In the second part he adds something that is questionable and not supported by data. Because of this syntaxis, the whole sentence radiates a sense of validity and authority. In this citation we can see that the first part of this sentence which relates to addiction is accurate and based on academic references, but the second part (in italics), which is related to patients with chronic pain, is not supported by valid data and seems to be based on wishful thinking.

Over a period of 25 years, with his publications and presentations, Portenoy has shaped a medical culture which normalised the use of opioid analgesics for patients with chronic non-malignant pain. Medical guidelines were shaped by Portenoy and his colleagues who were influenced by his pro-opioid education. Over time this narrative became problematic because it referred to a medical situation of close supervision by a physician, which was not in line with daily practices in the late 1990s and in the first decade of the 2000s. Because OxyContin and other similar drugs were not seen as addictive they were prescribed as if they were smarties. Patients were prescribed, in one consultation, a large amount of strong opioid painkillers for several months, which meant that they could use them without any form of medical supervision during that period.

The redefinition of addiction and specifically the differentiation between good (physically dependent) and bad (psychologically dependent) patients also played a crucial role in how the medical world, especially pain specialists, reacted to the developing opioid epidemic in the first decade of the 2000s. Patients who became addicted (that is, showing signs of aberrant behaviour), patients who overdosed, and patients who died a medicinal opioid-related death were labelled in one specific way: they were 'bad' patients, patients who did not stick to medical guidance. Pain specialists continued their mantra that 'addiction' among patients who followed the medical guidelines was rare, less than one percent.

How Rare Is Iatrogenic Addiction?

In the first decade of the opioid epidemic, its explanation did not focus on the addictive strength of the opioid analgesic. Besides the usual suspects of 'street addicts' and 'recreational users', the dominant explanation used the distinction between good patients and bad patients to blame the latter. This was contradicted by patients' narratives which became part of the public discussion in the 2010s. In these narratives, trajectories of addiction and overdose started with prescribed opioid analgesics. These narratives show that the distinction between 'good' and 'bad' patients is highly artificial and not in line with the daily experience of pain patients.

This comes to the forefront in a news report from Fauber and Gabler (2012) in the *Milwaukee Journal Sentinel* titled 'What happened to the poster children of OxyContin?'. In the article, the authors retraced five of seven people who participated in a video sponsored by the pharmaceutical industry titled *"I got my life back": Patients in pain tell their stories*, which was distributed to 15,000 physicians. Out of the five persons, two were still content with their pain medication, but three became addicted, of which two subsequently died. The latter three needed more medication to deal with their pain up to the point that they became physically and psychologically dependent on prescribed opioid analgesics.

When it was hard to ignore the developing opioid epidemic, medical researchers started to test whether iatrogenic addiction was indeed rare. Martell et al. (2007) exposed in a systematic review of the use of opioids for chronic back pain that between five and 24 percent showed aberrant behaviour. Fishbain et al. (2008) showed in a review that the addiction rate of people who were prescribed opioids was between three and four percent, and that aberrant behaviour was found in 11.5 percent. Research by Boscarino et al. (2011) among 2000 pain patients stated that 35 percent of the long-term opioid users met the DSM-criteria for opioid use disorder. A systematic review by Vowles et al. (2015) indicated that the weighted score for opioid misuse was between 21 and 29 percent, and the mean percentage for addiction was between eight and 12 percent. Though there is large variability in the results of these publications—mostly related to different definitions of addiction and medical treatment—it is clear that iatrogenic addiction was not as rare as stated in the pro-opioid narrative.

Conclusion

In this chapter I set out to describe and analyse the social construction of the pro-opioid narrative, and specifically the relabelling of addiction. I have indicated that there are two different phases within the development of the pro-opioid narrative. The first one (1970–1986) aimed to normalise the use of illegal drugs and the use of opioid analgesics for managing malignant pain and palliative care. Medical specialists resisted the label of the drug user as an 'addict' as it carried the stigma of moral weakness. The first narrative highlighted undertreatment, opiophobia and a new definition of addiction. The lack of sufficient pain management using opioids (undertreatment) was related to an illogical fear and stigma of these strong drugs (opiophobia). The narrative stated that dependency (and tolerance) should be separated from the concept of 'addiction', as the first does not automatically lead to the second. The first pro-opioid narrative explicitly related this to the context of legal and illegal drug use. With this new definition, the narrative could indicate that though patients in palliative care and with malignant pain were indeed dependent, they were as a rule not addicted (see also Noorani, this volume—Noorani outlines a similar redefining process here, in relation to the medical normalisation of psychedelics). Of course, in the context of a hospital setting and close medical supervision there is, as a rule, an adequate amount of opioids available. As a result, this way of reasoning had a high tautological quality. Still, with this new definition, campaigners could refer to studies in a hospital setting and state that addiction was rare. Thanks to the liberal and humanitarian campaigners who created this narrative, it is now common practice to use opioids in palliative care and to manage malignant pain.

The narrative created in the first period was used in the second period in which the aim was to normalise opioid pain killers for chronic non-malignant pain, such as back pain, arthritis, and chronic migraine. One issue which was highly problematic was the lack of rigorous research on the addictive reaction to the use of opioids for non-malignant pain. In the first period this could be studied in hospices and in hospitals, but there was not a population with non-malignant pain to be studied on the same scale—and in a similarly rigorous manner—outside the hospital setting. This problem was circumvented by constructing pro-opioid articles based on non-rigorous research and referring to other research publications in a misleading way. This produced fraudulent evidence that addiction (psychological dependency/aberrant behaviour) was rare (less than one percent). Other concepts were introduced, such as 'pseudoaddiction', and 'aberrant drug-related behaviour', through which opioid treatment for chronic pain became destigmatised. The pro-opioid narrative was highly successful and was embraced by the pain management community. This created a culture, in which opioid pain killers were prescribed in abundance. The pro-opioid narrative—supported by the aggressive and false marketing of pharmaceutical companies—paved the way for a massive increase in the use of opioid pain killers, which culminated in almost 90 prescriptions for opioids per 100 Americans in 2010.

When in the late 1990s the first signs of the opioid epidemic were noticeable, the labelling of 'good' and 'bad' addicts was used to ignore the problematic quality of OxyContin and other strong opioid painkillers. The rhetoric was that the opioid epidemic was caused by street addicts, recreational users and patients that did not stick to the medical guidelines. Pain specialists still embraced the notion that addiction was rare among patients who were 'good' addicts/patients and, if they showed signs of aberrant behaviour, this was labelled as pseudoaddiction and more drugs were prescribed. Patients' narratives and academic publications proved that the core themes of the pro-opioid narrative were wrong and based on wishful thinking: addiction was not rare, the differentiation between 'good' and 'bad' addicts was not in line with the everyday experience of patients taking opioid analgesics, and the "predisposing psychological, social and physiological factors" that cause addiction were *not* "uncommon in the heterogenous population of patients with chronic pain" (Portenoy, 1996, p. 210).

References

Altheide, D., Coyle, M., DeVriese, K., & Schneider, C. (2008). Emergent qualitative document analysis. In S. N. Hesse-Biber & P. Leavy (Eds.), *Handbook of emergent methods* (pp. 127–151). Guilford Press.

Berg, P. (Director). (2023). *Painkiller* [television series]. Netflix.

Blumberg, A. S. (1973). The politics of deviance: The case of drugs. *Journal of Drug Issues, 3*(2), 105–114. https://doi.org/10.1177/002204267300300202

Blumer, H. (1954). What is wrong with social theory? *American Sociological Review, 19*(1), 3–10. https://doi.org/10.2307/2088165

Boscarino, J. A., Rukstalis, M. R., Hoffman, S. N., Han, J. J., Erlich, P. M., Ross, S., Gerhard, G. S., & Stewart, W. F. (2011). Prevalence of prescription opioid-use disorder among chronic pain patients: Comparison of the DSM-5 vs. DSM-4 diagnostic criteria. *Journal of Addictive Diseases, 30*(3), 185–194. https://doi.org/10.1080/10550887.2011.581961

Center for Behavioral Health Statistics and Quality. (2012). *2011 national survey on drug use and health: Summary of national findings*. Substance Abuse and Mental Health Services Administration.

Chou, R., Fanciullo, G. J., Fine, P. G., Miaskowski, C., Passik, S. D., & Portenoy, R. K. (2009). Opioids for chronic noncancer pain: Prediction and identification of aberrant drug-related behaviors: A review of the evidence for an American pain society and American academy of pain medicine clinical practice guideline. *The Journal of Pain, 10*(2), 131–146. https://doi.org/10.1016/j.jpain.2008.10.009

Elander, J., Lusher, J., Bevan, D., Telfer, P., & Burton, B. (2004). Understanding the causes of problematic pain management in sickle cell disease: Evidence that pseudoaddiction plays a more important role than genuine analgesic dependence. *Journal of Pain and Symptom Management, 27*(2), 156–169. https://doi.org/10.1016/j.jpainsymman.2003.12.001

Fauber, J., & Gabler, E. (2012). What happened to the poster children of OxyContin? *Milwaukee Journal Sentinel*. https://eu.jsonline.com/story/news/investigations/2019/05/17/what-happened-poster-children-oxycontin/3705244002/

Fine, P. G., & Portenoy, R. K. (2007). *A clinical guide to opioid analgesia*. Vendome Group: Healthcare Division.

Fishbain, D. A., Cole, B., Lewis, J., Rosomoff, H. L., & Rosomoff, R. S. (2008). What percentage of chronic nonmalignant pain patients exposed to chronic opioid analgesic therapy develop abuse/addiction and/or aberrant drug-related behaviors? A structured evidence-based review. *Pain Medicine, 9*(4), 444–459. https://doi.org/10.1111/j.1526-4637.2007.00370.x

Foley, K. M. (1985). The treatment of cancer pain. *New England Journal of Medicine, 313*(2), 84–95. https://doi.org/10.1056/NEJM198507113130205

Foley, K. M. (1986). The treatment of pain in the patient with cancer. *CA: A Cancer Journal for Clinicians, 36*(4), 194–215.

Foley, K. M. (1988). The cancer pain patient. *Journal of Pain and Symptom Management, 3*, S16–S19. https://doi.org/10.1016/0885-3924(88)90207-2

Foley, K. M. (1989). Controversies in cancer pain medical perspectives. *Cancer, 63*(11), 2257–2265. https://doi.org/10.1002/1097-0142(19890601)63:11<2257::AID-CNCR2820631134>3.0.CO;2-6

Goffman, E. (1963). *Stigma: Notes on the management of spoiled identity*. Prentice-Hall.

Graeven, D. B., & Folmer, W. (1977). Experimental heroin users: An epidemiologic and psychosocial approach. *The American Journal of Drug and Alcohol Abuse, 4*(3), 365–375. https://doi.org/10.3109/00952997709002771

Greene, M. S., & Chambers, R. A. (2015). Pseudoaddiction: Fact or fiction? An investigation of the medical literature. *Current Addiction Reports, 2*, 310–317.

Guy, G. P., Jr., Zhang, K., Bohm, M. K., Losby, J., Lewis, B., Young, R., Murphy, L. B., & Dowell, D. (2017). Vital signs: Changes in opioid prescribing in the United States, 2006–2015. *Morbidity and Mortality Weekly Report, 66*(26), 697–704. https://doi.org/10.15585/mmwr.mm6626a4

Himmelstein, J. L. (1978). Drug politics theory: Analysis and critique. *Journal of Drug Issues, 8*(1), 37–52. https://doi.org/10.1177/002204267800800103

Kanner, R. M., & Foley, K. M. (1981). Patterns of narcotic drug use in a cancer pain clinic. *Annals of the New York Academy of Sciences, 362*(1), 161–172. https://doi.org/10.1111/j.1749-6632.1981.tb12804.x

Keefe, P. R. (2021). *Empire of pain: The secret history of the Sackler dynasty*. Doubleday.

Lurie, J. (2021) The untold story of Purdue pharma's cozy relationship with the American medical association. *Mother Jones*. https://www.motherjones.com/politics/2021/08/purdue-pharma-american-medical-association-relationship-opioid-crisis-public-health/

Macy, B. (2018). *Dopesick: Dealers, doctors and the drug company that addicted America*. Bloomsbury Publishing.

Marks, R. M., & Sachar, E. J. (1973). Undertreatment of medical inpatients with narcotic analgesics. *Annals of Internal Medicine, 78*(2), 173–181.

Martell, B. A., O'Connor, P. G., Kerns, R. D., Becker, W. C., Morales, K. H., Kosten, T. R., & Fiellin, D. A. (2007). Systematic review: Opioid treatment for chronic back pain: Prevalence, efficacy, and association with addiction. *Annals of Internal Medicine, 146*(2), 116–127.

Medina, J. L., & Diamond, S. (1977). Drug dependency in patients with chronic headaches. *Headache: The Journal of Head and Face Pain, 17*(1), 12–14. https://doi.org/10.1111/j.1526-4610.1977.hed1701012.x

Meier, B. (2018). *Pain killer: An empire of deceit and the origin of America's opioid epidemic*. Random House.

Meldrum, M. (2005). The ladder and the clock: Cancer pain and public policy at the end of the twentieth century. *Journal of Pain and Symptom Management, 29*(1), 41–54. https://doi.org/10.1016/j.jpainsymman.2004.08.004

Morgan, J. P. (1985). American opiophobia: Customary underutilization of opioid analgesics. *Advances in Alcohol & Substance Abuse, 5*(1–2), 163–172. https://doi.org/10.1300/J251v05n01_11

Müller, T. (2018). Artsen en moreel ondernemerschap: De casus van de normalisering van verslavende opioïde pijnstillers in de Verenigde Staten [Medical doctors and moral entrepreneurship: Normalisation of opioid painkillers in the US]. *Tijdschrift over Cultuur & Criminaliteit, 8*(3), 25–42. doi:https://doi.org/10.5553/TCC/221195072018008003003

Newman, R. G. (1983). The need to redefine addiction. *New England Journal of Medicine, 308*(18), 1096–1098. https://doi.org/10.1056/NEJM198305053081811

Perry, S., & Heidrich, G. (1982). Management of pain during debridement: A survey of US burn units. *Pain, 13*(3), 267–280. https://doi.org/10.1016/0304-3959(82)90016-1

Poitras, L. (Director). (2022). *All the beauty and the bloodshed* [film]. HBO.

Portenoy, R. K. (1990). Chronic opioid therapy in nonmalignant pain. *Journal of Pain and Symptom Management, 5*(1 Suppl), S46–S62.

Portenoy, R. K. (1996). Opioid therapy for chronic nonmalignant pain: A review of the critical issues. *Journal of Pain and Symptom Management, 11*(4), 203–217. https://doi.org/10.1016/0885-3924(95)00187-5

Portenoy, R. K., Dole, V., Joseph, H., Lowinson, J., Rice, C., Segal, S., & Richman, B. L. (1997). Pain management and chemical dependency: Evolving perspectives. *JAMA, 278*(7), 592–593. https://doi.org/10.1001/jama.1997.03550070084043

Portenoy, R. K., & Foley, K. M. (1986). Chronic use of opioid analgesics in non-malignant pain: Report of 38 cases. *Pain, 25*(2), 171–186. https://doi.org/10.1016/0304-3959(86)90091-6

Portenoy, R. K., Lussier, D., Kirsh, K. L., & Passik, S. D. (2005). Pain and addiction. In R. J. Frances, S. I. Miller, & A. H. Mack (Eds.), *Clinical textbook of addictive disorders* (pp. 367–395). The Guilford Press.

Porter, J., & Jick, H. (1980). Addiction rare in patients treated with narcotics. *New England Journal of Medicine, 302*(2), 123. https://doi.org/10.1056/nejm198001103020221

Robins, L. N., Davis, D. H., & Nurco, D. N. (1974). How permanent was Vietnam drug addiction? *American Journal of Public Health, 64*(12_Suppl), 38–43.

Rosenblum, A., Marsch, L. A., Joseph, H., & Portenoy, R. K. (2008). Opioids and the treatment of chronic pain: Controversies, current status, and future directions. *Experimental and Clinical Psychopharmacology, 16*(5), 405–416. https://doi.org/10.1037/a0013628

Schuchat, A., Houry, D., & Guy, G. P. (2017). New data on opioid use and prescribing in the United States. *JAMA, 318*(5), 425–426. https://doi.org/10.1001/jama.2017.8913

Sees, K. L., & Clark, H. W. (1993). Opioid use in the treatment of chronic pain: Assessment of addiction. *Journal of Pain and Symptom Management, 8*(5), 257–264. https://doi.org/10.1016/0885-3924(93)90154-N

Tafreshi, S., Steiner, A., & Sud, A. (2022). Shifting interpretations in evidence and guidance in pain and opioids research: A bibliometric analysis of a highly cited case series from 1986. *Journal of Evaluation in Clinical Practice, 28*(4), 509–519. https://doi.org/10.1111/jep.13680

Van Zee, A. (2009). The promotion and marketing of oxycontin: Commercial triumph, public health tragedy. *American Journal of Public Health, 99*(2), 221–227.

Vowles, K. E., McEntee, M. L., Julnes, P. S., Frohe, T., Ney, J. P., & Van Der Goes, D. N. (2015). Rates of opioid misuse, abuse, and addiction in chronic pain: A systematic review and data synthesis. *Pain, 156*(4), 569–576. https://doi.org/10.1097/01.j.pain.0000460357.01998.f1

Weaver, M. F., & Schnoll, S. H. (2002). Opioid treatment of chronic pain in patients with addiction. *Journal of Pain & Palliative Care Pharmacotherapy, 16*(3), 5–26. https://doi.org/10.1080/J354v16n03_02

Weissman, D. E., & Haddox, J. D. (1989). Opioid pseudoaddiction—An iatrogenic syndrome. *Pain, 36*(3), 363–366. https://doi.org/10.1016/0304-3959(89)90097-3

Zhang, S. (2017). The one-paragraph letter from 1980 that fueled the opioid crisis. *The Atlantic*. https://www.theatlantic.com/health/archive/2017/06/nejm-letter-opioids/528840/

7

Excessive Appetites and Disarming Innovations: The Shifting Socio-Materialities of Nicotine and Gambling Addiction

Mark Elam

The dramatic broadening of the concept of addiction in recent decades, or what Eve Sedgwick (1993, p. 135) famously christened the "epidemic of addiction and addiction attribution" has coincided with the growth of an excessive appetite model of addiction. This model is firstly associated with the work of Jim Orford (2000, 2001) and his psychological view of addictions but, broadly speaking, it can be said to inform leading neurobiological, sociological and historical understandings of addiction alike today. These are all prepared to move beyond a primary focus on drug-taking and drug dependence to connect addiction with an 'over-attachment' to any number of different objects and activities.

M. Elam (✉)
University of Gothenburg, Gothenburg, Sweden
e-mail: mark.elam@gu.se

B. M. Z. Cohen et al. (eds.), *Addiction and the Medicalisation of Conspicuous Behaviour*, The Politics of Mental Health and Illness,
https://doi.org/10.1007/978-3-032-06313-7_6

Mirroring the late nineteenth century disease concept of 'inebriety', addictions understood as excessive appetites are once more synonymous with 'morbid cravings'—powerful impulses and desires repeatedly leading appetitive behaviour astray. Just as behavioural neuroscientists now see 'wanting' and desire as progressively overriding and erasing 'liking' and pleasure during the course of addiction (Robinson et al., 2015), so sociologists like Gerda Reith wish to connect the contemporary proliferation of addictions with the abandon and excess of consumer capitalism more generally; insatiable appetites reveal the 'dark side of consumption' (Reith, 2019, p. 5) where consumers themselves risk being consumed and devoured by their own limitless desires. Similarly, for the historian David Courtwright (2019), the contemporary epidemic of addictions tells of the latest phase in the development of 'limbic capitalism' and of big businesses that purposively design and market their goods and services to interfere with the brain circuitry controlling appetitive behaviour.

As Orford (2001, p. 16) discusses, appetites become excessive as objects and activities which were once purely pleasurable mutate into enslaving necessities. Accounting for this transformation, neuroscientists point to how the mesolimbic reward pathway in our brains originally developed to reinforce behaviours guaranteeing our survival. However, over time, and in the context of the contemporary 'age of addiction' (Courtwright, 2019), this circuitry has become a double-edged sword and a persistent source of vulnerability. As Courtwright (2019, p. 9) charts, pleasure after pleasure has been *weaponized* and engineered in a fashion capable of triggering compulsive consumption. For this reason, continual caution and vigilance are called for if we are to prevent ourselves from being hijacked and led astray by addiction.

The 'loss of control' that has always been central to addiction has gradually changed in character with the ascendence of the excessive appetite model. During the mid-twentieth century, this was firstly connected with the consumption of intoxicating substances producing clearly distinguishable symptoms of physical dependence. Addicts were individuals palpably in the grip of drugs whose vivid symptoms helped to translate addiction into a genuine disease. This focus on the more dramatic symptoms of tolerance and withdrawal encouraged a distinction to be drawn between mere drug habits and true addictions. Therefore, when cigarette smoking first became a serious public health issue in the 1950s it was initially classified as a question of drug habituation. According to the US Surgeon General in 1964, the habitual smoker who continually reaches into their pocket for a cigarette bears no resemblance to the desperate heroin addict who regularly resorts to crime and "sometimes even murder" due to their physiological dependence on drugs (Advisory Committee to the Surgeon General of the Public Health Service, 1964, p. 352).

However, by the end of the 1980s, the same authority had changed its tune, concluding in its twentieth report on smoking and health that cigarettes are addicting and that the pharmacologic and behavioural processes determining tobacco addiction are like those determining addiction to heroin and cocaine (U.S. Department of Health and Human Services, 1988, p. 29). During the course of this turnaround the loss of control that addiction implies was re-envisaged as something comparatively commonplace and unspectacular. It shifted towards an inability to control an appetitive activity despite harmful consequences (see Orford, 2001, p. 18). While drugs remain at the heart of many cases of addiction today, these are now firstly defined as severe substance use disorders rather than matters of drug dependence. In other words, they have become what can be broadly defined as pathologies of consumption.

Cigarettes in many ways tipped the balance as, after the late 1980s, addiction was no longer confined to the margins of society and wedded with illicit drug trades. Instead, even low levels of consumption of a licit product sold in the trillions worldwide was established as a deadly source of addiction. Of course, alcoholic products have been broadly marketed and sold since the very discovery of addiction (Levine, 1978). However, with the shift to the excessive appetites model, the alcoholic is also no longer a marginal figure; no longer the habitual drunkard, but rather the regular drinker whose everyday consumption amounts to a severe risk of harm.

In this chapter my ambition is to elaborate further on the sociological and historical interpretation of the excessive appetite model of addiction. For Orford (2000, p. xi), excessive appetites are best thought of as 'over-attachments' to objects or activities. While fully agreeing with this relational approach I want to present processes of addictive attachment in broader socio-material terms, rather than narrower psychological and biobehavioural ones. This I shall do by drawing on the path-breaking research of Robert Proctor on the socio-materialities of nicotine addiction and of Natasha Dow Schüll on the technology of gambling addiction. Having outlined how addictive attachment can be envisioned as a broader question of technical mediation and innovation, I will turn to a subset of innovations that typically accompany the rise of particularly addictive technologies. These are what I call *disarming innovations* which can either serve to further elaborate processes of attachment or enable detachment from growing patterns of compulsive consumption. With reference to the examples of nicotine replacement therapies and responsible gambling devices, I will discuss the persistent ambiguity of disarming innovations which may be primarily concerned with allaying public fears regarding the safety of addictive technologies or, more disruptively, with breaking compulsive patterns of addictive consumption. As disarming innovations become more disruptive, they are likely to become closely entangled with scientific research and the medicalisation of different addictions. However, such disruption may ultimately have more to do with the modulation and rechannelling of addictive behaviour than its lasting restraint.

Socio-Materialities of Addictive Attachment

Envisioning addictions as excessive appetites also means viewing them as relational entities, as forms of *attachment*. Therefore, it can be somewhat misleading to set out a list of core addictions as Orford (2000, p. 3) does, as none of the objects and activities he identifies are innately addictive. The addictiveness of things like alcohol, cocaine, gambling, processed foods, and tobacco is something that arises through their repeated consumption in some particular manner. In similar fashion, no one is destined to become an addict. Rather, people become addicts as they are drawn into particular patterns of interaction with different objects and activities. In other words, addictions transform people and things alike by mediating the relations between them. Neither are the same after they enter an addictive relationship with each other (see for example, Latour, 1994, p. 33; Schüll, 2012, p. 20). People lose control of their consumption of things as these things simultaneously transform into objects of necessity for them.

If not intrinsically addictive, some objects and activities can still *afford* their addictive consumption, in the same way as some people, if not predestined, can still be socially and genetically *predisposed* to consuming them in this fashion. The social and material configuration of things and the genetic make-up of individuals matter as both are, to varying degrees, responsible for enabling or constraining addictive behaviour. As David Courtwright (2001, p. 14) has remarked in relation to the former, "the history of psychoactive substances resembles that of the arms race". It is the history of the weaponisation of pleasure and the continual redesign of pleasures to afford new qualities of attachment. The definitive example of this process remains the invention of the modern cigarette. As Robert Proctor has documented, a range of inventions were responsible for the triumph of the cigarette during the early twentieth century. However, the deadliest of these was the introduction of the 'flue-curing' process which produces a dried tobacco leaf with an increased sugar content (Proctor, 2011, pp. 31–35). This sweeter leaf yields a milder, less alkaline, tobacco smoke that affords its relatively easy inhalation into the lungs. Such deep inhalation affords in turn a uniquely rapid absorption of nicotine into the bloodstream, enabling it to reach the brain within seconds. Therefore, rather than the innate properties of nicotine, it is just the *inhalable* nature of cigarette smoke compared to other forms of tobacco smoke that Proctor sees as underlying the exceptional lethality of the human attachment to this drug.

However, in addition to a new quality of tobacco smoke a whole range of other mediators played vital roles in historically establishing the deadly global appetite for nicotine. Cigarettes were part of a larger 'packaged pleasure revolution' which combined innovations in production, packaging, and distribution (Cross & Proctor, 2014). This revolution served to capture, preserve, and concentrate a series of sensual experiences into a new range of portable, durable, cheap, and accessible products which could be universally marketed across boundaries of social class and physical space. Elaborating on Courtwright's notion of the weaponisation of pleasure, Cross and Proctor (2014, pp. 11–15) discuss this in terms of a process of 'tubularization'. Just as opium was industrially refined into morphine to be medically delivered through the newly invented hypodermic syringe from the 1850s, so a whole series of mass-produced 'tubes' emerged in the late nineteenth century specially designed to deliver new chemically refined sensations. The combination of flue-curing and automated cigarette-rolling machines gave rise to the tubularization of tobacco consumption in the same way as the rise of the food canning industry served to mechanise the production of standardised portions of preserved foods (Cross & Proctor, 2014, chapter 1). Bottling factories also emerged at the same time as the first Coca-Cola bottling plant opened in Chattanooga in 1899. The invention of the chocolate bar can be seen as a further example of tubularization as famous snacks like Hershey's, Toblerone, Cadbury's Dairy Milk, and Fry's Chocolate Cream were all introduced around the turn of the twentieth century.

New packaged pleasures were wrapped and/or labelled and marketed through new practices of branding. For example, the creation of brands like Camel in 1913, Pall Mall in 1899, Chesterfield in 1896, and Marlboro in 1924 afforded the mass marketing of cigarettes, serving again like inhalable tobacco smoke as vital (immaterial) mediators between the ever-expanding objects and subjects of nicotine addiction. Through its ability to render pleasures portable, durable and 'ready at hand', tubularization enabled the new combination of relations of both delayed and instantaneous gratification. Unlike in the past, new packaged pleasures were now able to be enjoyed almost anywhere, anytime, by anyone (Cross & Proctor, 2014, chapter 1). In relation to the instantaneous gratification provided by cigarettes, one further closely related case of tubularization was the invention of the safety match—aka the 'Swedish match'—in 1855 in Jönköping. Originally made by hand, production was soon mechanised including that of matchboxes. Evidencing their intimate connection, the Swedish tobacco industry and Swedish matchmaking were rolled into the one company, Swedish Match AB, during the mid-1990s—a company which, in February 2023, became completely owned by Philip Morris International (PMI).

Therefore, when Courtwright asserts that the history of psychoactive things resembles an arms race he is pointing to how technology is continually transforming these things and the ways in which they are consumed and delivered. It is always creating new attachments between the subjects and objects of addiction and revising the nature of both in the process. Hence, there are no core addictions as Orford describes, there are rather many shifting socio-material forms of addictive attachment leading to differing levels of harm.

As Proctor documents how the cigarette weaponised tobacco consumption, so Natasha Dow Schüll has charted how technology has transformed the experience of gambling, rendering it more addictive. Gambling machines emerged in the late nineteenth-century packaged pleasure revolution alongside other coin-operated machines dispensing food, snacks, cigarettes, and any number of "automated amusements" (Schüll, 2012, p. 80; see also Huhtamo, 2005). The difference was that gambling machines dispensed nothing other than the chance (or not) to win back more money than you fed into them. Through a series of design innovations these mass-produced machines successfully packaged the consumption of gambling as cigarettes did in relation to tobacco. In the place of inhalable smoke, what firstly transforms machine gambling into a form of necessity is the fine tuning of the schedules by which rewards are dispensed or withheld (Schüll, 2012, p. 108). As mechanical slot machines became electromechanical by the 1960s and electronic from the late 1970s, so the ability of reward schedules to reinforce gambling behaviour grew ever more advanced and sophisticated. This has resulted in the continuing proliferation today of multiline video slots where players wager on multiple lines of symbols. By offering small rewards more frequently these machines can keep players gambling by making them feel they are winning all the time, when they are only losing more and more (Schüll, 2012, p. 121).

However, the technology that has done most to increase gambling industry revenues in recent decades is behavioural tracking and analytics. This emerged together with loyalty programmes in US casinos where, to begin with, attendants simply watched players gamble and awarded them free gifts once they had spent a certain amount of money. Other early devices also included punch cards for collecting reward points before the first loyalty cards were introduced that customers could simply insert into slot machines to earn credits automatically as they played (Schüll, 2012, p. 144). A particularly influential loyalty card system was Harrah's Total Gold system established in the 1990s. As the former CEO of the company recounts in the *Harvard Business Review*, the gambling data deriving from this system showed that only 26 percent of the company's customers produced 82 percent of its revenues. Surprisingly, these big spenders were not classic high rollers, but rather regular slot machine players who preferred a $60 gift of gambling tokens to two free steak meals simply because they "enjoyed the anticipation and excitement of gambling itself" (Loveman, 2003, p. 111). By tracking gambling behaviour it became possible to calculate individual 'customer worth' and divide the customer base into different segments on which marketing experiments could be run, exploring if they could be incentivised to gamble more. As the CEO further reveals:

> We also set up a series of triggers in the database and analysed the customers' responses … If, for example, we discovered that a customer who spends $1000 per month with us hadn't visited us in three months, a letter or telephone call would invite him back. If we learned he lost money during his last visit, we invited him back for a special event. Our telemarketers were trained to listen for responses to specific offers (Loveman, 2003, p. 112).

Such data-driven practices have now become the cornerstone of the online gambling industry which has completely repackaged gambling by transforming your mobile phone or your laptop into a state-of-the-art gambling machine. As the Swedish online gambling group Kindred explains its commitment to personalized marketing:

> Our data-driven online world means that customers expect to feel recognized and remembered. Personalized engagement is psychologically powerful, and it goes a long way to encouraging our customers to continue playing with us. Big data in the form of behavioural, demographic, and

> contextual data gives us crucial information to tailor messages for specific audiences ... It also helps us to adapt to changes in individual habits, user journeys and expectations, information that's vital to be aware of if we are to keep customers engaged ... for example, most younger slots and roulette players belong to the high thrill seeking demographic that's drawn to themed games with high stakes along with high rewards or jackpots. (Dhaisne, 2019)

The internet has created a global infrastructure for 24/7 patterns of consumption and the endless elaboration of new forms of addictive attachment and identity. Packaged pleasures have evolved into platform and app-based pleasures where technological mediation is rendering the objects and means of addiction even harder to distinguish from each other. Provided you don't lose your phone or your internet connection these new pleasures are always immediately at hand, only a couple of taps away (Crary, 2014; Reith, 2019, p. 131). Receiving offers and alerts directly to your phone means it also becomes harder to resist impulsive purchasing, especially if you are already enabled to use different forms of electronic payment.

Always at your fingertips, mobile gambling is the perfect vehicle for integrating gambling into growing areas of everyday life. It becomes something to do on the bus, together with friends, during your coffee break, or at home alone with only one eye on the television. Just in many of those spaces where cigarette smoking is now prohibited so, thanks to mobile phones and networks, gambling has been enabled and is becoming more commonplace. Also, hand in hand with radical innovations in sports betting, gambling companies are continually expanding their sponsorship of sporting events and teams (Hing et al., 2023). Sports betting has become a more intensive form of gambling through the invention of 'in-play' and 'micro-events' betting formats. This means you can not only bet on the result of a sporting event before it takes place but also 'live' as it unfolds. Furthermore, you can continually bet on smaller events within a single match or race (Killick & Griffiths, 2019; Parke & Parke, 2019). For example, in a tennis match you can bet on who will win the next point, and/or the next game, and/or the next set, and/or whether the next point will be a serve ace or a double fault, and so on. In this way, a tennis match comes to resemble a multiline slot machine as money is continually won and lost through multiple bets. As any match or race ends, so a new range of global sporting events will be on offer for the sleepless gambler 24/7.

Disarming Innovations

If addictive technologies attract public criticism, it is typical for them to be modified through various processes of disarming innovation. In the first instance, such innovation aims to allay fears regarding basic safety and counter opposition to the continued development and diffusion of technologies. Therefore, innovation will be firstly incremental in character and dedicated to further elaborating the socio-material relations of attachment embedding addictive technologies in society. On the other hand, should concerns and criticisms persist amid growing evidence of harm, then disarming innovation is liable to take on another character. It will tend to become more disruptive, affording and enabling detachment rather than more elaborate relations of attachment. However, in similar style to technologies of attachment, those of detachment will also remain dependent on package deals of accompanying elements to secure their success. By facilitating detachment, a further risk is that disruptive technologies may only serve to redirect addictive consumption on to themselves and affiliated objects rather than lastingly away from such patterns of behaviour. In this way, the identification of technologies of detachment as medical or therapeutic innovations able to effectively treat and manage excessive appetites always remains fragile and uncertain.

The Many Faces of Nicotine Replacement

To provide an initial illustration of these two forms of disarming innovation we can refer to the actions taken in response to the health consequences of cigarette smoking. To start with these centred on the modification of cigarettes themselves, like the shift to filtered cigarettes during the 1950s and the development of 'light' and 'safe' cigarettes in the 1960s and 1970s (Proctor, 2011). Both changes were initiated by the tobacco industry and neither acknowledged that the ills of smoking ultimately derived from a problem of nicotine addiction. Thus, by the end of the 1970s, it had started to become apparent that 'less hazardous cigarettes' only served to further intensify cigarette consumption. To maintain their blood nicotine levels, addicted smokers were obliged to smoke more cigarettes, inhaling more deeply, and blocking filter ventilation holes with lips and fingers (Kozlowski et al., 1980).

The shift to more disruptive innovations attempting to detach smokers from cigarettes arose with the introduction of new technologies of nicotine replacement at the beginning of the 1970s. These technologies were pioneered in Sweden as they were directly connected to the unique history of tobacco consumption in this country (Elam, 2012, 2015). Cigarettes had always faced competition from a popular homegrown moist oral tobacco product called *snus*. By the end of the 1960s, the Swedish state-owned tobacco industry was on the verge of phasing out snus as an archaic product before deciding to relaunch it as a less hazardous alternative to cigarettes. Traditionally sold as a loose tobacco product, snus became available in pre-packaged sachet portions from 1973 as an attempt was made to translate it into a modern and more universally appealing item (Elam, 2015). However, the initial brand—simply called 'Smokeless'—proved a market failure as consumers saw it as 'too clinical' in orientation and no longer understandable as a pleasure product.

In parallel, the Swedish pharmaceutical industry embarked on its own project of developing a substitute for cigarettes (Elam, 2012; Fernö et al., 1973). The health consequences of smoking were seen to derive from a problem of contaminated drug delivery calling for the replacement of cigarettes by 'Nicorette', a platform delivering nicotine in the 'right way' (Fernö, 1994). Envisioning the creative destruction of the cigarette, Nicorette would move beyond the false promises of safe cigarettes and repackaged oral tobacco alike. However, for a pharmaceutical company to be able to legitimately pursue this vision, Nicorette would have to be developed as a medical product and a therapeutic aid to smoking cessation. This created many challenges, as nicotine was only known at the time as a lethal poison used in pesticides and was not recognized to possess any medicinal properties at all (Ahlin & Lundgren, 2002).

Ove Fernö, the research director at the LEO Pharmaceutical Company in Helsingborg was first interested in developing Nicorette as an aerosol, but the risks for nicotine poisoning were considered too difficult to control (Fernö, 1977). Instead, experiments were carried out with chewing gum mimicking the drug delivery of chewing tobacco and snus. Here the difficulty was controlling the release of nicotine added to gum to avoid again the serious risks of poisoning. The solution was found to be an ion exchanger enabling nicotine release over a period of 20–30 minutes, like oral tobacco (Fernö et al., 1973). However, Nicorette gum could still not be chewed like conventional gum, as drug delivery is only effective if it is alternately chewed like chewing tobacco and 'parked' between teeth and gums like snus. Further product development was also called for before commercial launch could be made possible, including the addition of a buffering agent capable of raising the pH of saliva to further assist nicotine absorption across the buccal membrane (Fernö, 1994). This again heightened Nicorette's mimicry of snus where similar buffers like potash had been used to heighten its pleasurable effects since the early nineteenth century (Elam, 2012).

However, when the first attempts were made to register Nicorette gum as a medical product in Sweden it was ruled that agents acting against the desire to smoke cannot be classified as medicines. Instead, the gum was classed as a foodstuff in the same fashion as oral tobacco. This provoked LEO to establish contact with the Swedish Tobacco Company in 1975 to explore whether Nicorette could be launched by them under license as a similar replacement product to new portion snus. Swedish Tobacco suggested some marketing scripts for Nicorette designed to moderate the 'clinical stamp' attached to it such as 'helping you to smoke less' and 'hygienic, fresh in the mouth and good for your teeth' (Elam, 2015). As the Swedish state-owned pharmacy rejected advances from LEO to consider selling Nicorette as a prescription-free healthcare item, the licensing of Nicorette to the Swedish Tobacco Company seemed increasingly likely. However, a motion in the Swedish Parliament opposing the free marketing of nicotine chewing gum in general stores put an end to such plans, leaving Nicorette gum outlawed in Sweden in 1977 (Elam, 2015; Fernö, 1994).

As it turned out, the way forward was a prolonged period of clinical testing which led to the eventual registration of Nicorette as a prescription medicine in Canada, the UK and Sweden by 1981. Of particular significance were the results of randomised double-blind trials published in the *British Medical Journal* (Jarvis et al., 1982) which opened the door to registration in the United States in 1984. This wave of clinical trials not only succeeded in demonstrating the usefulness of nicotine chewing-gum as a smoking cessation aid but also the reality of smoking as a manifestation of nicotine addiction. As 'tobacco dependence' appeared as a new diagnosis in the third edition of the American Psychiatric Association's *Diagnostic and statistical manual of mental disorders* in 1980 (the DSM-III; American Psychiatric Association, 1980), an explosion of nicotine psychopharmacological research followed, significantly inspired by the clinical experimentation that the invention of nicotine replacement therapy (NRT) had set in motion (Elam, 2012).

Over time the technological sophistication of NRTs has grown as new vapour and aerosol delivery systems have more closely imitated the drug delivery of cigarettes. In 2000, a new startup NRT firm called Niconovum was established in Helsingborg by several former employees of LEO who were involved in the development of Nicorette gum. Further exploring a path not taken during the 1970s, venture capital for the new firm was provided by the now private Swedish tobacco company Swedish Match. The aim was to develop faster acting and more effective NRTs which could be bought in pharmacies and general convenience stores (see www.niconovum.se). They would be marketed as not only smoking cessation tools but also smoking reduction devices as well as means for consuming nicotine in environments where smoking and vaping are prohibited. The new brand of NRTs was called 'Zonnic' and came to focus on two products: a faster-acting mouth spray and a nicotine pouch. The latter closely resembles a portion of snus except that it is tobacco free. While Swedish Match pulled out of Niconovum after a couple of years, the company was bought in 2009 by the US tobacco producer R. J. Reynolds which, in 2017, was acquired by British American Tobacco (BAT).

Starting out as an NRT, the tobacco free nicotine pouch has in recent years become a major new smokeless product for all the major tobacco companies. Rather than marketed as an NRT, the pouch is presented as a new enjoyable, reduced-risk product. Sales in the US increased by more than 500 percent between 2019 and 2022, with the Swedish Match brand Zyn conquering roughly 60 percent of the market (Majmundar et al., 2022). This market dominance has been consolidated by PMI's acquisition of Swedish Match in 2023. Although tobacco companies claim pouches are designed to enable habitual smokers to migrate to less harmful products, it appears as though they are attracting a new generation of 'clean nicotine' addicts. In comparison with traditional 'brown snus' products, 'white snus' pouches are advertised as avoiding stained teeth, bad breath, and even the taste of tobacco. Coming in a range of discreet formats, pouches vary in nicotine content from 1.5mg to 11mg with flavours as diverse as apple mint, black cherry, violet liquorice, peach and prosecco, and coffee and nougat.

Despite still selling 550 billion cigarettes in 2023, BAT presents sales of 5.4 billion pouches in the same year as helping them 'to build a smokeless world' (British American Tobacco, 2023). Their global pouch brand Velo is the market leader in 14 European markets including Sweden and has been successfully introduced into countries like Pakistan and Kenya. The identity of Velo as a tobacco free product has also enabled BAT to return to Formula 1 motorsport sponsorship with a new deal signed with McLaren in 2019.

Disarming Gambling Politics with Gambling Research?

Since the rise of online gambling in the mid-1990s there have emerged a collection of global gambling operators like Bet365, Entain, Flutter Entertainment plc and Kindred which dominate the gambling industry, as firms like BAT, Altria Group and Imperial Brands continue to rule over the tobacco industry. In the case of gambling, the growth of global operators has gone hand in hand with the rise of global gambling software developers. Some of these, like International Gaming Technology (IGT) and Aristocrat, were already leaders in the digitalisation of machine gambling, while others like Microgaming and Playtech were the original founders of online casino platforms and sportsbook products.

From the start, online gambling was largely an unregulated offshore industry where operators and technology developers congregated in locations like Antigua and Barbuda, Costa Rica, Malta, Gibraltar, and the Isle of Man. These locations remain vital hubs for the industry, but increasingly different countries have introduced licensing systems as ways of regulating some measure of the online gambling taking place within their borders. For example, the UK Gambling Commission currently licenses over 590 online casino, betting and bingo operations while the Swedish Gambling Authority licenses 55 companies (see respectively, www.gamblingcommission.gov.uk and www.spelinspektionen.se). As the granting of licenses is made dependent on the absence of links to organised crime and commitments to protecting consumers against excessive gambling, so the larger gambling operators have adopted a growing range of 'responsible' and 'sustainable' gambling measures. These are disarming innovations which are intended to further normalise online gambling in society through modifications to platforms mitigating the harms connected with their use. Such innovations also become important for established state-owned gambling companies, as they are obliged to update their product ranges in response to the new market situation. For example, state-owned Svenska Spel in Sweden now offers similar online casino and sports betting products to their new domestic competitors (see www.svenskaspel.se). This has led them into new collaborations with leading gambling technology suppliers including dynamic Swedish software developers such as Evolution Gaming, Yggdrasil and Play'n GO.

Responsible gambling measures clearly resemble the initial disarming innovations introduced in response to concerns over the health consequences of smoking like filters and safer cigarettes. Just as the development of the latter product modifications led to new forms of collaboration between science, government, and the tobacco industry (Berridge, 2007, 2014), so the development of responsible gambling tools and measures is weaving similar relations of connection, further embedding online gambling in society. The core technology which is subject to disarming modification in this instance is behavioural tracking and analytics. This technology out of which the enormous revenues of the gambling industry spring is presented by collaborative researchers as capable of producing 'a paradigm shift' in gambling research, supporting evidence-based policy (Shaffer et al., 2010). Conventionally, the empirical foundations of research have been self-reports of gambling behaviour. A classic example of this is the Swedish longitudinal gambling study Swelogs (see www.folkhalsomyndigheten.se/the-public-health-agency-of-sweden/living-conditions-and-lifestyle/andtg/gambling/swelogs/) which is one of the world's most comprehensive population studies of the relations between gambling and health. However, the strength of such studies hinges on the willingness of citizens to participate and on the accuracy/truthfulness of their reported gambling behaviour. This can be viewed as problematic, as a recognised symptom of disordered gambling is lying about the extent of your involvement in gambling (American Psychiatric Association, 2013).

Combatting this weakness of established gambling research, gambling companies can present a shift from self-reports to reliance on their own behavioural tracking data as an empirical move from unreliable memories and recollections to the equivalent of direct observations of actual gambling behaviour (Griffiths, 2009; Shaffer et al., 2010). In other words, close cooperation between science and industry is widely presented today as affording a new standard of scientific objectivity and a more accurate epidemiology of gambling harms than that dependent on the testimony of gamblers themselves.

A pioneering collaboration using industry data to map risks of gambling harm was established in 2005 between the online company bwin and Harvard Medical School. To start with, a longitudinal cohort of more than 40,000 online gamblers from over 80 countries was followed for a period of three years, resulting in a series of publications charting the basic contours of online gambling behaviour and seeking to identify 'behavioural markers' of high-risk gambling (see for example, Braverman & Shaffer, 2010; LeBrie et al., 2007; LaPlante et al., 2009). By mapping behavioural patterns preceding the development of excessive gambling, the aim was to lay the foundations for effective preventive and treatment strategies. Almost twenty years later—and after bwin has become part of the larger gambling group Entain—collaboration with Harvard researchers continues in the fine-tuning of the latter group's advanced responsibility and care (ARC) system (Entain, 2022). Compared to the behavioural tracking systems used in land-based casinos in the 1990s, the ARC system implements a more enlightened approach to maximising customer value and retention. Moving beyond the one-sided focus on triggers designed to accelerate gambling, new personalised interventions are intended to inform and moderate the behaviour of gamblers at risk of harm and even to exclude from platforms those customers who show clear signs of out-of-control gambling.

In similar fashion, the gambling group Kindred (2022) is publicly committed to reducing to zero the share of its revenue coming from high-risk players. To advance this goal the group has established a variety of research collaborations including with the psychologist Mark Griffiths, probably the most cited gambling and addiction researcher in the world. This latter collaboration deals with the use of Kindred's behavioural data to apply the DSM-5 criteria for gambling disorder (American Psychiatric Association, 2013) to actual gambling behaviour. Advancing such applications is seen as further strengthening the ability of gambling operators to accurately identify and predict harmful gambling behaviour online without recourse to self-report diagnostic screening instruments. As Catania and Griffiths (2022) argue in a recent article, many of the nine DSM-5 criteria for gambling disorder—such as a preoccupation with gambling, a loss of control, and 'chasing losses'—can be successfully operationalised using actual transactional data points. By experimentally doing so, it becomes possible to segment the whole of Kindred's gambling population in relation to a new set of scientific indicators of harm.

Such segmentation is well-attuned to Kindred's over-arching strategy of 'sustainable value creation' (Kindred, 2022). This strategy encompasses an unflinching commitment to excluding high risk players and informing them of treatment options while providing personalised behavioural coaching for loyal, high spending customers, so the advertised thrills and enjoyment of gambling do not visibly tip over into more spectacular levels of financial and emotional stress, courting public controversy and criticism (for a parallel discussion of disarming gambling innovations in Germany, see Möll, this volume).

Conclusions

Starting out as a psychological view of addictions, the excessive appetite model is closely associated with the neurobiology of addiction today. Moving away from a focus on physical dependence, neuroscience has re-envisaged addiction as a brain disease expressed through a lack of impulse control. Rather than simply opening for the recognition of new behavioural addictions, this recasts addiction as a quintessentially 'biobehavioural disorder' (Leshner, 2001, p. 76). Just as Parkinson's sufferers cannot control their trembling and schizophrenics their delusions, so addicts cannot restrain their consumption. However, addiction as a brain disease remains only half the story of excessive appetites. The other half is composed of what neuroscientists simplify as 'environmental factors' and the qualities of 'behavioural reinforcers'. To properly get to grips with these things, social and historical perspectives are required. These reveal addictions to be broader relational entities and forms of socio-material attachment. Therefore, if brains are 'hijacked' through addictions, this occurs not only as behaviours grow compulsive, but as people are drawn into intricate webs of socio-material relations which can be global in reach. The shift from voluntary behaviour to compulsion, and from pleasure to necessity, is also a matter of technical mediation where typically a highly diverse and heterogenous range of material and immaterial mediators are brought into play. These are the processes Schüll (2012) calls 'addiction by design', Courtwright (2019) names as the 'weaponization' of consumption, and Cross and Proctor (2014) see as 'packaging pleasure'.

As addictive designs provoke debates about harm, so they will be followed by a series of disarming innovations. Initially, these will be incremental in character, designed to allay fears and hostility towards pervasive new patterns of socio-material relations. They may be advertised as reducing palpable harms but will rather further elaborate the infrastructures embedding new forms of addictive behaviour in society. Such innovations are likely to be industry-led but can also encourage new collaborations between science, industry and government promoting the proto-medicalisation of addictions.

In the face of continuing controversy, disarming innovation and medicalisation will likely become more closely entangled as facilitating detachment from addictive technologies becomes as important as the further elaboration of relations of attachment. During this process, disarming innovations as seen in the cases of nicotine replacements and behavioural tracking in gambling may translate into vital new tools and infrastructures of addiction research. However, ambiguity and uncertainty in the identity of these innovations in between poison and cure will remain even as they come to be more closely associated with medical technologies and therapies. As demonstrated by the rise of the nicotine pouch and the growing sophistication of sustainable gambling tools, radical disarming innovations are likely to be as much about the strategic modulation and rerouting of addictive behaviour as its lasting restraint.

References

Advisory Committee to the Surgeon General of the Public Health Service. (1964). *Smoking and health: Report of the Advisory Committee to the Surgeon General of the Public Health Service* (No. 1103). US Department of Health, Education, and Welfare, Public Health Service.

Ahlin, J., & Lundgren, R. (2002). *Från leopiller till Nicorette* [From leo pills to nicorette]. Pharmacia.

American Psychiatric Association. (1980). *Diagnostic and statistical manual of mental disorders* (3rd ed.). American Psychiatric Association.

American Psychiatric Association. (2013). *Diagnostic and statistical manual of mental disorders* (5th ed.). American Psychiatric Association.

Berridge, V. (2007). *Marketing health: Smoking and the discourse of public health in Britain, 1945–2000*. Oxford University Press.

Berridge, V. (2014). Electronic cigarettes and history. *The Lancet, 383*(9936), 2204–2205.

Braverman, J., & Shaffer, H. J. (2010). How do gamblers start gambling: Identifying behavioural markers for high-risk internet gambling. *European Journal of Public Health, 22*(2), 273–278. https://doi.org/10.1093/eurpub/ckp232

British American Tobacco. (2023) *Building a smokeless world: Combined annual and sustainability report*. British and American Tobacco plc.

Catania, M., & Griffiths, M. D. (2022). Applying the DSM-5 criteria for gambling disorder to online gambling account-based tracking data: An empirical study utilizing cluster analysis. *Journal of Gambling Studies, 38*, 1289–1306. https://doi.org/10.1007/s10899-021-10080-9

Courtwright, D. T. (2001). *Forces of habit: Drugs and the making of the modern world*. Harvard University Press.

Courtwright, D. T. (2019). *The age of addiction: How bad habits became big business*. Harvard University Press.

Crary, J. (2014). *24/7: Late capitalism and the ends of sleep*. Verso.

Cross, G. S., & Proctor, R. N. (2014). *Packaged pleasures: How technology and marketing revolutionized desire*. University of Chicago Press.

Dhaisne, C. (2019). The importance of personalized online gambling experiences. *Kindred*. https://www.kindredgroup.com/news%2D%2Dinsights/2019/the-importance-of-personalised-online-gambling-experiences/

Elam, M. (2012). Pharmaceutical incursion on cigarette smoking at the birth of the brain disease model of addiction. In J. Netherland (Ed.), *Critical perspectives on addiction* (pp. 53–75). Emerald Group Publishing.

Elam, M. (2015). Nicorette reborn? E-cigarettes in light of the history of nicotine replacement technology. *International Journal of Drug Policy, 26*(6), 536–542. https://doi.org/10.1016/j.drugpo.2015.02.002

Entain. (2022). *Moments of excitement: Annual report*. Entain plc.

Fernö, O. (1977). The development of a chewing gum containing nicotine and some comments on the role played by nicotine in the smoking habit. In J. Steinfeld, W. Griffiths, K. P. Ball, & R. M. Taylor (Eds.), *Smoking and health II* (pp. 569–573). U.S. Department of Health, Education and Welfare.

Fernö, O. (1994). Conversation with Ove Fernö. *Addiction, 89*(10), 1215–1226. https://doi.org/10.1111/j.1360-0443.1994.tb03300.x

Fernö, O., Lichtneckert, S. J. A., & Lundgren, C. E. G. (1973). A substitute for tobacco smoking. *Psychopharmacologia, 31*, 201–204. https://doi.org/10.1007/BF00422510

Griffiths, M. D. (2009). The implications of real time behavioural tracking. *Casino and Gaming International, 5*(3), 99–104.

Hing, N., Rockloff, M., & Browne, M. (2023). A bad bet for sports fans: The case for ending the "gamblification" of sports. *Sport Management Review, 26*(5), 788–812. https://doi.org/10.1080/14413523.2023.2260079

Huhtamo, E. (2005). Slots of fun, slots of trouble: An archaeology of arcade gambling. In J. Raessens & J. Goldstein (Eds.), *Handbook of computer game studies* (pp. 3–21). MIT Press.

Jarvis, M., Raw, M., Russell, M., & Feyerabend, C. (1982). Randomised controlled trial of nicotine chewing gum. *British Medical Journal, 285*(6341), 537–540. https://doi.org/10.1136/bmj.285.6341.537

Killick, E. A., & Griffiths, M. D. (2019). In-play sports betting: A scoping study. *International Journal of Mental Health and Addiction, 17*, 1456–1495. https://doi.org/10.1007/s11469-018-9896-6

Kindred. (2022). *Creating long-term value. Annual and sustainability report and accounts*. Kindred plc.

Kozlowski, L., Frecker, R., Khouw, V., & Pope, M. (1980). The misuse of "less hazardous" cigarettes and its detection: Hole-blocking and ventilated filters. *American Journal of Public Health, 70*(11), 1202–1203.

LaPlante, D. A., Kleschinsky, J. H., LeBrie, R. A., Nelson, S. E., & Shaffer, H. J. (2009). Sitting at the virtual poker table: A prospective epidemiological study of actual internet poker gambling behavior. *Computers in Human Behavior, 25*(3), 711–717. https://doi.org/10.1016/j.chb.2008.12.027

Latour, B. (1994). On technical mediation. *Common Knowledge, 3*(2), 29–64.

LeBrie, R. A., LaPlante, D. A., Nelson, S. E., Schumann, A., & Shaffer, H. J. (2007). Assessing the playing field: A prospective longitudinal study of internet sports gambling behavior. *Journal of Gambling Studies, 23*(3), 347–363. https://doi.org/10.1007/s10899-007-9067-3

Leshner, A. I. (2001). Addiction is a brain disease. *Issues in Science and Technology, 17*(3), 75–80.

Levine, H. G. (1978). The discovery of addiction: Changing conceptions of habitual drunkenness in America. *Journal of Studies on Alcohol and Drugs, 39*(1), 143–174. https://doi.org/10.15288/jsa.1978.39.143

Loveman, G. (2003). Diamonds in the data mine. *Harvard Business Review, 81*(5), 109–113.

Majmundar, A., Okitondo, C., Xue, A., Asare, S., Bamdi, P., & Nargis, N. (2022). Nicotine pouch sales trends in the US by volume and nicotine concentration levels from 2019–2022. *JAMA Network Open, 5*(11), e2242235. https://doi.org/10.1001/jamanetworkopen.2022.42235

Orford, J. (2000). *Excessive appetites: A psychological view of addictions* (2nd ed.). John Wiley & Sons Ltd..

Orford, J. (2001). Addiction as excessive appetite. *Addiction, 96*(1), 15–31. https://doi.org/10.1046/j.1360-0443.2001.961152.x

Parke, A., & Parke, J. (2019). Transformation of sports betting into a rapid and continuous gambling activity: A grounded theoretical investigation of problem sports betting in online settings. *International Journal of Mental Health and Addiction, 17*(6), 1340–1359. https://doi.org/10.1007/s11469-018-0049-8

Proctor, R. N. (2011). *Golden holocaust: Origins of the cigarette catastrophe and the case for abolition*. University of California Press.

Reith, G. (2019). *Addictive consumption: Capitalism, modernity and excess.* Routledge.
Robinson, M. J. F., Fischer, A. M., Ahuja, A., Lesser, E. N., & Maniates, H. (2015). Roles of "wanting" and "liking" in motivating behavior: Gambling, food, and drug addictions. In E. H. Simpson & P. D. Balsam (Eds.), *Behavioral neuroscience of motivation* (pp. 105–136). Springer.
Schüll, N. D. (2012). *Addiction by design: Machine gambling in Las Vegas.* Princeton University Press.
Sedgwick, E. K. (1993). *Tendencies.* Duke University Press.
Shaffer, H. J., Peller, A. J., LaPlante, D. A., Nelson, S. E., & Labrie, R. A. (2010). Toward a paradigm shift in internet gambling research: From opinion and self-report to actual behavior. *Addiction Research and Theory, 18*(3), 270–283. https://doi.org/10.3109/16066350902777974
U.S. Department of Health and Human Services. (1988). *The health consequences of smoking: Nicotine addiction—A report of the surgeon general.* Office on Smoking and Health.

8

'Addiction' and Agency at the Threshold of Infinite Pornographic Access

Kris Taylor

Is pornography viewing a conspicuous behaviour? On one hand, viewing pornography could be considered inconspicuous: the preferences that people have, the acts of self-pleasure that presumably accompany pornography viewing, and the moral and ethical difficulties that might arise are rarely spoken about. Indeed, as I learned through interviewing pornography-viewing men as part of my PhD research in 2018, there are few avenues to discuss it without the perceived risk of personal disclosure, embarrassment, or the potential for ridicule. On the other hand, talk about watching pornography is seemingly everywhere in popular culture. As an example, pornography viewing has been made conspicuous through representations in mainstream media, where such viewing is often shown as a sexual rite of passage for boys and young

K. Taylor (✉)
Waipapa Taumata Rau/University of Auckland, Auckland, New Zealand
e-mail: kris.taylor@auckland.ac.nz

B. M. Z. Cohen et al. (eds.), *Addiction and the Medicalisation of Conspicuous Behaviour*, The Politics of Mental Health and Illness,
https://doi.org/10.1007/978-3-032-06313-7_7

men (Boyle, 2010). Crucially, we should note here that discussion and representation of men's and women's porn viewing are often quite different. While women have also been addressed as viewers of pornography in such media (although this is a recent trend; Goldstein, 2021), women's relationships with pornography, when they are shown at all in such media, have acted as grounds for eroticisation and objectification (Boyle, 2010). In other words, boys and men's pornography viewing has been shown as something natural to men and boys, and deviant or salacious in the case of girls and women (a dynamic that can present complex negotiations for women who watch pornography; see Chadwick et al., 2018; Gurevich et al., 2017). Thus, we can see a tension between popular representation of pornography viewing for men as normative (or else as a joke), and my experience of speaking to men about the difficulties in reflecting seriously on their pornography viewing experiences.

However, boy's and men's pornography viewing have also been subject to a specific form of scrutiny. In an example of pornography viewing as conspicuous, discussions of 'pornography addiction' in both mainstream and social media, have described pornography viewing as becoming 'out of control' and interfering with 'real life' relationships and responsibilities (see for example, McKee, 2006; Taylor, & Gavey, 2020). Pornography addiction too has featured in mainstream films and television, as well as publicly confessed to by celebrities and legislated against in governmental policies (in the US and UK at least, with varying levels of success; for review see Taylor, 2019). Further, pornography addiction has been described by health professionals in the language of an 'epidemic', implicated as causal to a wide array of possible adverse outcomes, including sexual dysfunction, marriage problems, the warping of sexual desire, and criminal sex offending (see for example, Taylor, 2019, 2020). As I have observed in my own research, pornography *addiction* can act as a powerful discursive tool for making the inconspicuous (the negative side of otherwise normative pornography viewing) conspicuous through the language of medicalisation and diagnosis. As I see it, there is a clear gap here between understanding pornography viewing as *either* 'normal' and part of everyday life (for young men at least) *or* as a diagnosable ailment in the form of an addiction.

Between these two conceptions of pornography viewing 'done right' and pornography viewing 'gone wrong' lies a wide range of complex, multifaceted, and even contradictory experiences in need of deeper consideration. This chapter works within this gap, outlining how the language of medicalisation (namely, 'addiction') has become the dominant, most conspicuous way of making sense of pornography viewing 'gone wrong' (whatever that might mean). That is, while pornography viewing could be understood as enmeshed within complex negotiations of pleasure, gender, shame, ethics, morals, politics, and other considerations, currently these behaviours are almost exclusively interpreted through the quasi-medical lens of 'pornography addiction'. Yet, by its very nature, the label 'pornography addiction' cannot provide anything more than a binary understanding of pornography viewing as a behaviour that is either appropriate or pathological. To this end, the central focus of this chapter is on how pornography viewing and accounts of pornography viewers themselves defy the superficial convenience of such categorisation. Accordingly, my specific focus here is on the particular question of 'threshold', and specifically the space between access to infinite pornographic content, the self-perceived risks of excess, and the way that we make judgments about when pornography viewing might cross over between the pleasures of ready access and the threat of personally dilemmatic excess.

I begin by addressing two of the critical factors that make the concept of pornography addiction possible: 1) sociocultural anxieties about excessive consumption, and 2) the convenient vagaries of the pornography addiction concept. I then turn to how these factors inform understandings of pornography viewing through a few brief case studies, drawing on my interviews conducted with men about their pornography viewing experiences. I conclude by discussing sociocultural anxieties about excess and self-control and how these work in tandem with the visibility of the pornography addiction concept to produce a self-diagnostic *par excellence*: a discretionary label which ostensibly describes deviance from a norm *despite* the norm and the nature of said deviance remaining poorly defined, relying instead on idiosyncratic and subjective assessments of one's violation of a self-ascribed threshold. In other words, I ask that if there is a line to draw between 'normal' and 'addictive' pornography then where is this line, who draws it, how do they draw it, and why?

Access/Excess, Agency/Addiction

Today, we live in a world where access to consumer products and immediate entertainment are only a few clicks away. On the one hand, this appears to be the realisation of a utopian vision of the future, with the internet democratising pleasure and luxury and opening up new avenues for human exploration and fulfilment. On the other hand however, the assumption that increased access leads by virtue to consumer freedom (and, in turn, increased well-being) becomes more complicated when we consider how increased choice (and virtually limitless choice at that) creates a burden of responsibility on every one of us. As Reith (2004) has argued, historically the proliferation of access to consumer goods has presented the public with an obligation to be vigilant of our choices and to monitor our behaviour in order to avoid slipping into excessive consumption. Today, the internet's opening of new avenues for consumption and its encroachment into everyday life has created a responsibility to consume *correctly.*

Concepts like pornography, shopping, or gaming addiction exemplify this tendency to view the dark side of freedom as the slippery slope towards excess. In this sense, an onus to make correct choices of what to consume lays the conceptual foundations for popularising a concept like 'behavioural addiction' (see Taylor, 2024). Following Foucault (1990), while the promise of increased sexual agency (to learn about, talk about, and watch sex) could be seen as liberalising our understandings of sex and sexual behaviour, such increased sexual autonomy counter-intuitively produces new dictates. In short, if we understand sex and sexuality as parts of 'natural' human expression, then the way that we speak about and perceive sex also expresses our desire to identify the boundaries or uniform truths of sex. In the case of pornography, as access has increased—along with a discourse of pornography addiction—pornography viewers must understand their viewing within a matrix of virtually unlimited free access *and* the possibility of excess/addiction engendered by that same access: how much is too much? What forms are normal? What is and is not permissible?

Crucially, while these anxieties about pornography viewing are openly expressed (in terms of how frequent, how long, what kind, and so on), the actual line of such transgression is unclear. Indeed, as the case of quantifying appropriate frequency illustrates, pornography viewing is mediated by a range of idiosyncratically derived factors. For example, as Twohig et al. (2009, p. 263) suggest, "[i]f viewing [pornography] is contrary to an individual's values or moral base, then even one instance would be experienced as problematic". In turn, attempts to quantify where and when pornography goes wrong (and for whom) have produced a dizzying constellation of theories and conceptual frameworks which fail to add up to anything resembling a coherent nosology (Ley et al., 2014; Taylor, 2020). Consider criticisms of previous attempts to translate the physiological symptoms of substance abuse (namely, habituation and tolerance) into conceptions of behavioural addiction (Starcevic, 2016). Attempts to locate a boundary in the physiology of pornography viewers has been hampered by the fact that self-assessment of tolerance to viewing pornography is not analogous to dose escalation in drug dependence (and we might again ask whether it would be frequency, duration, or content that indicate tolerance), and negative emotional responses are not comparable to withdrawal symptoms accompanying the cessation of substance use (see Starcevic, 2016). As such, while there is a concern for access creating excess online, the actual *threshold* of where pornography viewing crosses over from normal to abnormal, from enjoyable to problematic, or from agentic to addictive cannot be easily described, let alone operationalised (beyond a subjective sense of 'losing self-control', whatever that might mean). Indeed, there is no consistent symptom profile, no robust measure, and no theoretically coherent explanation of pornography addiction that goes beyond the criterion of losing self-control. The pornography addiction diagnosis is interesting in this regard in that it operates outside of fields of diagnostic credibility (it is absent from both the American Psychiatric Association's *Diagnostic and Statistical Manual of Mental Disorders* and the World Health Organization's *International Classification of Diseases*) yet seemingly retains a sense of authority within popular culture (Taylor, 2020).

I do not want to get hung up on an argument about measurement here because I have a more fundamental critique of the pornography addiction concept that makes the search for accurate measurement essentially redundant: namely, at a conceptual level, labelling pornography viewing as an addiction can only offer a closed loop of explanation. Research and discussion of pornography viewing 'gone wrong' routinely and predictably focuses on the *what* of such pornography viewing (for example, the symptoms, the consequences, the putative programmes of treatment; see Ley et al., 2014; Taylor, 2020). However, these efforts fail to address the ways that viewers of pornography make sense of their pornography viewing, or the *why* of prospective self-diagnosis. As an analogy, in understanding obsessive-compulsive spectrum disorders, a focus on repetitive behaviours themselves (the symptoms) tells us nothing of the function or cause of these behaviours (Starcevic, 2016). In pornography addiction, the heterogeneity of psychological and social explanations for self-diagnosed pornography addiction (for example, sexual shame, guilt, trauma, social anxiety, sexual exploration/curiosity, high libido, intimacy problems, relationship difficulties, and emotional dysregulation; to say nothing of other established explanatory taxonomies such as obsessive-compulsive spectrum disorders, depression, mania, and so on) are rarely addressed and are more frequently conceptualised as symptoms rather than playing a causal role in self-diagnosis. As such, rather than looking at the *what* of pornography addiction (as most accounts seem to do), to help people struggling with their pornography viewing we must understand the *why* of their diagnosis.

Why Pornography Addiction?

As I have outlined, one popular explanation for the *why* of pornography addiction maintains that pornography is uniquely addictive because of the accessible and affordable (indeed, often free) nature of the content.

Such a construction of pornography addiction often suggests that internet pornography causes addiction because human biology cannot compete with technological advances. As I have highlighted elsewhere such accounts are also frequently, perhaps unsurprisingly, either amnesic or else openly nostalgic about pre-internet pornography (see Taylor, 2021). However, the popularisation of the pornography addiction diagnosis is not *only* the result of more/harder pornography on the internet impacting our brains but a consequence of how we understand sexuality, the internet, and pornography as a genre. Here, then, we must explore the spaces between access and excess to ask how we can conceptualise the shape of pornography addiction beyond a binary, and specifically interrogate the *why* of its aetiology.

The uptake of a self-diagnosed pornography addiction is part of a larger social change in which the responsibilities of maintaining health and conformity are no longer the sole jurisdiction of clinical authorities (see Conrad & Bergey, 2014; Conrad & Schneider, 1992). Thus, to understand more fully the *why* of pornography addiction, we need to consider the ways that pornography viewers themselves make sense of pornography addiction as a sociocultural phenomenon. Indeed, pornography is seemingly only made 'addictive' at the point at which a viewer determines their behaviour to be personally problematic in some way or another (see Grubbs et al., 2015; Twohig et al., 2009). In this vein, some empirical research on pornography addiction avoids the theoretical and taxonomic quagmire of describing pornography addiction as a sort of 'natural kind' by instead investigating the 'perception' of being addicted to pornography (Grubbs & Perry, 2019; Grubbs et al., 2015; Wéry et al., 2019). This body of literature is less interested in measuring pornography addiction in a realist sense and more interested in the ways that pornography may cause personal dilemmas, which can in turn be explained by viewers as indicative of pornography addiction. Echoing Twohig et al.'s (2009) observation about problematic pornography viewing (as occurring at the point of breaching a moral threshold), such research suggests that the reported adverse outcomes of viewing pornography arise as a direct result of the moral work done by its viewers. For example, in their review of research on moral incongruence and pornography viewing, Grubbs and Perry (2019) suggest not only that moral self-perceptions can predict adverse outcomes for some pornography viewers but also that such perceptions can predict a self-diagnosis of pornography addiction.

For our purpose here, then, we will consider the *why* of pornography addiction as arising in idiosyncratic ways through the transgression of self-established boundaries of viewing, rather than pornography addiction representing some specific, measurable psychological or physiological state. In other words, I suggest that the pornography addiction concept is more productively approached as a grassroots label taken up as a result of lay people's assessment of their problematic pornography viewing (as arrived at by a subjective sense of social transgression) rather than as an iatrogenic diagnosis created by health professionals. Here, the presumed inability of pornography viewers to correctly moderate their viewing and to identify this for themselves is at the centre of the pornography addiction concept. To be sure, increased access *has* created the conditions for a struggle for moderation, but what this self-control looks like and how it is formulated is the focus of the following section. The centrality of self-control to the concept of pornography addiction—and, as I will argue, pornography viewing in general—raises significant questions as to how pornography viewers distinguish between problematic and non-problematic viewing and *why* they might describe problematic viewing as addictive.

Case Studies: Thresholds of Pornography Viewing

Up to this point, I have sketched the parameters of three points of argument: 1) that the pornography addiction concept allows pornography viewing to be made conspicuous and has become the dominant way to describe pornography viewing gone wrong; 2) that the concept is a product of our unease about unlimited access to content via the internet; and 3) that the label is only made popular if pornography viewers feel a sense of personal responsibility to avoid crossing an idiosyncratic and subjectively assessed boundary of viewing from ostensibly 'normal' to 'pathological'. It is in this space of increased personal responsibility and the self-monitoring of perceived sexual transgression that I want to situate the following brief case studies. How might pornography viewers make sense of their self-ascribed thresholds of pornography viewing, and how do they relate these thresholds to addiction self-attribution? Thus, my focus in the following case studies is not on the claims of the biological power of novelty or any other speculative criteria for pornography addiction but instead on the way that pornography viewers themselves make sense of the boundary between their viewing and their perception of transgression as addictive risk.

The following extracts are drawn from interviews conducted with 30 pornography-viewing men in Aotearoa New Zealand, whose self-described pornography viewing ranged from a positive self-perception through to those struggling with their viewing in some form or other (including those who described themselves as 'addicts'). These men were recruited through a survey that was included in an article about the current research in the *New Zealand Herald* (a national newspaper). In the recruitment article I stressed that the only criteria for participation was that the respondents identify as men and that they had viewed pornography previously. The men were aged between 18 and 71 (the median age was 46), 90 percent were Pākehā/NZ European (a local indicator of ethnicity which often, though not always, describes European heritage), with 83 percent describing themselves as irreligious, atheist or agnostic (17 percent were Christian), and with a relatively broad range of sexual diversity (57 percent heterosexual, 26.5 percent bisexual, and 16.5 percent homosexual). The interviews were semi-structured wherein I worked to facilitate an open and conversational context, conveying minimal judgment and making room for wide ranging discussion. This study received ethical approval from the University of Auckland's Human Participants Ethics Committee (for further details of recruitment and participants, see Taylor, 2020).

In what follows, it is not my intention to present a representative sample or to compare the ways that men who described themselves as 'addicts' talked about pornography viewing differently to those who did not, but instead to present extracts that help to illustrate the tension and ambivalence of viewing pornography and the ways that these pornography viewers recount their experiences of personal transgression. In other words, I present the following extracts as examples of how an amorphous conception of pornography addiction can inform a person's accounting of their viewing and how a variety of subjective assessments of what *counts* as a transgression informs different conceptions of addiction.

Thresholds and Frequency

Perhaps unsurprisingly, the majority of interviewees suggested that access to pornography had become easier and that with increased access, the possibilities to view more diverse content had also increased. The framing of this change varied between participants, with both positive and negative descriptions depending on the viewer's self-perception of being able to 'control' the quantity of pornography viewed. As the following extract illustrates, this sense of self-control and autonomy was readily invoked, even in cases of those describing ostensibly non-problematic viewing:

> (Interviewee B.—51 years old, Pākehā, bisexual, single, non-religious)
>
> Kris Um, what do you think about your own pornography use currently?
>
> B. Um, I think it's, well, acceptable.
>
> Kris Yeah. [laughing]
>
> B I don't think that it's um- I- I'm not addicted. I don't ne- I don't have to watch pornography, you know. Like I'm- and many cases, I've just gone oh nah, and just stopped watching it- consciously stopped watching it. Like not just, oh, didn't get round to it kind of thing. Like I'm, no, no, I'm not gonna watch any porn, I'm just gonna do without it for X amount of time period that I think I want to, and then if or when it crosses my mind again then I might indulge in it, but that's about it. Um, and … because I'm a single guy, it's assumed that I watch pornography and, especially being an older single guy. And um, you know, the creepy old guy [both laugh]. And it's like, well, that's- I- I- I'm comfortable with that, like people that assume that. It's like because I'm comfortable enough to know that I'm in control of what I'm doing and watching and, you know, and it's like I don't feel like I, um, have to race home to watch porn, you know.

While B. describes himself as "not addicted" because of his ability to "consciously" abstain from pornography, this account illustrates a seemingly fraught relationship with pornography in that he describes his pornography viewing as "acceptable" and that he is "comfortable" with being "in control" of what he is watching, suggesting that he also understands the potential risk of losing self-control. This is not to say that he does not view it, but instead that his viewing is informed by multiple considerations: the normative expectation that he must watch pornography because he is an older single guy, the stigma of being seen as a "creepy old guy", along with the possibility that pornography viewing could become uncontrollable at some point. Here, B. has seemingly accepted the description of pornography viewing as *potentially* addictive while also distancing himself from the possibility of addiction by virtue of his ability to set personal limits ("I'm in control of what I'm doing").

Other interviewees also described pornography as threatening to become a problem premised on a conflict between pornography's availability and a sense of self-control. In these cases, like B. above, the actual content of pornography was subordinate to an inability to control one's behaviour:

(Interviewee A.—35 years old, Pākehā, heterosexual, married, non-religious)

A. It's just too- ya know ya know, if ya want to look up- or you find your horny in the day and your partner's not around you can go to a porn site like *that* [snaps fingers] it's just way too easy.

Kris But, sorry, what I mean is, why is that a problem? Like why is that something that would cause you distress?

A. Cos I'm a control freak, and I'm losing control.

Kris Right, because you want to…

A. Yeah, I-I- one part of me needs to watch- to do that, and the rest of me is saying 'fuck don't do it'.

Kris Right, okay.

A. Does that make sense?

Kris So I'm really interested in what it is-

A. So it's the guilty- it's the guilty-

Kris So, I'm saying that you have that part of you that says 'don't do it', but I'm interested in why you would *not* want to?

A. Aww, why I'd not want to?

Kris Well, you know you said-

A. Because I overthink things and think 'this is not good'. I'm not in control here; there's something else that's saying, 'go and do something bad.'

Here, A. describes his struggle against viewing pornography arising from "that part of" him that considers abstaining without going on to explain *why* part of him might not want to watch pornography. In this sense, A.'s 'problem' with pornography viewing arises principally from his feeling of "guilt" for being out of control. In other words, here, the risk of pornography addiction becomes synonymous with a negotiation of self-control, as A. describes his simultaneous "need to watch" pornography coming into conflict with his statement of being a "control freak". In this sense, pornography viewing is described here as a problem of availability that hails him to "do something bad", which is balanced by a moderating threshold of viewing 'too much'. Here, then, the *why* of a potential pornography addiction is about controlling the frequency and flow of pornography and the risk of viewing it too much or for too long.

Thresholds of Content

Besides the claims that pornography's danger seemingly resides in its availability—and thus the need to restrict one's volume of access—other interviewees described the need to moderate their pornography viewing in terms of the content itself. Most commonly, interviewees accounted for their decisions to view or avoid certain content by describing their ability to 'draw a line', creating a personal boundary that partitioned personally dilemmatic (or not pleasurable) pornography viewing from their preferred preferences:

(Interviewee M.—52 years old, Pākehā, heterosexual, married, non-religious)

M. Yeah, but I think that, for me, you bounce around in a box. So, you'll try one boundary, and then you'll cross the boundary and say I don't particularly wanna go there. I'm gonna explore something else. Wh- when you go back to this boundary, you don't step straight over to where you were before. The boundary almost resets

> itself back to where your original boundary was. The reason that you're- you're getting titillation out of crossing a line that you know is there, but you don't end up- for me, you don't end up on the other side of the line, but you come back again.

Such a process of erecting a threshold of viewing content (not volume) and the ongoing assessment of one's behaviour in relation to this boundary were evident across interviews in varying ways. For example, some of the men who had seen forms of pornography that they described as unwanted or disturbing echoed M.'s description above, describing the establishment of boundaries against seeing that type of pornography again. At the same time, there was a tension throughout the interviews wherein the availability of different kinds of pornography allowed the men to explore content for pleasure in ways that they also found personally dilemmatic, raising internal conflicts. For example, in the following extract, J. describes himself as, at turns, both an agentic pornography seeker *and* a passive audience member depending on the type of pornography he watches:

(Interviewee J.—18 years old, Pākehā, heterosexual, in a relationship, non-religious)

Kris: So you've never umm, maybe like ventured into areas of like pornography that was a bit more umm [pause]

J.: Like hard out?

Kris: Yeah, hard-core, you know like BDSM or like, something like that you know, how we were talking about the exceptions to the mainstream earlier-

J.: Yeah, nah, I actually haven't, but I like, I dunno, I- for me? I'm quite like- I'm quite conscious about how I watch it, especially lately. I mean, so when I first got into it I was just kind of like experimenting and like, 'aww yeah, like what's this? What's this?' Like just like on the basic stuff, and then I'd start- I-I discovered that like I-I start like- all this stuff like a guy with a huge dick like it's just completely destroying a woman, you know what I mean? And that's like, I don't really like- I mean A. it's like unrealistic and B. it's like, it- clearly, the woman- I mean sex, I find is quite a mutual thing, so like clearly the woman's not getting anything out of it, I mean- so probably the-the worst I've got would be just like a guy with a huge dick, and I'm like, I'm not- I'm on it for like 20 seconds- *Although* I find that [sigh] you- when you're like horny and such, and you go and look at pornography like, it's easier- I-I found sometimes I'm on videos of these chicks who are mud ugly but like old- older women and this sort of stuff and then like obviously I use it and afterwards I look back and I'm like- like- like I wouldn't find that girl attractive.

Here J. not only describes a process of initial exploration, where he would see, and ostensibly avoid, pornography that he describes as extreme (namely, men with large penises and women "being destroyed") but goes on to describe viewing pornography that would later give him pause. Curiously, J. describes himself as both conscious of the pornographic content that he watches before going on to describe the viewing when he is "horny" in a curiously passive way ("I've found sometimes I'm on videos of these chicks"). Later on in the interview, J. worked to explain how his negotiation between agentic and pleasurable viewing and less-pleasurable unconscious viewing might work, describing it as "when you're horny, your brain is just pushing you", constructing himself as both an active consumer of pornography at one time, and somehow not in full control of his decisions at others.

In this sense, interviewees deployed the concept of threshold to pronounce a mastery over viewing certain content at certain times while simultaneously acknowledging the challenges of being in full control of viewing other content at other times. While J.'s example above speaks to what might be considered a more trivial example of this, consider the example of the following final extract in which G. describes seeking images of naked children along with a similar description of physiological drives in the brain:

(Interviewee G.—71 years old, Pākehā, heterosexual, married, Christian)

Kris Have you ever seen extreme pornography?

G. [Pause] Um, occasionally I've stumbled across, um, something with some violence in it, not- not extreme violence, but where someone's being forced against their will, but I'm not- I don't like it, and I tend to shy away if I accidentally come across one of that kind. I've never seen any child sexual pornography; I've looked at images of children naked but not involved in any sexual acts.

Kris So, following on from this, do you think that pornography is always pleasurable, or do you think that there are aspects of using pornography that can be more complicated?

G. I think it can be complicated, um obviously one of the reasons that um men anyway do it is for the dopamine hit and the- and obviously the excitement of the pleasure centres in the brain ahh and so that's a very strong element, but it's more complex than that and certainly in my case I was well aware that I was medicating ah- at least that was I started looking at it on any particular occasion um medicating for uh technically childhood wounding and my perceived deficient- personality deviancies or um so on.

It is interesting to compare this account of being steered away from certain types of pornography ("extreme violence") and drawn to others (via "dopamine") with J.'s account above, in which J. also describes his pornography viewing as a product of his "brain" pushing him to view pornography. Here, G. uses a series of self-justifications for viewing images of naked children: these images are different to "child sexual pornography", the action of "dopamine" causes the seeking, and the need for a form of self-medication for past traumas. In this sense, G. distances himself from the moral import of his pornography viewing by appealing to the physiological mechanisms contributing to his viewing of pornography that he finds personally dilemmatic. Such an account illustrates a sort of outsourcing of moral authority through a narrative of personal harm, as described by Thomas (2016), whereby a confession to pornography addiction is a preferable explanation for personally dilemmatic pornography viewing than an acceptance of one's repeated violation of a personally (or in G.'s case, socially and legally) derived threshold. Accordingly, throughout the interviews, interviewees routinely took up more passive subject positions in their accounts of seeing personally dilemmatic pornography by describing their personal transgressions through a medicalised lens. Thus, taken together, we can see that the *why* of a self-diagnosed pornography addiction (that is, why someone might describe themselves as such) may be that it acts as a discursive tool through which to describe transgressive pornography viewing in a way that sidesteps a personal moral accounting and locates it somewhere else.

Discussion

In the introduction, I described the problem with a focus on the *what* of problematic pornography viewing and a seeming disinterest in the *why*. My interest in researching men's pornography viewing has not really been focused on 'pornography addiction' per se, but the limited range of ways that we have to describe and explore the complexity of the pornography viewing experience. It has been into this discursive vacuum that the pornography addiction label has stepped. Yet, considering that the discussion in this chapter has focused on pornography addiction, here I should address the relative lack of addiction self-attribution in the extracts above. First, it is worth noting although I have not signposted which participants, half of the men above described themselves as 'pornography addicts'. Arguably, that a reader could interpret any of the above accounts as describing the testimony of a pornography addict (apart from B. perhaps, who describes himself as "not addicted") corroborates the argument that pornography addiction is easily graphed onto any problematic behaviour related to pornography, offering a "simplification of a complex individual's psychological functioning with limited clinical relevance" (Wéry et al., 2019, p. 124; see also Starcevic, 2016). In this sense, if the central diagnostic criteria of pornography addiction is defined in popular culture as simply a loss of self-control, then *all* the above extracts speak to the presence of addiction. Second, and accordingly, throughout the extracts we can see the different ways that these men make sense of their own boundary crossing, not through an addiction attribution, but *in relation to the possibility* of pornography addition. Even while B. disavows addiction, his viewing is still set in relation to the suggestion that pornography could indeed *be* addictive. Indeed, in the introduction I described the value of the pornography addiction concept (namely, *why* someone might describe themselves as addicted to pornography) as resting upon both the visibility of the label in popular culture, and the utility of the label as a culturally meaningful explanation for when viewing crosses from ostensibly 'normal' to 'pathological'. As the extracts above show, these ranged from viewing too much pornography, overstepping a loosely defined personal boundary, seeking personally dilemmatic forms of pornography, and more extreme cases of seeking child pornography (which are later disavowed as a physiological response outside of conscious control). Here, watching pornography was routinely set against various personally derived thresholds of self-control, where 'normal' pornography viewing is viewing that one can control.

What is difficult to reconcile here is that the link between self-control and pleasure is not a straightforward proposition because watching pornography (and sexual behaviour more generally) involves a level of losing self-control. Indeed, throughout the extracts are a range of self-problematisations that suggest that losing self-control is not symptomatic of pornography addiction *per se*, but rather a fundamental part of the pornography viewing experience itself. For example, while the extracts all suggest that the reason pornography viewing can be problematic is the crossing of personal boundaries, M. above also states that the why of *pornography viewing itself* is the crossing of a line "that you know is there". Here, while losing self-control can be personally problematic, we must ask if it is also part and parcel of the experience that makes watching pornography appealing, and further if the appeal of the pornography addiction concept lies (in part) in its ability to describe this transgression of self-control. In other words, if pornography addiction describes a sense of losing self-control, and the very thing that makes pornography appealing is that it *is* transgressive, then what pornography addiction really diagnoses is a personally derived uneasiness arising from *choosing* transgression, trying to pick the right type or amount of transgression from an infinite supply, and bearing the responsibility to consume correctly where no model for correct consumption exists.

To conclude, I argue that the path towards better helping those who struggle with their pornography viewing is not to simplify these experiences down to a binary proposition of either controlled or not, healthy or not, addictive or not. Instead we have to work towards understanding these negotiations as nuanced and distinct personal reactions towards a provocative and intentionally challenging genre of media. Applying an 'addiction' lens manages to obfuscate the seemingly inherently complex and contradictory nature of browsing for the 'correct' type, or else regulating the 'right amount' of pornography. Moreover, using the lens of pornography addiction puts in place an explanatory framework that somehow turns the act of watching pornography into a simplistic continuum between acceptable and unacceptable viewing and avoids the stickier questions of what we imagine moderate/acceptable pornography viewing to look like. As a result, the diversity and complexity of viewing pornography, and thus the *why* of the pornography addiction self-diagnosis, are negated by the diagnosis itself. Moreover, we must understand that these negations play out against the backdrop of our sociocultural contexts, which often frame excessive consumption as pathological sexual behaviour (and thus a medical concern) yet fail to outline what the agreed norms of pornography viewing actually are. To be clear, I am *not* suggesting that we need to draw these lines more clearly to finally construct a robust clinical category for pornography viewing gone wrong, but I am concerned that our understandings of pornography viewing seemingly bend towards a wilful ignorance of the messiness and complexity of the behaviour that we seem so fascinated by, if not frightened of. From media reporting and public discussion to academic research and clinical encounters, in my view, our understanding of pornography viewing will remain in a state of arrested development for as long as we concentrate on debates about operationalisation, quantification, and problematisation. Instead, understanding pornography viewing, and its challenges, requires a more nuanced investigation of what people do with pornography, how they feel about it, and *why* they feel the way they do.

References

Boyle, K. (2010). Porn consumers' public faces: Mainstream media, address and representation. In K. Boyle (Ed.), *Everyday pornography* (pp. 134–146). Routledge.

Chadwick, S. B., Raisanen, J. C., Goldey, K. L., & van Anders, S. (2018). Strategizing to make pornography worthwhile: A qualitative exploration of women's agentic engagement with sexual media. *Archives of Sexual Behaviour, 47*(6), 1853–1868. https://doi.org/10.1007/s10508-018-1174-y

Conrad, P., & Bergey, M. R. (2014). The impending globalization of ADHD: Notes on the expansion and growth of a medicalized disorder. *Social Science & Medicine, 122*, 31–43. https://doi.org/10.1016/j.socscimed.2014.10.019

Conrad, P., & Schneider, J. W. (1992). *Deviance and medicalisation: From badness to sickness*. Temple University Press.
Foucault, M. (1990). *The history of sexuality: An introduction, volume I*. Vintage.
Goldstein, A. (2021). Learner, laugher, lover, critic: Young women's normative and emerging orientations towards pornography. *Porn Studies, 8*(1), 5–20. https://doi.org/10.1080/23268743.2020.1736608
Grubbs, J. B., Exline, J. J., Pargament, K. I., Hook, J. N., & Carlisle, R. D. (2015). Transgression as addiction: Religiosity and moral disapproval as predictors of perceived addiction to pornography. *Archives of Sexual Behaviour, 44*(1), 125–136. https://doi.org/10.1007/s10508-013-0257-z
Grubbs, J. B., & Perry, S. L. (2019). Moral incongruence and pornography use: A critical review and integration. *The Journal of Sex Research, 56*(1), 29–37. https://doi.org/10.1080/00224499.2018.1427204
Gurevich, M., Brown-Bowers, A., Cosma, S., Vasilovsky, A. T., Leedham, U., & Cormier, N. (2017). Sexually progressive and proficient: Pornographic syntax and postfeminist fantasies. *Sexualities, 20*(5–6), 558–584. https://doi.org/10.1177/1363460716665785
Ley, D., Prause, N., & Finn, P. (2014). The emperor has no clothes: A review of the 'pornography addiction' model. *Current Sexual Health Reports, 6*, 94–105. https://doi.org/10.1007/s11930-014-0016-8
McKee, A. (2006). The aesthetics of pornography: The insights of consumers. *Continuum, 20*(4), 523–539. https://doi.org/10.1080/10304310600988310
Reith, G. (2004). Consumption and its discontents: Addiction, identity and the problems of freedom. *The British Journal of Sociology, 55*(2), 283–300. https://doi.org/10.1111/j.1468-4446.2004.00019.x
Starcevic, V. (2016). Behavioural addictions: A challenge for psychopathology and psychiatric nosology. *Australian & New Zealand Journal of Psychiatry, 50*(8), 721–725. https://doi.org/10.1177/0004867416654009
Taylor, K. (2019). Pornography addiction: The fabrication of a transient sexual disease. *History of the Human Sciences, 32*(5), 56–83. https://doi.org/10.1177/0952695119854624
Taylor, K. (2020). Nosology and metaphor: How pornography viewers make sense of pornography addiction. *Sexualities, 23*(4), 609–629. https://doi.org/10.1177/1363460719842136
Taylor, K. (2021). 'Accessing something that's meant to be inaccessible': Pornography viewers' reconciliation between early pornographic memories and pornography's perceived risk. *Porn Studies, 8*(1), 39–57. https://doi.org/10.1080/23268743.2020.1736609

Taylor, K. (2024). The social diagnoses of digital addictions: Technophobic ambivalences, the limits of the natural and imperatives of self-governance in the information age. *Sociology of Health & Illness, 46*(S1), 18–36. https://doi.org/10.1111/1467-9566.13624

Taylor, K., & Gavey, N. (2020). Pornography addiction and the perimeters of acceptable pornography viewing. *Sexualities, 23*(5–6), 876–897. https://doi.org/10.1177/1363460719861826

Thomas, J. N. (2016). The development and deployment of the idea of pornography addiction within American evangelicalism. *Sexual Addiction & Compulsivity, 23*(2–3), 182–195. https://doi.org/10.1080/10720162.2016.1140603

Twohig, M. P., Crosby, J. M., & Cox, J. M. (2009). Viewing internet pornography: For whom is it problematic, how, and why? *Sexual Addiction & Compulsivity, 16*(4), 253–266. https://doi.org/10.1080/10720160903300788

Wéry, A., Schimmenti, A., Karila, L., & Billieux, J. (2019). Where the mind cannot dare: A case of addictive use of online pornography and its relationship with childhood trauma. *Journal of Sex & Marital Therapy, 45*(2), 114–127. https://doi.org/10.1080/0092623X.2018.1488324

Part III

Conspicuous Behaviours as 'Addictions'

9

Wellness, Addiction and Temperance

Richard Hammersley

Across the second half of the twentieth century and into the twenty-first, modern societies have increasingly promoted individual wellness as a central trend. Here, it is proposed that the behaviours known as 'addictions' are defined and caused by the unintended consequences of this. Understanding addiction as the unfortunate by-product of a broader aspect of society helps to explain why the addiction concept is resilient despite substantial evidence that it poorly fits the well-established facts of substance use, problematic use and recovery (for detailed debate, see Heather et al., 2022). Blaming addiction primarily on drugs' properties does not fit the facts, including that there have been quite rapid historical changes regarding the status of various psychoactive substances as wellness aids, controlled medicines, or powerful causes of addiction. Consequently, it is impossible to tackle addiction whilst simultaneously promoting liberal use of wellness aids, because they are the same substances in different settings.

R. Hammersley (✉)
University of Hull, Hull, UK

B. M. Z. Cohen et al. (eds.), *Addiction and the Medicalisation of Conspicuous Behaviour*, The Politics of Mental Health and Illness,
https://doi.org/10.1007/978-3-032-06313-7_8

So, to genuinely prevent addictions, the wellness agenda would need to be toned down and regulated, for if people *should* take and do things to feel better, then some people *will* take or do things to excess. Moreover, all things that make people feel better have the potential to be used excessively and problematically, although this is more common for some things than others. The alternative to both wellness and addiction is temperance and moderation in everything, not just substance use. This chapter will discuss drugs and alcohol, but similar arguments could be made for the behavioural addictions (see for example, Brossard et al., this volume).

What Is Wellness?

A non-profit organisation aiming to support wellness businesses, the Global Wellness Institute (2023) proposes that 'wellness' can be understood as "the active pursuit of activities, choices and lifestyles that lead to a state of holistic health". While, according to Global Wellness Day (2023), wellness is:

> an active process of becoming aware of and making choices towards a healthy and fulfilling life. It is more than being free from illness, it is a dynamic process of change and growth. A good or satisfactory condition of existence; a state characterized by health, happiness, and prosperity; welfare.

Similarly, the World Health Organization defines wellness as "a state of complete physical, mental, and social well-being, and not merely the absence of disease or infirmity" (cited in Global Wellness Day, 2023; for further discussion on definitions and approaches to wellness, see for example, Carlisle et al., 2009; Davies, 2015; Goodwin, 2023; Searle et al., 2021). Here, 'wellness' will be used to refer to the industries rather than academic understandings. There are also critiques of happiness (Davies, 2015; Cabanas & Illouz; 2019), often implied to be the goal of wellness activities along with holistic health. As will be seen in this chapter, the industry of wellness and the states of well-being and of happiness are distinct. Well-being and happiness are distinct because many things that make us happy are not good for us, including substance use, over-eating and over-indulging in foods high in fat, fermentable carbohydrate or salt (see U.S. Centers for Disease Control and Prevention, 2023). Also, some things good for our well-being are not universally enjoyed; for example, some 37 percent of UK adults do not deliberately exercise (Department for Digital, Culture, Media and Sport, 2024). Moreover, Ruggeri et al. (2020) point out that "[w]ell-being is more than happiness and life satisfaction" Furthermore, holistic well-being is not just at the human level, but is influenced by biology, as well as social and economic forces. Making deliberate wellness choices is not the same thing as achieving well-being or happiness, as some common wellness choices—such as taking vitamins and dietary supplements—have little or no measurable effects on our psychological condition (Zhang et al., 2020).

Wellness assumes that it is relative to individual capabilities, and that it cannot simply be imposed by social or economic engineering. For example, Cabanas and Illouz (2019) are critical of the positive psychology movement because it emphasises a positive individual mindset and downplays socioeconomic forces. However, positive psychology and other so-called 'third wave' cognitive behavioural therapies including compassion-focused therapy, acceptance and commitment therapy, dialectical behaviour therapy and mindfulness (see Kennedy & Pearson, 2020) focus on a positive and compassionate mind set because a person can more easily change how they think than their socioeconomic and political situation. Nonetheless, there are recent moves by psychologists to become more political and act as agents of social change (Johnstone et al., 2018).

Perfectionism is often problematic (Shafran & Mansell, 2001) and many people seeking help are anxious or depressed because they have been unable to achieve or sustain the high standards that they have set themselves in life. One set of such standards concerns wellness, including distressing concerns about their appearance, their deficient athletic ability and fitness, their inability to always feel happy, fulfilled or self-actualised, and making possibly inappropriate choices of friends and partners. One toolkit of psychotherapy is to explore the realism of people's expectations that feeling good should be an enduring state and to reconstruct expectations to recognise that people can become more resilient if they have overcome adversity (Cyrulnik, 2009). Many people recovering from mental health problems say that coping with the problems made them 'better people' (see for example, Substance Use and Mental Health Services Administration, 2023). Indeed, life experience itself seems to increase wellness—older people tend to be happier, report better health, and to be more content with themselves, than those in middle age, despite objectively having more health challenges, often more severe negative life events, and generally being less healthy and beautiful than when they were younger (Becker & Trautmann, 2022).

Implicitly, in what Manuel Castells (2000) called the 'network society', wellness is a personal aspiration based on personal choices. The person needs to do some things and avoid others to achieve and maintain wellness: eat fruit and vegetables rather than highly processed foods; take vitamins and dietary supplements, avoid 'addictive' drugs; exercise, but avoid repetitive strain and other injuries; maintain a healthy body weight, but do not take dietary restraint to extremes; keep the mind active, but do not ruminate; be able to relax, but do not watch screens too much; be mindful in the moment, but also organise your day efficiently. And so on.

Although major factors that prevent wellness are outside individual control and might be alleviated by state-level interventions, the roles of the state and the global economy in developing the conditions for wellness are generally downplayed (Cederström & Spicer, 2015). Most obviously, these include a society's economic inequality, food insecurity, poor infrastructure and housing, poor health care systems, and violence, conflict and war. Alexander (2008) would add dislocation, where people are separated and alienated from their social and physical environment and left to negotiate their own individual relationships with social and economic forces (Beck, 1992; Castells, 2000). This chapter is not about the potential governmental enhancement of wellness, or reduction of risk, but about wellness as a common moral and ideological code, exploited by corporate marketing, that inadvertently promotes substance use and addiction in the guise of medicating wellness.

Why Has Wellness Increased?

The rise in wellness is possibly due to our relationships to illness and death having changed considerably over about the last 150 years. This change is evidenced for instance by the plots of many pre-twentieth century novels. Before health advances (including in hygiene, the understanding of infectious disease, antibiotics, and analgesia), people became unexpectedly ill and sometimes died, especially children and women in childbirth (Porter, 2006). What are now minor and repairable injuries were often fatal. People's attitudes to their own lives and those of their loved ones must have been very different, for illness and death could happen at any time, unexpectedly, and derail whatever plans and expectations had been made. Many more people than now took ideas of an afterlife seriously and concepts of morality were usually connected to seeking redemption in heaven. In parallel, noble and heroic self-sacrifice for the greater good, even if fatal, was highly valued, whereas nowadays, for example, even in war, the death or disability of a small number of military personnel is portrayed as tragic. One particularly personalised example is Perkins (2021), who describes the loss of 32 Welsh soldiers in Afghanistan, praising the qualities of each one in detail. Another example is Blevins (2021), who retrospectively personalises those who fought in Vietnam, acknowledging that at the time they were referred to as 'grunts', demonstrating that attitudes have changed markedly in 50 years.

Things are still changing. Nowadays, in peaceful and relatively affluent places, people can anticipate relatively long lives, children who generally grow to adulthood and mothers who usually survive childbirths (Office for National Statistics, 2017; Sheingold & Hahn, 2014). Over the same time, in many countries, belief in an afterlife, God and religion are declining rapidly (Duffy et al., 2023), with half or less of people in the UK and some other countries believing. Even in countries where religious beliefs are more prevalent—notably the US—people have increased expectations of the quality of their lifestyle and well-being now rather than after death. These expectations are encouraged by the well-being industries. Changes are illustrated by the history of self-help books in the US. According to Effing (2009), before the mid-twentieth century these texts focused on industry and effort (to be rewarded in the afterlife), then moved on to leisure and ease. Finally at the end of the century they shifted to self-mastery and self-knowledge. Perhaps in the twenty-first century the latter two themes have merged into wellness.

The founders of psychology, most explicitly William James, thought that one of its key tasks was to find empirical evidence for life after death (Knapp, 2017), which was widely believed in. Nowadays psychology's core questions are more likely to be about the optimisation of the person both intellectually and emotionally, including how to organise society and to avoid discriminatory practices, and how to train, nurture and maintain our brains so that everyone lives the best lives that they can. This ties into the self-help literature and wellness. The current motto of the American Psychological Association (2025) is "[w]e promote psychological science and knowledge to benefit society and improve lives", which illustrates the wellness agenda and is modernist, positive, and applied, with no trace of spirituality, metaphysical wondering, or overt challenging of the social status quo. However, psychologists are beginning to recognise that this does not sit well with late or post-modern concerns about discrimination, inequality and global warming.

One example is the movement to replace the psychiatric diagnosis of mental health problems with formulation (Johnstone et al., 2018). In diagnosis, the clinician uses a checklist or flow chart approach to deciding what is wrong with a person, then selects appropriate interventions based on generic current guidelines, such as the UK's National Institute for Health and Care Excellence (NICE) guidelines (see https://www.nice.org.uk/about/what-we-do/our-programmes/nice-guidance/nice-guidelines). In contrast:

> Formulation can be defined as the process of co-constructing a hypothesis or 'best guess' about the origins of a person's difficulties in the context of their relationships, social circumstances, life events, and the sense that they have made of them. It provides a structure for thinking together with the client or service user about how to understand their experiences and how to move forward. (Johnstone et al., 2018, p. 32).

Formulation is collaborative between client and therapist and develops a personalised model of what concerns them, why it concerns them/why they are seeking help now, the positive aspects of their life, what makes their problems worse, and what in the past may have contributed to the current problems. An action plan is then drawn up by client and therapist. The formulation is revised as therapy progresses and more information comes available.

Wellness and Substance Use Today

The central proposal of this chapter is that anything that is supposed to make people feel better also has the potential to be used to excess, and wellness-seeking and problematic use cannot be differentiated with a catalogue of 'good' and 'bad' substances or activities. Wellness is a huge global industry estimated to be worth US$4.3 trillion in 2020 (Statista, 2023b; for consistency, statistics from Statista are used in this discussion whenever possible, but all such figures are informed best guesses). The World Health Organization (2012) defines quality of life—an evidence-based relative of wellness—as having four domains: physical health; psychological health; social relationships; and environment. Many products that are only marginally related to any of those domains are marketed for their wellness-providing properties. The marketing websites quoted earlier in this chapter describe wellness as an aspiration that leads to unmet consumer needs, rather than being something generally achieved. Aspirations are good for marketing, because they tend to generate needs that can be met repeatedly; last year's product won't do.

Four examples from the wellness industry can help illustrate the above point: (1) the magazine *Men's Health* routinely markets products that allegedly produce a highly muscular 'ripped' body, although the research evidence suggests that far more moderate levels of exercise suffice for health and well-being (Yang, 2019) as well as being more achievable for overweight or obese adults who now make up the majority of the population in many countries (Lobstein et al., 2023). (2) Apps and gadgets that allegedly train one's cognitive skills and prevent or reduce dementia are a growing market, despite insufficient evidence of efficacy (Simons et al., 2016). (3) Social prescribing (that is, GPs and other practitioners guiding patients to a wide variety of groups, clubs and social activities) is promoted and popular in the UK, despite limited evidence that such interventions improve well-being (as well as the major difficulties for researchers in defining 'social prescribing' and gathering evidence on its effectiveness, see for example, Husk et al., 2019). (4) Wellness tourism is globally worth US$476.1 billion (Statista, 2024), despite often harming and degrading the wellness-promoting environments that the tourists seek (see for example, Torsney & Buckley, 2023).

The wellness market is vast; as a contrast, the United Nations Office on Drugs and Crime (UNODC) (2012) estimates the global illegal drug trade to be worth US$32 billion (the UNODC webpage is copyrighted 2023, so this appears to remain their best guess). So, while drugs are huge, they are not as huge as wellness, and perhaps only slightly larger than the global market for vitamins and supplements (US$29.02 billion according to Statista, 2023a)—the latter another wellness market where evidence for efficacy is extremely variable and often inadequate. Most discourse about illegal drugs constructs drug use as utterly separate from wellness, even as its complete opposite. Yet, many illegal drugs—from cannabis to heroin—began as medicines and wellness aids (Berridge & Edwards, 1987). Likewise, alcohol is currently marketed as promoting wellness (Alcohol Change UK, 2024), as were cigarettes in their heyday (Altman et al., 1987).

Moreover, the widespread but misleading concept of 'responsible drinking' is often mentioned in passing, whilst the main body of the advertising and marketing focusses on brand awareness and suggesting different aspects of wellness (see for example, Clegg Smith et al., 2014). More recently, the Australian NGO, Foundation for Alcohol Research and Education (2020), analysed 107 alcohol adverts on Facebook and

Instagram for one hour on one Friday during the COVID-19 pandemic. Of six messages identified, two were "[u]se alcohol to cope, 'survive', or feel better" (16 percent) and "[c]hoose 'healthier' alcohol products" (14 percent). More commonly adverts also emphasised easy access, saving money and buying more, as well as drinking during the pandemic. These are just two of a myriad of examples.

Substance use in general, not just alcohol, is central to wellness, for the so-called addictions are residual problematic consequences of the accepted and encouraged use of substances and to the general message that substances can and should enhance wellness. Attempts to separate out alcohol, caffeine, nicotine, medicines, over-the counter analgesics, vitamins and supplements from addictive drugs on the basis of their psychopharmacology do not work because drug harms depend not just on the drug but also on the mindset of the user and the socioeconomic, legal and political setting of use (Zinberg, 1984). Alcohol, which facilitates socialisation and increases confidence, also ranks first in terms of harms to the self and others, followed by heroin and crack cocaine (Nutt et al., 2010). Heroin and other opiates are not uniquely addictive (Shewan et al., 1998), while most cocaine users are able to quit without help (Waldorf et al., 1991).

Equally lacking evidence is the recent movement of cannabis products, especially CBD (Cannabidiol-based) products, into the wellness space. CBD is an interesting case because it appears to have multiple effects modulating cognitive processing and reducing psychotic-type brain functioning (Batalla et al., 2021). These effects are apparently universally accepted as beneficial and benign to the extent that they are defined as not constituting 'psychoactive' effects at all (Advisory Committee on Novel Foods & Processes, 2023). As of October 2023, the UK Food Standards Agency lowered the recommended daily intake of CBD from 70 mg to 10 mg due to concerns about long term damage to the liver and thyroid. There was still no concern about its psychological effects, as these have been arbitrarily defined as non-psychoactive. This includes no concern regarding drowsiness, despite the Advisory Committee on Novel Foods & Processes (2023, p. 4) stating that "somnolence effects were noted at doses ≥10 mg/kg". Somnolence, or drowsiness, is however of concern for opiates and other illegal drugs. A current UK patient information leaflet (Aspar Pharmaceuticals, 2022) states "Co-Codamol [more commonly known as codeine and paracetamol], can affect your ability to drive as it can make you sleepy or dizzy." But CBD is not a drug, so drowsiness is not a hazard and there is no information leaflet. Similarly, opiates' superb pain-relieving properties are viewed with increasing alarm because they are addictive, although very few people continue using opiates for acute pain once the pain stops (Klimas et al., 2019). In the UK, over-the-counter Co-codamol comes with the following large print warning: "[c]an cause addiction. For three days' use only." Yet, it would be hard to find a contemporary addiction expert who believed that addiction to opiates after three days use was possible. France has made all codeine products prescription only (Cracknell, 2017). There is no evidence that CBD products can cause addiction, but only because so far, to my knowledge, nobody is looking for any. Substances that facilitate wellness are thought about and treated differently from those that are supposedly addictive, dangerous drugs. This distinction is inappropriate.

Wellness can be considered the obverse of risk, which is well-documented as driving modern societies in general (Bauman, 2006; Beck, 1992) and addiction policies and practices in particular (Hammersley, 2008). As with risk, individuals must make their own judgements regarding how to achieve wellness, under conditions of uncertainty, including a general lack of evidence. Also, as with risk, faith in modernity has deteriorated, so even things that only *might* promote wellness are widely espoused and promoted. Many popular magazines include monthly articles reporting the latest wellness aids; the latest exercises, foods, settings, mental attitudes and holidays. Not forgetting the potential benefits of alcohol, now often marketed to make the consumer feel good about themselves. For example, at Naked Wines (2024) one can become an 'angel' and support and interact with independent wine makers. It would be lovely if being an angel with good intentions reduced one's risks of alcohol harms, but it does not.

In contrast, illegal drugs are commonly offered as a canonical example of behaviour that should be banned or heavily controlled because they lead to death, crime and social harm (see for example, Department for Levelling Up, Housing & Communities, 2022). The UK strategy is to treat those who have serious dependency problems and prosecute those who supply or traffic illegal drugs. In reality, in England in 2021, there were officially 4,859 deaths from drug poisoning, 20,970 alcohol-related deaths and 227 deaths from paracetamol overdose; paracetamol does not count as a 'drug' in UK government rhetoric, nor does alcohol, although, as well as being a cause of death, it can lead to very serious problems including domestic violence and other violent crime (Commission on Alcohol Harm, 2020). The bifurcation of substances is neatly illustrated by the continued separation of alcohol from other drugs in UK policy, probably influenced by the effective lobbying of the alcohol industry (McCambridge et al., 2013). Other than tobacco in its heyday and nicotine vapes today, it is difficult to imagine any other 'drug' being sold 24 hours a day from petrol stations. CBD, vitamins and caffeine products are not generally considered to be drugs at all.

Substance use is integral to wellness, and risky- and wellness-promoting use cannot be effectively differentiated. Over the decades, substances move in and out of riskiness and wellness. For example, benzodiazepines were initially hailed as marvellous mood enhancers that were much safer than previous anti-depressants such as barbiturates. 30 years later, it was discovered that they could be taken chronically in large quantities leading to inebriation, sedation and feelings of dependence (Wick, 2013). More dishonestly, Oxycontin was marketed as a safe non-addictive analgesic, suitable for use for chronic pain and widely promoted to and offered by doctors, initiating the current US opioid epidemic (Volkow, 2014; see also Müller, this volume).

The wellness market offers a myriad of products and methods for individuals to achieve wellness. Many of them have little or no efficacy. Many products are marketed implying that they will confer wellness upon their owners; TV adverts for cars and for perfumes are two often ludicrous illustrations. Wellness can also be achieved by consuming substances of many kinds, including foods, drinks, vitamins and supplements, medicines and 'drugs'—substances known to have psychoactive effects. Very generally, it is relatively plausible that a specific diet, or a medicine, might enhance wellness, even if in many cases they do not. This possibility raises a widespread and often urgent social demand to differentiate wellness-creating substances and substance use practices from those that are dangerous, contra-wellness, and addictive. In the UK medical cannabis has been legally prescribed (under quite strict conditions) since 2018, yet apparently sometimes the police decide medical cannabis is an illegal drug because of the characteristic smell (Busby, 2023).

The need to differentiate wellness products from addictive drugs generates the need and desire to discover properties of some substances, interacting with people's central nervous systems, that cause and define addiction, and which are separate from the properties that make people feel better when taking them. Unfortunately, the search is grounded in a fundamental misunderstanding of how people become addicted to things. People do not become dependent solely due to the addictive properties of a substance, whatever those are hypothesised to be, but also due to their mindset whilst using and to the setting of use (Zinberg, 1984). What about medicines for chronic conditions? Are insulin, blood pressure medication, or anti-depressants addictive because patients need to keep taking them? If addiction is an obverse of wellness, then this question becomes meaningless.

A key aspect of setting is socioeconomic deprivation, which is associated with substance use problems, but not with the prevalence of use itself (see for example, Karriker-Jaffe, 2011). Depending on survey methods and definitions, substance use (alcohol, tobacco, illegal drugs) may be more prevalent amongst more affluent people. The setting of use extends to the proximal social and physical environment, right across to social and governmental policies. It is easier to become addicted in conditions of squalor, with peers who also use, have little social capital to damage by use, and when the drugs (or alcohol) to be used are readily accessible 24 hours a day. Benzodiazepines are more widely prescribed in more deprived areas (Soyombo et al., 2020) and more widely abused, having leaked from prescriptions or been stolen, within a polydrug abusing lifestyle (Roe, 2020).

Another example (as of October 2023), is the controversy regarding vaping devices, available to buy over-the-counter in many countries. Aerosol delivery of nicotine was developed as an effective aid to smoking cessation (Hartmann-Boyce et al. 2021; see also Elam, this volume). It is still considered to be a less harmful alternative to tobacco (and probably marijuana, for aerosol THC (Tetrahydrocannabinol) or CBD products) smoking. However, an enormous and weakly regulated market has since developed for vape products, with myriads of flavours and attractive gadgets. As previously with tobacco and other drugs, there are now concerns that vaping adolescents may become dependent on nicotine and that the inhaled substances may be affecting their neuropsychological development and harming their lungs, especially if they vape products containing THC (Striley & Nutley, 2020). Vaping is moving into being an addictive problem.

From Wellness to Addiction

This historical path from medicine to popular substance, to be used with complacency to dangerous and addictive drug, has been taken many times. Sometimes the pathway is circular, for instance cannabis is currently moving from dangerous and addictive drug to medicine and popular substance to be used with complacency, as it was in some countries prior to the twentieth century. With vaping, it may turn out that it is not harmful after all. Or it may be driven into the unregulated black market.

Tobacco began as a dangerous substance sanctioned by the death penalty, moved to being a popular substance, then endemically popular once machine rolled cigarettes were invented, then it was recommended for 'nerves', then finally its addictiveness and harmfulness was discovered by epidemiological research. In reality, the harms of smoking cigarettes were known and documented from soon after the outset of mass cigarette smoking, and there were additional concerns about them promoting immorality (for a summary see Borio, 2020). Nonetheless they were popular and profitable, so use escalated and became big business, with the tobacco industry downplaying its harms to the best of its ability.

Opiates began as essential medicines for pain relief which could be purchased freely (Berridge & Edwards, 1987). In the UK, addicts were relatively rare up until the mid-twentieth century and tended to be managed by prescribing opiates (see Strang & Sheridan, 1997). This changed with the heroin epidemics, such as those in the US in the 1970s and 1980s and the UK in the 1980s and 1990s. Opiates were now addictive and dangerous. Medical use continued, but such are the concerns about addiction that there are now trials of opioid free surgery (for further discussion, see Hammersley, 2022). The cycle has not turned to complacent popularity yet.

These are examples of how the same substance, even the same pattern of behaviour, can be constructed at different times as either 'addictive' or 'safe' (which is commonly used, if illogical, as the opposite of addictive). Because collective memory is short, these changes tend to be presented as due to the discovery of new evidence, when often the now forgotten old evidence already pointed to the same conclusions. All psychoactive drugs that are not physically poisonous at normal doses can be both safe and addictive depending upon both how they are used, and how they are thought about and judged. One theory is that the fewer the physical, social, psychological, moral and economic constraints on use, the more likely is addiction (Hammersley, 2014). Consider cigarette smoking in its heyday when they could be purchased and consumed almost everywhere at all times, for there were cigarette vending machines in the streets.

Some people take drugs as a form of self-harm or self-destructiveness, but I have previously listed (see Hammersley, 2008, p. 134) the positive reasons that people take drugs (including legal substances not currently stigmatised as 'drugs'), namely: (1) because they enjoy the effects; (2) because drugs affect their arousal or cognitive performance in ways that seem pleasurable or beneficial; (3) for other instrumental reasons, including to alleviate pain, to reduce anxiety, to sleep, to stay awake, to enhance sex and to dance more enthusiastically; (4) because they seem like the appropriate thing to do in the social setting where they are; (5) because, if they do not take the drugs, they expect unpleasant things will happen to them (for example, people believe from experience that if they do not take heroin they will have unpleasant withdrawal effects, so they seek out more heroin and take it (Johnson et al., 1985); generally, they do this before withdrawal kicks in); (6) as a form of escape from the problems of their everyday life; (7) because mind-altering effects of drugs are, for some people, enjoyable in their own right; (8) as a part of religious or spiritual rituals. All but perhaps reason number four could be classified as wellness-oriented activities.

If a substance promotes wellness, then demand for it increases, then it becomes more widely available, then more people can use it, more heavily. Its popularity then suggests that it is relatively safe, so more people use the substance with more complacency. This generates more people who use very heavily and exhibit signs of dependence. Some heroin injectors report that they started use not knowing that the powder was heroin, but being in a place where it was widely available and being told that it would make them feel better and help them to forget their problems, which it did (Hammersley et al., 2016). A more mundane example is the rise of high caffeine, high sugar energy drinks such as Red Bull, followed by reports of people taking large quantities with adverse effects to their mental health (Richards and Smith, 2016) and then voluntary age restrictions being introduced on their purchase (at least in the UK), repeating the common pattern of society having most concern about the substances that young people take.

Nonetheless, some substances are easier to become dependent upon than others, but dependence potential just modulates the basic process. For, belief in the dependence potential of a substance is a common reason for maintaining temperate use, or avoiding use entirely (Hammersley et al., 2020; Shewan & Dalgarno, 2005). Whereas belief that a substance is safe can lead to unrestricted use and dependence. At some point in the transition from wellness promoter to addictive drug, there is often political awareness that the substance might be problematic. As Bauman (2006) documents, 'might be' is good enough to trigger the usual response, which is to legislate against it, usually by banning the substance and imposing penalties for its use. Banning substances may work for those for which there is little or no popular demand, but when there is demand, then bans usually generate a black market that is even more profitable—without regulations, price controls or taxation—than a legal market. Thus, a problematic illegal drug has been generated from a substance that was previously a medicine or a wellness aid.

In November 2023 nitrous oxide was made a Class C drug in the UK. The language of the Home Office news item (Philp & Braverman, 2023) quite clearly suggests that the drug is to be banned because young people take it, often in public, and because it creates littering, rather than because it is genuinely dangerous or has addiction potential. For every nitrous oxide container littering a park, there will be multiple alcohol and soft drink containers. It seems likely that the ban is entirely political and expedient to seem tough on substance use and disorder, appealing to older voters who are most likely to be anti-drugs. There is not much else left to ban, for alcohol is politically untouchable.

The transition from drug to wellness aid is much more difficult, although cannabis is currently making that transition and perhaps some hallucinogens are moving back to being therapeutic medicines (see Noorani, this volume). Tobacco made this transition in the late nineteenth/early twentieth century, causing terrible damage to long-term health (Borio, 2020). One aspect of this transition is that any harmful consequences of wellness aids are side effects to be managed (for instance, yoga injuries, drowsiness after medical marijuana), whereas harmful consequences of addictive drugs or behaviours are evidence of addiction and rationales for regulation or banning them.

The form of substance use problems and the social and medical responses to them are constructed within wellness discourse. Forms of problematic substance use were recognised and of concern long before modern health and well-being were developed materially and constructed into what has become wellness. Famous examples include veterans' widespread addiction to morphine after the American Civil War (Jones, 2020), the 'gin craze' in the early 1700s in the UK (Mitchell, 2019), the historical use of tobacco (Borio, 2020), and concerns (eventually unfounded) about the endemic use of cannabis products in Imperial India (Indian Hemp Drugs Commission, 1894). Older examples are less well documented. Yet, with a different morality and expectations about health and mortality, these were not seen so much as problems to be redressed for individual well-being—which would come in heaven—but practical problems affecting society. Concerns commonly included immorality, corrupting others, neglect of duties (especially being unable to work effectively), expenditure, and dangers to health. But those reasonable concerns were not attributed to the unmanageable and uncontrollable (addictive) effects of the substance. As Aaron and Musto (1981, p. 1) state of drunkenness during such times, it "was condemned and punished, but only as an abuse of a God-given gift. Drink itself was not looked upon as culpable, any more than food deserved blame for the sin of gluttony. Excess was personal indiscretion."

How things have changed; as of the 2020s food is being blamed, but for obesity and food addiction rather than gluttony. In its early years, the American temperance movement was opposed to excessive drinking (hence temperance, not abstinence), but there were varying views about whether alcohol was utterly hazardous or merely something that was often taken to excess (Aaron & Musto, 1981). Excessive drinking was not yet blamed upon alcohol's properties.

Temperance as an Alternative to Wellness and Addiction

Due to the historical fluctuations in whether a substance is a wellness aid, a controlled medicine, or an addictive drug, it is impossible to promote temperance or abstinence for potentially addictive drugs whilst simultaneously promoting liberal use of wellness aids because they are the same substances in different settings. The message that it is a good thing to take substances to feel better and to aspire to maximum wellness also generates the message that heavy substance use can be good, which can lead to excessive use. Yet, wellness aids can become addictive drugs, especially if widely available, widely tolerated and used daily. Beyond its common usage regarding alcohol, temperance is about self-restraint. The unrestrained pursuit of wellness can turn into dependence, as in the examples discussed above.

A modern temperance would involve rejecting the idea that wellness can be limitless and should be sought after by extensive consumption behaviour or other extensive activities. Rather, for temperance we need to promote the idea that excessive use of anything is potentially problematic. However, the wellness industry is vast, industrialised, and motivated by profit, making temperance unlikely as a widespread corporate or societal message. This includes the pharmaceutical and other medical industries. At the same time, there are increasing concerns about the over-prescribing of such pharmaceuticals (Department of Health and Social Care, 2021). Arguments can also be made for the legalisation of all controlled drugs in common use (Dalgarno et al., 2021) so that they can be regulated and taxed. Perhaps regulation should extend to evidence of safety and efficacy being actively required for all ingestible substances, although given the plethora of ingestible products this might be impractical.

While this chapter has focused on substance use it is worth noting that, in 2023, intemperate use of natural resources, including energy from non-renewable sources, is a much larger problem for humanity than addiction. So is intemperate eating, especially of highly processed foods, often overtly marketed for their allegedly wellness-promoting properties. McDonalds in the UK, for example, has been advertising their 'Breakfast Done Properly', with the Campaign Director stating that, "we wanted to show, *whatever the mood or occasion*—McDonald's is there to provide a little moment of enjoyment and proper satisfaction at breakfast time" (cited in Leo Burnett UK, 2021, emphasis added).

Rather than the lack of breakfast, wellness is often challenged by global environmental, social and political factors that the individual cannot control. The sociology of risk has documented that locating risk management in the individual, then offering them consumer products to cause enjoyment, satisfaction and other aspects of wellness, is partly a diversionary activity to evade the issue that national and local governments cannot really control global factors either (Castells, 2000). Temperance involves accepting that there are things that the person cannot change or offset by their individual efforts at wellness and accepting that trying to compensate for or redress life's challenges by consumption can have harmful effects, including substance dependence.

References

Aaron, P., & Musto, D. (1981). Temperance and prohibition in America: A historical overview. In M. H. Moore & D. R. Gerstein (Eds.), *Alcohol and public policy: Beyond the shadow of prohibition* (pp. 127–181). National Academies Press.

Advisory Committee on Novel Foods & Processes. (2023). *Joint position paper from the Advisory Committee on Novel Foods and Processes (ACNFP) & Committee on Toxicity (COT) on establishing a provisional acceptable daily intake (ADI) for pure form (≥98%) cannabidiol (CBD) in foods, based on new evidence.* https://doi.org/10.46756/sci.fsa.zcg392

Alcohol Change UK. (2024). Alcohol marketing. *Alcohol Change UK.* https://alcoholchange.org.uk/policy/policy-insights/making-sure-alcohol-is-marketed-responsibly

Alexander, B. K. (2008). *The globalisation of addiction: A study in poverty of the spirit.* Oxford University Press.

Altman, D. G., Slater, M. D., Albright, C. L., & Maccoby, N. (1987). How an unhealthy product is sold: Cigarette advertising in magazines, 1960–1985. *Journal of Communication, 37*(4), 95–106. https://doi.org/10.1111/j.1460-2466.1987.tb01010.x

American Psychological Association. (2025). [Home page]. www.apa.org

Aspar Pharmaceuticals. (2022). *Patient information leaflet for Co-Codamol 8mg/500mg tablets (Codeine Phosphate and Paracetamol).* Aspar Pharmaceuticals.

Batalla, A., Bos, J., Postma, A., & Bossong, M. G. (2021). The impact of cannabidiol on human brain function: A systematic review. *Frontiers in Pharmacology, 11*, 618184. https://doi.org/10.3389/fphar.2020.618184

Bauman, Z. (2006). *Liquid fear.* Polity.

Beck, U. (1992). *Risk society: Towards a new modernity.* Sage.

Becker, C. K., & Trautmann, S. T. (2022). Does happiness increase in old age? Longitudinal evidence from 20 European countries. *Journal of Happiness Studies, 23*(7), 3625–3654. https://doi.org/10.1007/s10902-022-00569-4

Berridge, V., & Edwards, G. (1987). *Opium and the people: Opiate use in nineteenth century England.* Yale University Press.

Blevins, V. B. (2021). A 'Grunt' in the Vietnam war. *The Daily Advocate.* https://www.dailyadvocate.com/2021/07/07/a-grunt-in-the-vietnam-war/#:~:text=%E2%80%9CGrunts%E2%80%9D%20was%20a%20common%20expression,for%20being%20grievously%20wounded%20there

Borio, G. (2020). Tobacco history. *Tobacco Collectibles.* https://tobaccocollectibles.co.uk/the-history-of-tobacco

Busby, M. (2023). 'They put handcuffs on me': UK users of medical cannabis tell of raids and arrests. *The Guardian.* https://www.theguardian.com/uk-news/2023/nov/06/they-put-handcuffs-on-me-uk-users-of-medical-cannabis-tell-of-raids-and-arrests?CMP=Share_AndroidApp_Other

Cabanas, E., & Illouz, E. (2019). *Manufacturing happy citizens: How the science and industry of happiness control our lives.* Polity.

Carlisle, S., Henderson, G., & Hanlon, P. W. (2009). 'Wellbeing': A collateral casualty of modernity? *Social Science and Medicine, 69*(10), 1556–1560. https://doi.org/10.1016/j.socscimed.2009.08.029

Castells, M. (2000). *End of millennium, volume III: The information age: Economy, society and culture*. Wiley.

Cederström, C., & Spicer, A. (2015). *The wellness syndrome*. Polity.

Clegg Smith, K., Cukier, S., & Jernigan, D. H. (2014). Defining strategies for promoting product through 'drink responsibly' messages in magazine ads for beer, spirits and alcopops. *Drug and Alcohol Dependence, 142*, 168–173. https://doi.org/10.1016/j.drugalcdep.2014.06.007

Commission on Alcohol Harm. (2020). 'It's everywhere'—Alcohol's public face and private harm. *The Report of the Commission on Alcohol Harm*. https://ahauk.org/wp-content/uploads/2020/09/Its-Everywhere-Commission-on-Alcohol-Harm-final-report.pdf

Cracknell, C. (2017). Codeine now restricted to prescription-only. *The Connexion*. https://www.connexionfrance.com/article/French-news/Codeine-now-restricted-to-prescription-only

Cyrulnik, B. (2009). *Resilience*. Penguin.

Dalgarno, P., O'Rawe, S., & Hammersley, R. (2021). Illegal drugs in the UK: Is it time for considered legalisation to improve public health? *Drug Science, Policy and Law, 7*. https://doi.org/10.1177/20503245211005351

Davies, W. (2015). *The happiness industry: How the government and big business sold us well-being*. Verso.

Department for Digital, Culture, Media and Sport. (2024). Ethnicity facts and figures: Physical activity. *GOV.UK*. https://www.ethnicity-facts-figures.service.gov.uk/health/diet-and-exercise/physical-activity/latest/

Department for Levelling Up, Housing & Communities. (2022). From harm to hope: A 10-year drugs plan to cut crime and save lives. *GOV.UK*. https://www.gov.uk/government/publications/from-harm-to-hope-a-10-year-drugs-plan-to-cut-crime-and-save-lives/from-harm-to-hope-a-10-year-drugs-plan-to-cut-crime-and-save-lives

Department of Health and Social Care. (2021). Good for you, good for us, good for everybody: A plan to reduce overprescribing to make patient care better and safer, support the NHS, and reduce carbon emissions. *UK Government*. https://assets.publishing.service.gov.uk/media/614a10fed3bf7f05ab786551/good-for-you-good-for-us-good-for-everybody.pdf

Duffy, B., May, G., Voas, D., Wright, J., Harsanyi, R., Hewlett, K., & Stoneman, P. (2023). *Lost faith? The UK's changing attitudes to religion*. https://doi.org/10.18742/pub01-134

Effing, M. M. (2009). The origin and development of self-help literature in the United States: The concept of success and happiness, an overview. *Atlantis, 31*(2), 125–141. https://www.jstor.org/stable/41055368

Foundation for Alcohol Research and Education. (2020). *Alcohol ad every 35 seconds during COVID. Foundation for Alcohol Research and Education*. https://fare.org.au/alcohol-ad-every-35-seconds-during-covid-19/

Global Wellness Day. (2023). What is wellness? *Global Wellness Day*. https://www.globalwellnessday.org/about/what-is-wellness/

Global Wellness Institute. (2023). What is wellness? *Global Wellness Institute*. https://globalwellnessinstitute.org/what-is-wellness/

Goodwin, J. (2023). Chasing a feeling: The modern wellness journey and the role of digital media. *Vox Media*. https://www.voxmedia.com/2023/1/4/23539451/chasing-a-feeling-the-modern-wellness-journey-and-the-role-of-digital-media

Hammersley, R. (2008). *Drugs and crime: Theories and practices*. Polity.

Hammersley, R. (2014). Constraint theory: A cognitive, motivational theory of dependence. *Addiction Research & Theory, 22*(1), 1–14. https://doi.org/10.3109/16066359.2013.779678

Hammersley, R. (2022). Addiction is a human problem, but brain disease models divert attention and resources away from human level solutions. In N. Heather, M. Field, A. C. Moss, & S. Satel (Eds.), *Evaluating the brain disease model of addiction* (pp. 176–186). Routledge.

Hammersley, R., Dalgarno, P., McCollum, S., Reid, M., Strike, Y., Smith, A., Wallace, J., Smart, A., Jack, M., Thompson, A., & Liddell, D. (2016). Trauma in the childhood stories of people who have injected drugs. *Addiction Research & Theory, 24*(2), 135–151. https://doi.org/10.3109/16066359.2015.1093120

Hammersley, R., Holmes, N., & Reid, M. (2020). Testing the constraint theory of addiction: Cannabis constraints discriminate users from nonusers and heavy from light users. *Journal of Addiction, 1*, 3427270. https://doi.org/10.1155/2020/3427270

Hartmann-Boyce, J., Lindson, N., Butler, A. R., McRobbie, H., Bullen, C., Begh, R., Theodoulou, A., Notley, C., Rigotti, N. A., Turner, T., Fanshawe, T. R., & Hajek, P. (2021). Electronic cigarettes for smoking cessation.

Cochrane database of systematic reviews, 11. https://doi.org/10.1002/14651858.CD010216.pub7

Heather, N., Field, M., Moss, A., & Satel, S. (Eds.). (2022). *Evaluating the brain disease model of addiction*. Routledge.

Husk, K., Elston, J., Gradinger, F., Callaghan, L., & Asthana, S. (2019). Social prescribing: Where is the evidence? *British Journal of General Practice, 69*(678), 6–7. https://doi.org/10.3399/bjgp19X700325

Indian Hemp Drugs Commission. (1894). *Report of the Indian Hemp Drug Commission, 1893–94*. Government Central Printing Office.

Johnson, B. D., Goldstein, P. J., Preble, E., Schmeidler, J., Lipton, D. S., Spunt, B., & Miller, T. (1985). *Taking care of business: The economics of crime by heroin abusers*. Lexington Books.

Johnstone, L., Boyle, M., Cromby, J., Dillon, J., Harper, D., Kinderman, P., Longden, E., Pilgrim, D., & Read, J. (2018). *The power threat meaning framework: Towards the identification of patterns in emotional distress, unusual experiences and troubled or troubling behaviour, as an alternative to functional psychiatric diagnosis*. British Psychological Society.

Jones, J. S. (2020). Opiate addiction in the Civil War's aftermath. *Virginia Museum of History and Culture*. https://virginiahistory.org/learn/opiate-addiction-civil-wars-aftermath

Karriker-Jaffe, K. J. (2011). Areas of disadvantage: A systematic review of effects of area-level socioeconomic status on substance use outcomes. *Drug and Alcohol Review, 30*(1), 84–95. https://doi.org/10.1111/j.1465-3362.2010.00191.x

Kennedy, F., & Pearson, D. (2020). *Integrating CBT and third wave therapies: Distinctive features*. Routledge.

Klimas, J., Gorfinkel, L., Fairbairn, N., Amato, L., Ahamad, K., Nolan, S., Simel, D. L., & Wood, E. (2019). Strategies to identify patient risks of prescription opioid addiction when initiating opioids for pain: A systematic review. *JAMA network open, 2*(5), e193365. https://doi.org/10.1001/jamanetworkopen.2019.3365

Knapp, K. D. (2017). *William James: Psychical research and the challenge of modernity*. University of North Carolina Press.

Leo Burnett UK. (2021). McDonald's and Leo Burnett London celebrate the most important meal of the day. *Creative*. https://lbbonline.com/news/mcdonalds-and-leo-burnett-london-celebrate-the-most-important-meal-of-the-day

Lobstein, T., Jackson-Leach, R., Powis, J., Brinsden, H., & Gray, M. (2023). World Obesity Atlas 2023. *World Obesity Federation*. https://s3-eu-west-1.amazonaws.com/wof-files/World_Obesity_Atlas_2023_Report.pdf

McCambridge, J., Hawkins, B., & Holden, C. (2013). Vested interests in addiction research and policy: The challenge corporate lobbying poses to reducing society's alcohol problems: Insights from UK evidence on minimum unit pricing. *Addiction, 109*(2), 199–205. https://doi.org/10.1111/add.12380

Mitchell, D. (2019). The 18th-century craze for gin. *History Extra*. https://www.historyextra.com/period/georgian/gin-craze-panic-18th-century-london-when-came-england-alcohol-drinking-history/

Naked Wines. (2024). The wine club that works for you. *Naked Wines*. https://www.nakedwines.co.uk/angels

Nutt, D. J., King, L. A., & Phillips, L. D. (2010). Drug harms in the UK: A multicriteria decision analysis. *The Lancet, 376*(9752), 1558–1565.

Office for National Statistics. (2017). Causes of death over 100 years. Office for National Statistics. https://www.ons.gov.uk/peoplepopulationandcommunity/birthsdeathsandmarriages/deaths/articles/causesofdeathover100years/2017-09-18

Perkins, L. (2021). The Welsh soldiers who died in Afghanistan. *Wales Online*. https://www.walesonline.co.uk/news/wales-news/welsh-soldiers-who-died-afghanistan-21331179

Philp, C., & Braverman, S. (2023). Nitrous oxide to be illegal by end of the year. *GOV.UK*. https://www.gov.uk/government/news/nitrous-oxide-to-be-illegal-by-end-of-the-year

Porter, R. (Ed.). (2006). *The Cambridge history of medicine*. Cambridge University Press.

Richards, G., & Smith, A. P. (2016). A review of energy drinks and mental health, with a focus on stress, anxiety, and depression. *Journal of Caffeine Research, 6*(2), 49–63. https://doi.org/10.1089/jcr.2015.0033

Roe, L. (2020). *Echoes of endlessness: Time, memory, and experience for heroin users in Scotland*. Doctoral thesis, University of St Andrews. https://doi.org/10.17630/10023-20384

Ruggeri, K., Garcia-Garzon, E., Maguire, Á., Matz, S., & Huppert, F. A. (2020). Well-being is more than happiness and life satisfaction: A multidimensional analysis of 21 countries. *Health and Quality of Life Outcomes, 18*, 1–16. https://doi.org/10.1186/s12955-020-01423-y

Searle, B. A., Pyjett, J., & Alfaro-Simmonds, M. J. (Eds.). (2021). *A modern guide to wellbeing research*. Edward Elgar.

Shafran, R., & Mansell, W. (2001). Perfectionism and psychopathology: A review of research and treatment. *Clinical Psychology Review, 21*(6), 879–906. https://doi.org/10.1016/S0272-7358(00)00072-6

Sheingold, B. H., & Hahn, J. A. (2014). The history of healthcare quality: The first 100 years 1860–1960. *International Journal of Africa Nursing Sciences, 1*, 18–22. https://doi.org/10.1016/j.ijans.2014.05.002

Shewan, D., & Dalgarno, P. (2005). Low levels of negative health and social outcomes among non-treatment heroin users in Glasgow (Scotland): Evidence for controlled heroin use. *British Journal of Health Psychology, 10*(1), 33–48. https://doi.org/10.1348/135910704X14582

Shewan, D., Dalgarno, P., Marshall, A., Lowe, E., Campbell, M., Nicholson, S., Reith, G., McLafferty, V., & Thomson, K. (1998). Patterns of heroin use among a non-treatment sample in Glasgow (Scotland). *Addiction Research, 6*(3), 215–234. https://doi.org/10.3109/16066359808993304

Simons, D. J., Boot, W. R., Charness, N., Gathercole, S. E., Chabris, C. F., Hambrick, D. Z., & Stine-Morrow, E. A. (2016). Do "brain-training" programs work? *Psychological Science in the Public Interest, 17*(3), 103–186. https://doi.org/10.1177/1529100616661983

Soyombo, S., Stanbrook, R., Aujla, H., Capewell, D., Shantikumar, M., Kidy, F., Todkill, D., & Shantikumar, S. (2020). Socioeconomic status and benzodiazepine and Z-drug prescribing: A cross-sectional study of practice-level data in England. *Family Practice, 37*(2), 194–199. https://doi.org/10.1093/fampra/cmz054

Statista. (2023a). Vitamins & minerals—Worldwide. *Statista*. https://www.statista.com/outlook/cmo/otc-pharmaceuticals/vitamins-minerals/worldwide#revenue

Statista. (2023b). Wellness industry—Statistics & facts. *Statista*. https://www.statista.com/topics/1336/wellness-and-spa/#topicOverview

Statista. (2024). Global market size of the wellness tourism industry in 2022 and 2030. *Statista*. Retrieved from: https://www.statista.com/statistics/1018497/global-market-size-of-the-wellness-tourism-industry/

Strang, J., & Sheridan, J. (1997). Heroin prescribing in the "British system" of the mid 1990s: Data from the 1995 national survey of community pharmacies in England and Wales. *Drug and Alcohol Review, 16*(1), 7–16.

Striley, C. W., & Nutley, S. K. (2020). World vaping update. *Current Opinion in Psychiatry, 33*(4), 360–368. https://doi.org/10.1097/YCO.0000000000000617

Substance Use and Mental Health Services Administration. (2023). Living well with serious mental illness. *Substance Use and Mental Health Services Administration*. https://www.samhsa.gov/serious-mental-illness

Torsney, A., & Buckley, Y. M. (2023). Visitor demographics, site-type and activities determine the occurrence and severity of environmental impacts at nature-based tourist destinations. *Ecological Solutions and Evidence, 4*(1), e12207. https://doi.org/10.1002/2688-8319.12207

U.S. Centers for Disease Control and Prevention. (2023). Lifestyle Risk Factors. *U.S. Centers for Disease Control and Prevention.* https://www.cdc.gov/environmental-health-tracking/php/data-research/lifestyle-risk-factors.html?CDC_AAref_Val=https://www.cdc.gov/nceh/tracking/topics/LifestyleRiskFactors.htm

United Nations Office on Drugs and Crime. (2012). Drug trafficking: A $32 billion business affecting communities globally. *UNODC.* https://www.unodc.org/southasia/frontpage/2012/August/drug-trafficking-a-business-affecting-communities-globally.html

Volkow, N. D. (2014). Prescription opioid and heroin abuse. *National Institute on Drug Abuse.* https://www.nih.gov/sites/default/files/institutes/olpa/20140429-senate-testimony-collins.pdf

Waldorf, D., Reinarman, C., & Murphy, S. (1991). *Cocaine changes: The experience of using and quitting.* Temple University Press.

Wick, J. (2013). The history of benzodiazepines. *The Consultant Pharmacist, 28*(9), 538–548. https://doi.org/10.4140/TCP.n.2013.538

World Health Organization. (2012). *WHOQOL user manual.* World Health Organization.

Yang, Y. J. (2019). An overview of current physical activity recommendations in primary care. *Korean Journal of Family Medicine, 40*(3), 135–142. https://doi.org/10.4082/kjfm.19.0038

Zhang, F. F., Barr, S. I., McNulty, H., Li, D., & Blumberg, J. B. (2020). Health effects of vitamin and mineral supplements. *BMJ, 369*, m2511. https://doi.org/10.1136/bmj.m2511

Zinberg, N. (1984). *Drug, set and setting: The basis for controlled intoxicant use.* Yale University Press.

10

Using Sports: Constructing Extremity as Addiction

Lars Arntsen and Nancy D. Campbell

Risk societies (Beck, 1992) regularly present situations that exceed individual capacities for control, certainty, expertise, and knowledge—ranging from toxic exposures to climate change to legalised gambling to high-dose pharmaceuticals. Risk markets—licit and illicit, regulated and unregulated—deliver intense and potentially lethal experiences on the ragged edge of regulation. This chapter offers a new conceptual frame for 'risk regulatory societies', which order time and space in ways that emphasise safety, compliance, and insurance to anchor social norms and routines of risk avoidance while simultaneously promoting "cultivated risk-taking … in which danger and its resolution are bound up in the same activity" (Giddens, 1991, p. 133). This chapter examines how 'cultivated risk-taking' is curated for display in lifestyle markets promoted through mass and social media.

L. Arntsen • N. D. Campbell (✉)
Rensselaer Polytechnic Institute, Troy, NY, USA
e-mail: campbn2@rpi.edu

B. M. Z. Cohen et al. (eds.), *Addiction and the Medicalisation of Conspicuous Behaviour*, The Politics of Mental Health and Illness,
https://doi.org/10.1007/978-3-032-06313-7_9

Concrete risk situations "make possible the display of daring, resourcefulness, skill and sustained endeavour, where people are only too aware of the risks involved in what they are doing, but use them to create an edge which routine circumstances lack" (Giddens, 1991, pp. 132–133). This chapter centres a purposely self-defined edge-working population that seeks to avoid the dullness of routine by cultivating risk to a consensually extreme degree. Extreme athletes also participate in a "mass consumption phenomenon" (Raggiotto, 2020, pp. 10–11). This chapter considers the question of whether the regular courting of risk and extremity may be seen accurately as a form of addictive consumption (Reith, 2019). Are extreme athletes using sports as others use drugs?

Arising from anti-capitalist youth subcultures (Raggiotto, 2020, pp. 10–11), extreme sports span the poles of athlete and spectator, professional and amateur. A broad social base participates in extreme sports when such activities as BASE jumping, BMX, kite surfing and wing-suiting, rock climbing, skydiving, snowboarding, big wave surfing, triathlon, Iron Man and other endurance sports are considered; even consumers, spectators, or fans of extreme sports are assessed for 'psychological drivers' and 'managerial implications' of repeat attendance (Raggiotto, 2020; Raggiotto et al., 2019). Yet these activities are *made deviant* by contrast to regulatory norms of seeking safety and avoiding risk. The safety imperative of risk society labels those who suffer negative emotional, social, or physical consequences of repeated engagement in extreme sports to the exclusion of other activities and relationships as engaged in forms of 'addictive consumption' (Reith, 2019). This chapter discusses extreme sports in relation to substance and non-substance 'use disorders'.

Addiction attributions provide a familiar and convenient vocabulary of motive for cultivated risks in risk regulatory societies. As lifestyle innovations such as GoPro cameras make subjective experiences of risk and agility widely available on social media, they also increase experiential intensity and invite mass participation in, or consumption of, extreme events. These technologies widen vicarious participation in extreme sports beyond elite participants via platformed vehicles such as Instagram, replete with accounts depicting extreme sports from user perspectives. At the same time, 'adrenaline junkies' are understood to tap into the same brain-reward pathways emphasised in today's 'substance-related and addictive disorders' (American Psychiatric Association, 2013, pp. 543–665). Yet the expansive spillover of the conceptual framing of 'addiction'—currently defined as a 'substance use disorder' (SUD)—has been 'normalised' as a subject position in late modern society (Park, 2024). Interpreting extreme sports as fitting the addiction frame buys into the notion that experiences of extremity are used for their drug-like effects.

This chapter explores the various psychological, sociological, behavioural, and neuroscientific frames that assume that extreme sports are 'addictive'. We interviewed two social workers who specialise in couples counselling as a way to get at the therapeutic frames operating in this discursive arena. We analysed a dominant approach to behavioural addictions, based on addiction neuroscience, that spills out from the latest edition of the American Psychiatric Association's *Diagnostic and Statistical Manual of Mental Disorders* (DSM-5; American Psychiatric Association, 2013) into mass and social media and the scholarly literature on extreme sports (an umbrella term for a genre of diverse activities that demand participants engage with risk in unique, skill-based ways). Social scientists have sought to make sense of the drive to engage in 'stress-seeking' (Klausner, 1968), 'sensation-seeking' (Zuckerman, 1971, 1983a, 1983b, 1986, 1994, 2007), 'novelty-seeking' (Ebstein, 1997), 'risky' behaviour or 'edgework' (Lyng, 1990), and the demand for "intensified self-control" (Reith, 2019, p. 138). As we learned from the semi-structured interview we conducted with two couples counsellors—who had noticed an uptick in the extent to which extreme sports participation played a role in couples initiating therapy in a small northeastern US city—intensified self-control may be viewed as addictive behaviour in and of itself. They saw people 'using' sports to navigate their lives as drug users 'use' drugs to navigate theirs. This chapter explores the implications of incorporating an addictive behaviour framework for making legible the significance of extreme sports participation in everyday life within risk regulatory societies.

Aliveness and Control in Risk Regulatory Societies

Regulatory societies govern risk by promulgating consumer protection into social norms of seeking safety and avoiding risk. As symbolic and institutional weight has shifted towards safety, an ethos of deviance tinges appetites focused on risky activities. When patterns of use appear to escalate extremity—along the classic progression of getting 'hooked' on the 'rush' (getting 'high' as 'positive reinforcement'), becoming 'tolerant' (escalating use to gain similar effects), and 'hitting bottom' ('negative consequences' such as withdrawal or suicidality)—this vernacular repertoire draws on the conveniently available addiction frame. We explore what it means to suggest that people 'use' sports to navigate their lives, as drug users 'use' drugs to navigate theirs. 'Users' carry deviant and stigmatised meanings that are subsumed into "addiction … [defined as] a state marked by caring too much about the wrong things, and not enough about the right things" (Keane, 2002, p. 38). As Jaeyoon Park writes in *Addiction Becomes Normal: On the Late-Modern Subject* (2024, p. 125), addiction signifies a "complex state in which one's level of engagement is sustained at unusually high levels by an array of inner and outer forces that do not vitiate, but overpower, one's conscious wishes and intention." In risk regulatory societies, intense engagement is supposed to be channelled into socially sanctioned, productive activities such as work or stress-relieving recreation. When someone uses participation in extreme sports to the degree that risky activities interfere with activities and relationships of everyday life, they may be *made deviant*—called out for using sports as others use drugs, or identifying as such.

Although athletes' motivations, actions, and experiences for participating in extreme sports vary, many resort to the framing language of addiction to make their actions legible to non-participants: in mass and social media they use the discourse of getting 'high', mapping heightened or unnatural arousal onto such sports, or breaking the tedium of everyday life. But they do not typically exhibit the impaired control that resides at the core of definitions of SUD. Rather, the social contexts within which extreme sports participation take place "demand intensified self-control" (Reith, 2019, p. 138). Adventure and extreme activities also appear in wilderness or adventure therapy and in therapeutic community (TC) treatment programmes that incorporate elements that mimic the 'free-fall experience' of skydiving, which is said to resemble the 'rush' produced by heroin (Zuckerman, 1994, p. 252). Adventure sports programmes for therapeutic purposes substitute differing types of extremity as alternative reinforcers, are often aimed at youth, and have been shown to be "moderately effective in facilitating positive short-term change in psychological, behavioural, emotional, and interpersonal domains and that these changes appear to be maintained in the longer-term" (Bowen & Neill, 2013, p. 42). Such programmes, which show reduced depression and suicidality (Bowen et al., 2016), operate on the assumption that alternative reinforcers can stimulate subjective effects of comparable intensity to those of participants' 'drug of choice'.

Engaging in sports is naturalised as healthy until participation interferes with other aspects of life such as stable partnerships, family relations, or work-life balance. Concerns with 'addiction' arise when participants appear to be "out of control with being in control", as our interviewees put it. Control is central to definitions and diagnosis of the use disorders in risk regulatory societies, with 'impaired control' being linked to "gradual use-related damage to brain circuits controlling reward sensitivity, motivation, self-regulation, negative emotional states, and stress tolerance" (Koob et al., cited in McLellan et al., 2022, p. 749). But the intense mode of self-control required for skilful participation in extreme sports may detract from other aspects of an athlete's lifeworld, including intimate and parental relationships (Melody, 2003). If 'aliveness' is associated with extreme sensations or skilled activities, suggested one of our interviewees, this association may substitute for the intensity derived from "long term emotionally committed relationships where the emotional exchange is intense enough to satisfy the need to feel alive". The exquisite interaction between aliveness, intensity, and control must be maintained within normative bounds lest it slip into the category of "use-related damage" as defined by addiction neuroscientists Koob et al. (2015) and treatment researchers McLellan et al. (2022). Yet risk regulatory societies produce and promote extremity not solely as damage but as an attractive way to 'do' identity (Giddens, 1991)—one that has increasingly been made material by psychological science.

Breaking Boundaries: Addiction Spillover

When extreme sports are provisionally categorised as addictive disorders, they most resemble 'gambling disorder' (GD), the one non-substance-related behavioural disorder that appears in the DSM-5 (American Psychiatric Association, 2013). Gambling with their lives, extreme athletes conduct exemplary negotiations of risk and exquisite control—seeing themselves not as impaired or limited but as expansively competent. Whereas rational inhabitants of risk regulatory societies are supposed to seek risk reduction by acting within social constraints, those who deliberately seek out risky or extreme situations cut against the grain. There is perceived to be something pathologically enlarged, singular, unique, and even heroic about their moral character, social behaviour, or increasingly, their bodies or brains (Paruk et al., 2020). They are often tested, scanned, or studied to see what makes them tick by contrast to 'sedentary' or less accomplished controls (Showstark et al., 2022). Neuropsychologists studying elite athletes have sought to establish differences in brain structure and function, relying on studies showing differential responses to fear and brain region activation in similar areas to those studied by addiction neuroscientists.

Social science researchers, too, have sought to understand repeated engagement in risky activities in relation to the conceptual apparatus of 'addiction', documenting 'tolerance' to, or 'withdrawal' from, extreme sports (Franken et al., 2006), importing neuropharmacological terms like 'anhedonia', 'dysphoria', 'craving', 'hypophoria' and 'negative affect' to signal the presence of addiction. A key indicator for behavioural use disorders is whether withdrawal appears as a dose-related effect of abstinence. The accumulation of negative consequences said to accrue to individuals engaged in high-risk behaviour is cast as an "attract[ion to] embodied pleasures of such high intensity that they often have addictive consequences" (Lyng, 2005, p. 18).

Drawn from Hunter S. Thompson's experiential descriptions of drug use in *Fear and Loathing in Las Vegas* (1971) and his proto-ethnographic work in *Hell's Angels* (1967), 'edgework' has been used to describe expansive, experimental, 'anarchic' and extreme states of self. Voluntary risk-taking appeared to be "*necessary* for well-being" for some people, becoming crucial to the "socially constituted self in a historically specific social environment" (Lyng, 1990, pp. 852–853, emphasis in original). Many of Lyng's edgeworkers resorted to other high-risk lexicons in order to convey what they had experienced. No matter how they incurred risk—skydiving, scuba diving, downhill skiing, mountain climbing, race-car driving, wartime combat, or business entrepreneurship—Lyng's edgeworkers defined themselves as working on the boundary between "life versus death, consciousness versus unconsciousness, sanity versus insanity, an ordered sense of self and environment versus a disordered self and environment" (Lyng, 1990, p. 857). An elitist orientation towards skilled performance surfaced in edgeworkers' refusal to undertake risk reduction in aspects of their experience that remained under their control—Lyng (1990) did not find them gambling, going on amusement-park rides, or engaging in artificial risky activities because these shifted the locus of control to unknown variables rather than to their skills.

Drug users, too, negotiate modernity's twin imperatives to exercise self-control and to consume to excess (Reith, cited in Lyng, 2005, p. 228). Structural conditions have produced cultures of consumption that encourage participation in risky behaviours, but paradoxically emphasise control, safety, moderation, and harm reduction. There is abundant evidence in mass and social media and scholarly literature on the topic that individuals who cultivate capacity for edgework do not experience themselves as uncontrolled, chaotic, or 'impaired'. Rather the subjective experience is akin to Lyng's "instinctively acting entities, which leaves them with a purified and magnified sense of self" (1990, p. 860) that retains "cognitive control over the essential 'objects' in the environment or a feeling of identity with these objects" (Lyng, 1990, p. 861). One effect of doing things that you like a lot is the development of skill, expertise, 'flow', and tacit knowledge—all of which are affirmed and rewarded in other arenas of risk regulatory societies, yet are somehow withheld when activities become labelled 'unhealthy' and 'addictive'.

Gambling, Behavioural Addictions, and the Reworking of the Addiction Frame in the DSM-5

Conceptual framing and empirical study of 'addiction', 'impulse control disorders', or 'use disorders' has undergone many redefinitions. This section examines a brief history of their appearance in the DSM, and how that framing has shifted over time in response to the composition of the working groups convened to define diagnostic criteria for behavioural addictions (Petry, 2016). Gambling was initially classified as an impulse control disorder in the DSM-III (American Psychiatric Association, 1980). Gerda Reith astutely points to the 'capricious' language through which gambling entered the DSM, which shifted from "'compulsive' to 'pathological' to 'disordered' … as attention moved from the mind to the body of the afflicted individual and began to focus on its similarities with substance dependency and addiction" (2019, p. 135). As the only recognised non-substance addictive disorder (American Psychiatric Association, 2013, 2022), GD joins substance-related disorders in a taxonomy grouped around overlapping 'classes' of substances that have similar neural and subjective effects (American Psychiatric Association, 2013, p. 481). More recent iterations of the DSM, including the DSM-5-TR (American Psychiatric Association, 2022)—which did not fundamentally change the SUD entry—accord primacy to the activation of the brain reward system and its reinforcing effects, augmented by reinforcing memories, as the necessary condition to qualify for a use disorder diagnosis.

Conceptually, any substance or activity that activates the brain-reward system can become the basis for an addictive disorder, but according to the DSM-5 (American Psychiatric Association, 2013, p. 481) the activation must be "intense" or "direct" to count as "disordered". This discourse suggests that "adaptive" behaviours leading to pleasure in the pursuit of "normal activities" stimulate the brain-reward system "indirectly", and thus are not classified as "addictive" or a "disorder". "Intense" or "direct" activation of reward pathways leads problematically to "feelings of pleasure, often referred to as a 'high'", whereas "indirect" activation of the reward system produces non-problematic behaviour (American Psychiatric Association, 2013, p. 481). Normative judgments about proper and improper bodies, brains, substances, and behaviours are embedded in the DSM-5 paragraphs that we are analysing here. These are as much moral, social, and political as they are neurochemical or neurophysiological (Fraser et al., 2014; Keane, 2002; Valverde, 1998). Non-substance-related addictive disorders are continually defined as pathological in relation to their purportedly "direct" activation of brain-reward pathways in the kind of addiction neuroscience that has influenced the DSM-5 (American Psychiatric Association, 2013). While participants in an activity have no way to discern whether or not the activation of their brain-reward pathways is direct or indirect, neurotransmitters and metabolites may be extracted and assessed (for a summary of such studies, see Zuckerman, 1994) so that accurate determinations can be made. As a standard-setting diagnostic manual, the DSM-5 defines use disorders primarily on the basis of their direct or indirect action upon the neural pathways that comprise the brain-reward system, and secondarily on behavioural grounds, but does not acknowledge how the politics of neuroscientific and/or behavioural expertise are situated within the moral calculations and social norms that underlie addiction attributions in the social worlds of users.

Overall, definitions of addictive disorders smooth over several conceptual problems. One of these is that the intensity of emotional energy with which social activities are pursued may be enhanced or decreased by social organisation and ritual solidarity (Collins, 2004). Lack of attention to the design of social environments created to elicit and reinforce repetitive behaviours (for example, casinos, duty-free stores, and bars) pervades the scientific literature on sensation and thrill seeking—it is as if risky activities are occurring in a social vacuum. Yet GD is held to be the only behavioural addiction said to "reflect evidence that gambling behaviors activate reward systems similar to those activated by drugs of abuse and produce some behavioral symptoms that appear comparable to those produced by the substance use disorders" (American Psychiatric Association, 2013, p. 481). While leaving open the door to listing such syndromes in the future, the DSM-5 stated that non-substance-related behaviours other than gambling did not exhibit clear enough peer-reviewed evidence that other "excessive behavioral patterns, such as Internet gaming," sex addiction, exercise addiction, or shopping addiction qualified as mental disorders (American Psychiatric Association, 2013, p. 481; see also Petry, 2016).

Regular or even heavy participation in extreme sports does not currently count as an addictive disorder, much less a mental disorder—indeed, few peer-reviewed studies on the subject have been published in the specific literatures of behavioural pharmacology and addiction neuroscience (a rare exemption is offered by Meyer et al., 2015). Yet a wide range of people, including those with lived experience of extreme sports and the clinicians who treat them, philosophers of sport, and sports psychologists, respond to extreme sports participants as if they are 'addicted'. Severity of an addictive disorder is judged by how many symptoms are present and how often they appear in the dimensional diagnosis made available in the DSM-5, which resorts to the relative intensity of the activation of a brain-reward system—something that cannot be determined by anyone other than a behavioural neuroscientist—as the defining feature of addictive disorders. In summary, the DSM-5 defines disorder use as engaging in behaviours that directly and intensively activate the brain reward system in ways that reinforce persistent behaviours and produce memories that cause significant impairment or distress. This dominant definition has leaked into many social domains, including the approaches taken to study extreme sport 'users' in risk regulatory society. As this section has shown, this historically and culturally specific framing of behavioural 'addictions' emerged among a small group of behavioural scientists and neuroscientists who study addiction as an effect of intense activation of neural substrates that manifest in behaviours. This group sought evidence-based definitions for SUD and exercised definitional control over the DSM-5's Work Group on substance-related disorders. Despite the dominance of the DSM-5 for framing substance and non-substance-related use disorders, the next section explores other frames used to approach the social psychology of extreme athletes.

Multiple Pathways to Understanding the Social Life of 'Extreme Sports'

Stress, Sensation-Seeking, 'Rush' and Thrill

Among the earliest empirical explorations of individuals using extreme sports to cope with 'internal disequilibria' in stressful situations was ego psychologist Samuel Z. Klausner's pioneering studies of sports parachutists. Klausner noticed that some subjects repeatedly pursued intense arousal to such a degree that "stress-seeking [had] become an end in itself" (Klausner, 1968, p. 141). Far from reckless, Klausner's subjects returned "again and again to the stressful situation" (1968, p. 143). They were so concerned with safety procedures that Klausner considered them obsessive in their 'drive to repeat', a quality that enabled them to "jump from higher and higher altitudes, each time increasing free-fall time and attempting more complex maneuvers" (1968, p. 145). These 'stress-seekers' were bored on the ground; they exhibited a rhythmic 'arousal jag' that motivated the next jump. The move from 'stress-seeking' to 'sensation-seeking' was framed within the language of behavioural reinforcement.

Behavioural scientist Marvin Zuckerman developed the first 'sensation-seeking scale' in the 1960s, elaborating concepts such as 'thrill and adventure seeking' (TAS) and considering the idea that "optimal levels of stimulation and arousal" might vary between individuals in ways that could be correlated with biosocial behaviour, information processing, neurochemistry, and psychophysiology (1994, pp. 18–19). This work included genetic and behavioural studies of sensation- and novelty-seeking, underpinned by biochemical and neurochemical studies of noradrenergic and dopaminergic limbic systems. Sensation-seeking appeared to be a "trait defined by the *seeking* of varied, novel, complex, and *intense* sensations and experiences, and the willingness to take physical, social, *legal*, and *financial* risks for the sake of such experience" (Zuckerman, 1994, p. 27; emphasis original). Unsurprisingly, selective participation in high-risk sports was associated with high sensation-seeking in multiple studies.

Conflations of 'peak', thrill, and euphoria are subsumed into current drug use vernacular for the 'rush' experienced during initial, non-tolerant drug experiences. Desire for 'peak' experiences (Reith, 2019, p. 143) or time in the so-called 'zone', an "affective, trance-like condition in which gamblers' surroundings, the passage of time, the value of money, and even their sense of self are dissolved by the immersion in intensive play" (Reith, 2019, p. 130; see also Schüll, 2012) are commonly attributed to both drug and non-drug experiences. Experiential states of 'euphoria' or 'rush' have been explored in recent work on drugged pleasures (Dennis, 2017; Dennis & Farrugia, 2017; Duff, 2008; O'Malley & Valverde, 2004; Race, 2009; Treloar & Holt, 2008). Rush has been monetised as motivation for participating in skilled adventure tourism and formalised as a "combination of thrill and flow" experienced as the combined effects of skill, training, intensity, and a "hormonal component" (adrenaline) (Buckley, 2012). "From the participant perspective", observed Buckley (2012, p. 967),

> rush is a unified, intense and emotional psychological experience. According to the popular literature, rush is not a universal experience, but a rather rare one, available only to exponents who have invested time in acquiring particular skills. There is thus an element of elitism.

By this account, rush is a matter of expertise, of tacit knowledge, of know-how—a phenomenological experience available to elite participants rather than to amateurs.

Edgework

Edgework was remade as an academic concept by Lyng and Snow (1986; Lyng, 1990) to describe liminality in relation to lethality. As Buckley (2012, p. 964) explains it, "[t]he basic concept of edgework is that some people like to see how close they can get to death but still escape." In distancing rush from escape, edgework, or pleasure, Buckley frames it as an 'addiction' and invokes the concept of tolerance: "[I]f a person continues to repeat the same activity at the same level of skill and difficulty, rush may turn to boredom: as with most addictions, a person needs ever-increasing doses to maintain the same degree of response" (Buckley, 2012, p. 967). Increasing skill is translated via the vocabulary of addiction into a form of tolerance that must be broken through if a person is ever to attain the intensity of rush again. Shifting from thinking about lived experience of risk to the phenomenology of flow, Hardie-Bick and Bonner (2016, p. 373) recast edgework as "sensations gained from maintaining control over the seemingly uncontrollable" in the face of the threat of death or serious injury. The experience of emotional control in the face of transgressive experiences interests Hardie-Bick and Bonner (2016, p. 384), who found that,

> The majority of skydivers and climbers in our research projects did not deliberately set out to increase the risks by placing themselves in increasingly dangerous situations. Our research has emphasized how skydivers and climbers enjoy the challenge of managing rather than maximizing the risks associated with these pursuits.

Emphasis on risk management may also be seen as actions taken to minimise—rather than maximise—risk, stress, sensation, and thrill.

Rush was imported from drug user vernacular to explain motivations of extreme athletes. Creation of a 'rush experience scale' (Tez, 2023) allowed comparisons between peak experiences, with Tez (2023) finding that "[t]he phenomenologies of participation in extreme sports and substance abuse have some similarities, and parallels have been drawn between the personality traits of extreme sports participants and substance abusers", including high levels of impulsivity. "Furthermore", states Tez (2023), "extreme sports participants often describe their experiences as a 'rush' or 'peak', and these experiences are similar to those of drug users". Tez (2023) notes that the,

> addictive component of extreme sports could be the rush felt by participants, which can be either a combination of thrill and flow or a combination of skill and thrill. If this is the case, it could explain why high-thrill but low-skill activities such as bungee jumping or intense theme park rides do not create the same behavioural addictions as extreme sports.

There is something addictive about skill and something phenomenologically different about the peak experiences of experienced practitioners of extreme sports and those who are casual, inexperienced, low-skill consumers of them (Raggiotto, 2020).

Because positive effects attributed to intense experiences seem to wear off with familiarity and repetition via neuroadaptive processes akin to tolerance, rush cannot become routine. A more typically encountered key determinant of behavioural addictions are negative withdrawal states. To determine whether rock climbers felt withdrawal, Sripada (2021) purposely formulated plain-language questions and avoided 'withdrawal terminology' such as 'craving' or 'anhedonia'. But the withdrawal repertoire is widely available as a frame for making sense of feelings, affective states, and neurophysiological symptoms of displeasure. Sripada's subjects drew upon the lexicon of withdrawal, with high-ability rock climbers speaking of "more frequent and intense craving states and negative affect than average-ability climbers" (2021, p. 332). High-ability climbers appeared "to experience withdrawal symptoms when abstinent" from rock climbing similar to individuals with substance and behavioural addictions (Sripada, 2021, p. 332). Three key pieces of evidence led Sripada (2021, p. 338) to conclude that "addiction severity increases with exposure to the stimuli." These were: (1) anhedonia, characterised as a state in which "nothing compares" to climbing such that individuals were "desensitized" to all other activities; (2) "craving" or "effects of cue exposure" motivated individuals to structure their daily lives around "the stimulus" at the expense of all other activities; and (3) negative affect was more severely expressed as a stressor by the high-ability climbers (Sripada, 2021, pp. 336–337). Although this study took steps to avoid putting words in subjects' mouths, there was no recognition of the 'boundless' migration of the addiction frame and the consequent proliferation of its conceptual vocabulary.

Learning from Attending to Extreme Athletes' Experiences

Online accounts offered by extreme athletes, including Instagram accounts, documentaries, writing and YouTube videos posted by extreme athletes, yield plenty of anecdotal evidence that addiction and withdrawal frames are both widely used and contentious. Explorations of negative consequences were spoken of as "hitting rock bottom" in the vernacular of addiction treatment and recovery (Kirouac & Witkiewitz, 2017). These implicitly render extreme sports as addictive—being unable to stop a behaviour and persisting in the face of negative consequences is one of the criteria for SUD. For instance, professional BMX rider Dave Mirra was estimated to have "had at least 100 concussions" during his career (Higgins, 2022) and was one of the most decorated BMX stars in the history of the sport; retiring from BMX at the age of 35, his focus shifted to rally car racing, and triathlon and Iron Man training. Mirra's life revolved around his dedication to extremes, a commitment that could be considered a leading factor contributing to his unexpected suicide in 2016. Steph Davis, a well-known rock climber, wingsuiter, and BASE jumper, was one of the innovators of tandem BASE jumping. In *The American adrenaline narrative* (2020) by Kristin Jacobson, Davis explained how she "understood immediately how people dropped their lives into" skydiving and compared the rush to what she suspected heroin felt like (Jacobson, 2020, p. 176). Davis had lost both her career and her marriage prior to this interview. Jacobson described Davis' use of skydiving as a mechanism that "jolts her out of her funk" (2020, p. 176). Mirra and Davis had two different trajectories in their lives, highlighting unique aspects of the extreme athlete experience.

A postmortem study of Mirra's brain identified definitive evidence of chronic traumatic encephalopathy (CTE) and confirmed him as the "first action sports athlete with CTE" (Roenigk, 2020). CTE develops in the brains of individuals who have suffered from repeated concussions and sub-concussive contact to the head (VanItallie, 2019). Mirra pushed through persistent negative consequences; it is difficult to pinpoint whether it was the accolades, the 'rush', or financial pressure that kept him competing. Steph Davis was married to an expert BASE jumper, Mario Richard, who died in Italy in 2013 while BASE jumping with Davis (2015, p. 446). Prior to Richard's death, he and Davis ran a business offering the world's first tandem base-jumping experience (Davis, 2015, p. 438). Davis (2015, p. 438) shared a story of how a sexual assault victim wrote Richard a letter explaining how the experience made her feel strong and free "for the first time in her life." Richard himself described the experience of jumping as a temporary magical state that someone will go through great lengths to get back to (Davis, 2015, p. 459). These athletes' stories reflect how captivating and dangerous a life of extreme sports can be.

Athletes like Mirra, Davis, and Richard tend to 'stack' their lives with various extreme sports, as if starting with one sequentially invites another in turn as in the sequential stages hypothesised to lead to more extreme drug use (Kandel et al., 1992). 'Polydrug use' applies to individuals using multiple drugs to heighten positive effects. Extreme sports athletes employ similar patterns by being more open to engaging in other risky behaviours or combining different activities into one. Another idea from the world of substance use research is the belief that something is missing in the brains of extreme athletes, for which they are substituting or 'self-medicating'—a notion that shows up both in terms of mood disorders and cognitive deficits as vocabularies of motive for engaging in substance use. For example, an anonymous Instagram comment from an extreme athlete reflects on this deficit model: "[r]ecent studies show that we [in] the extreme crowd are weak before we even enter the sport. We go to adrenaline sports to compensate for the things our brains lack. In order to enjoy life we need the rush" (Dirty Habits, 2023).

The well-publicised struggles of extreme athletes to come up with ways to monetise continued involvement in extreme sports through sponsorships and social media patronage also illustrates persistence beyond negative consequences. Athletes often experience 'negative consequences'; while the tedium and stability of mainstream forms of work are displaced, relationships may be strained by irregular divisions of labour, variable commitments and perceptions, and constant reactivation of fear-based trauma for the partner. The behavioural concept of reinforcement as used in research on substance use is tightly linked to compulsive or repetitive activity and intermittent reward (Schüll, 2012). Extreme athletes embrace highly positive patterns of purposeful activity such as honing high-level skills, expertise, and capacity to endure sensations of intense absorption. Partners and family members, however, do not experience these intermittent rewards and may struggle to comprehend the cultivation of such risks within the parameters of normalcy. They may instead frame continued participation in risky activities and endurance sports as forms of compulsion, addiction, or 'impaired control'. Addiction attribution overrides the exquisite control exercised by extreme athletes, disregarding their unique role in contesting the over-regulation of risk implied by the over-emphasis on safety and compliance in risk regulatory societies.

Summary and Conclusion

Addiction attributions provide a familiar and convenient vocabulary of motive for understanding how some people build identities that cultivate risk despite living in risk-avoidant societies. This chapter has considered extreme athletes as embodying the notion of "cultivated risk" (Giddens, 1991, p. 133). For these individuals, self-identity is produced in activities that involve both danger and its resolution. The discussion focused on the question of whether this regular courting of risk may be seen accurately as a form of addictive consumption or addictive behaviour. In reviewing various approaches to risk, sensation-seeking, novelty-seeking, and edgework in the social psychological literature, this chapter has considered the limitations of transposing the addiction framework to make sense of conspicuous behaviours that appear to depart from dominant social norms. The spectacularised culture surrounding extreme sports, which is often viewed as 'reckless' and criticised for perpetuating unrealistic standards of athleticism, heroism, and bravery, leads to formal and informal labelling of extreme sport athletes as 'addicts', often explained through the diagnostic framework of SUD or as an endogenous version of 'addiction to adrenaline'.

Extreme sports athletes challenge the norms of a modern risk society by embracing risk rather than avoiding it. When jumping out of an airplane at 10,000 feet or traveling down a mountainside at 20 miles-per-hour on a bicycle, an athlete feels a heightened state of control over their physical well-being. Feeling as if they are granting themselves a sense of freedom and agency, they inhabit a world where individuals are increasingly bound by the societal constraints associated with risk aversion.

Holding individuals who are pushed to be self-expressive and personally autonomous to a set of risk regulatory standards gives rise to inherent contradictions and tensions. These contradictions may be the source of the societal need for the extreme sports community's unwanted pathologisation and even medicalisation. One might argue that in a society that is divided by race, wealth, and beliefs, extreme sports allow some edgeworkers to transcend these barriers by unifying strong bonds between people who share a passion for testing the limits of risk. Yet this form of solidarity also tests the boundlessness of 'addiction' as a social construct that is both meaningful and contested.

References

American Psychiatric Association. (1980). *Diagnostic and statistical manual of mental disorders* (3rd ed.). American Psychiatric Association.

American Psychiatric Association. (2013). *Diagnostic and statistical manual of mental disorders* (5th ed.) American Psychiatric Association.

American Psychiatric Association. (2022). *Diagnostic and statistical manual of mental disorders* (5th ed.) text rev. American Psychiatric Association.

Beck, U. (1992). *Risk society: Towards a new modernity*. Sage.

Bowen, D. J., & Neill, J. T. (2013). A meta-analysis of adventure therapy outcomes and moderators. *The Open Psychology Journal, 6*(1), 28–53. https://doi.org/10.2174/1874350120130802001

Bowen, D. J., Neill, J. T., & Crisp, S. J. R. (2016). Wilderness adventure therapy effects on the mental health of youth participants. *Evaluation and Program Planning, 58*, 49–59. https://doi.org/10.1016/j.evalprogplan.2016.05.005

Buckley, R. C. (2012). Rush as a key motivation in skilled adventure tourism: Resolving the risk recreation paradox. *Tourism Management, 33*(4), 961–970. https://doi.org/10.1016/j.tourman.2011.10.002

Collins, R. (2004). *Interaction ritual chains*. Princeton University Press.

Davis, S. (2015). *Learning to fly*. Simon and Schuster.

Dennis, F. (2017). Conceiving of addicted pleasures: A 'modern' paradox. *International Journal of Drug Policy, 49*, 150–159. https://doi.org/10.1016/j.drugpo.2017.07.007

Dennis, F., & Farrugia, A. (2017). Materialising drugged pleasures: Practice, politics, care. *International Journal of Drug Policy, 49*, 86–91.

Duff, C. (2008). The pleasure in context. *International Journal of Drug Policy, 19*(5), 384–392. https://doi.org/10.1016/j.drugpo.2007.07.003

Ebstein, R. P. (1997). Saga of an adventure gene: Novelty seeking, substance abuse and the dopamine D4 receptor exon III repeat polymorphism. *Molecular Psychiatry, 2*(5), 381–384. https://doi.org/10.1038/sj.mp.4000315

Franken, I. H., Zijlstra, C., & Muris, P. (2006). Are nonpharmacological induced rewards related to anhedonia? A study among skydivers. *Progress in Neuro-Psychopharmacology and Biological Psychiatry, 30*(2), 297–300. https://doi.org/10.1016/j.pnpbp.2005.10.011

Fraser, S., Moore, D., & Keane, H. (2014). *Habits: Remaking addiction*. Palgrave Macmillan.

Giddens, A. (1991). *Modernity and self-identity: Self and society in the late modern age*. Stanford University Press.

Dirty Habits. (2023). Mental health in extreme sports—We need to talk. [Video]. *YouTube*. https://www.youtube.com/watch?v=zBCxypVJIN8&t=925s

Hardie-Bick, J., & Bonner, P. (2016). Experiencing flow, enjoyment and risk in skydiving and climbing. *Ethnography, 17*(3), 369–387. https://doi.org/10.1177/1466138115609377

Higgins, M. (2022). The last days of Dave Mirra. *Outside Online*. https://www.outsideonline.com/outdoor-adventure/biking/last-days-dave-mirra/

Jacobson, K. J. (2020). *The American adrenaline narrative*. University of Georgia Press.

Kandel, D. B., Yamaguchi, K., & Chen, K. (1992). Stages of progression in drug involvement from adolescence to adulthood: Further evidence for the gateway theory. *Journal of Studies on Alcohol and Drugs, 53*(5), 447–457. https://doi.org/10.15288/jsa.1992.53.447

Keane, H. (2002). *What's wrong with addiction?* New York University Press.

Kirouac, M., & Witkiewitz, K. (2017). Identifying "hitting bottom" among individuals with alcohol problems: Development and evaluation of the noteworthy aspects of drinking important to recovery (NADIR). *Substance Use and Misuse, 52*(12), 1602–1615. https://doi.org/10.1080/10826084.2017.1293104

Klausner, S. Z. (1968). *Why man takes chances: Studies in stress-seeking*. Doubleday.

Koob, G. F., Kandel, D., Baler, R. D., & Volkow, N. D. (2015). Pathophysiology of addiction. In A. Tasman, J. Kay, J. A. Lieberman, M. B. First, & M. B. Riba (Eds.), *Psychiatry* (4th ed., pp. 359–381). Wiley. https://doi.org/10.1002/9781118753378.ch22

Lyng, S. H. (1990). Edgework: A social psychological analysis of voluntary risk taking. *American Journal of Sociology, 95*(4), 851–886.

Lyng, S. H. (2005). Edgework and the risk-taking experience. In S. H. Lyng (Ed.), *Edgework: The sociology of risk taking* (pp. 3–16). Routledge.

Lyng, S. H., & Snow, D. (1986). Vocabularies of motive and high-risk behaviour: The case of sky-diving. *Advances in Group Processes, 3*(157), 79.

McLellan, A. T., Koob, G. F., & Volkow, N. D. (2022). Preaddiction—A missing concept for treating substance use disorders. *JAMA Psychiatry, 79*(8), 749–751. https://doi.org/10.1001/jamapsychiatry.2022.1652

Melody, P. (2003). *Facing codependence: What it is, where it comes from, how it sabotages lives*. Harper and Row.

Meyer, V. J., Lee, Y., Böttger, C., Leonbacher, U., Allison, A. L., & Shirtcliff, E. A. (2015). Experience, cortisol reactivity, and the coordination of emotional responses to skydiving. *Frontiers in Human Neuroscience, 9*, 138. https://doi.org/10.3389/fnhum.2015.00138

O'Malley, P., & Valverde, M. (2004). Pleasure, freedom and drugs: The uses of 'pleasure' in liberal governance of drug and alcohol consumption. *Sociology, 38*(1), 25–42. https://doi.org/10.1177/0038038504039359

Park, J. (2024). *Addiction becomes normal: On the late-modern subject*. University of Chicago Press.

Paruk, T., Rauch, L., Jankiewicz, M., Van Breda, K., Stein, D. J., & King, M. (2020). Structural brain differences between ultra-endurance athletes and sedentary persons. *Sports Medicine and Health Science, 2*(2), 89–94. https://doi.org/10.1016/j.smhs.2020.05.004

Petry, N. M. (2016). Introduction to behavioral addictions. In N. M. Petry (Ed.), *Behavioral addictions: DSM-5® and beyond* (pp. 1–5). Oxford University Press.
Race, K. (2009). *Pleasure consuming medicine: The queer politics of drugs*. Duke University Press.
Raggiotto, F. (2020). *Consuming extreme sports*. Springer Link.
Raggiotto, F., Scarpi, D., & Mason, M. C. (2019). Faster! More! Better! Drivers of upgrading among participants in extreme sports events. *Journal of Business Research, 102*, 1–11. https://doi.org/10.1016/j.jbusres.2019.04.047
Reith, G. (2019). *Addictive consumption: Capitalism, modernity and excess*. Routledge.
Roenigk, A. (2020). Wife of Dave Mirra, first action sports athlete with CTE, discusses his last weeks and legacy. *ESPN*. https://www.espn.com/action/story/_/id/15613973/wife-dave-mirra-first-action-sports-athlete-cte-discusses-last-weeks-legacy
Schüll, N. D. (2012). *Addiction by design: Machine gambling in Las Vegas*. Princeton University Press.
Showstark, M., Bahadursingh, R., Zhang, S., Fry, A., Kozminski, B., Lundstam, P., & Putrino, D. (2022). Comparison of hemodynamic brain responses between big wave surfers and non-big wave surfers during affective image presentation. *Frontiers in Psychology, 13*, 800275. https://doi.org/10.3389/fpsyg.2022.800275
Sripada, C. (2021). Impaired control in addiction involves cognitive distortions and unreliable self-control, not compulsive desires and overwhelmed self-control. *Behavioural Brain Research, 418*, 113639. https://doi.org/10.1016/j.bbr.2021.113639
Tez, Ö. Y. (2023). Measuring the rush experiences: Development and validation of a short psychometric scale. *Journal of Outdoor Recreation and Tourism, 42*, 100590. https://doi.org/10.1016/j.jort.2022.100590
Thompson, H. S. (1967). *Hells angels*. Penguin Books.
Thompson, H. S. (1971). *Fear and loathing in Las Vegas: A savage journey to the heart of the American dream*. Random House.
Treloar, C., & Holt, M. (2008). Pleasure and drugs. *International Journal of Drug Policy, 5*(19), 349–352.
Valverde, M. (1998). *Diseases of the will: Alcohol and the dilemmas of freedom*. Cambridge University Press.
VanItallie, T. B. (2019). Traumatic brain injury (TBI) in collision sports: Possible mechanisms of transformation into chronic traumatic encephalopathy

(CTE). *Metabolism—Clinical and Experimental, 100*, 153943. https://doi.org/10.1016/j.metabol.2019.07.007

Zuckerman, M. (1971). Dimensions of sensation seeking. *Journal of Consulting and Clinical Psychology, 36*(1), 45–52. https://doi.org/10.1037/h0030478

Zuckerman, M. (1983a). Sensation seeking and sports. *Personality and Individual Differences, 4*(3), 285–292. https://doi.org/10.1016/0191-8869(83)90150-2

Zuckerman, M. (1983b). Sensation seeking: The initial motive for drug abuse. *Etiological Aspects of Alcohol and Drug Abuse*, 202–220.

Zuckerman, M. (1986). Sensation seeking and the endogenous deficit theory of drug abuse. *NIDA Research Monograph Series, 74*, 59–70.

Zuckerman, M. (1994). *Behavioral expressions and biosocial bases of sensation seeking*. Cambridge University Press.

Zuckerman, M. (2007). *Sensation seeking and risky behavior*. American Psychological Association.

11

From Medicalisation to Cultural Embrace: Drug Foundationalism Versus Techné in the Psychedelic Revival

Tehseen Noorani

The word 'psychedelic' was coined by Humphry Osmond in 1956 and is usually translated as 'mind-manifesting'. Naming sets in motion habits of thought and of association. The idea of mind-manifesting certainly takes us away from understanding these substances and experiences as mimicking psychosis, or 'psychotomimetic'—the older term that Osmond sought to supplant (Bisbee et al., 2018). However, mind-manifesting fails to speak to the ways psychedelic experiences exceed purely mental operations, taking us into the realms of lesser-known translations of *psyke*: the soul, the spirit, and the breath, let alone the bodily ecstasies through which psychedelic effects can manifest. Demarcating what counts as (a) psychedelic also remains contested, offering to bring into proximity varied substances and technologies, under particular conditions, and at specific doses or

T. Noorani (✉)
Waipapa Taumata Rau | University of Auckland, Auckland, New Zealand
e-mail: tehseen.noorani@auckland.ac.nz

B. M. Z. Cohen et al. (eds.), *Addiction and the Medicalisation of Conspicuous Behaviour*, The Politics of Mental Health and Illness,
https://doi.org/10.1007/978-3-032-06313-7_10

degrees (see for example, Tupper & Labate, 2014). Often the term refers to the most well-known tokens of a certain pharmacological class of hallucinogens that Western scientific practice has established to produce perceptual, affective, and cognitive alterations in conscious awareness through their effects upon the neurotransmitter serotonin's 2A receptor (for example, lysergic acid diethylamide (LSD), psilocybin, mescaline, and/or the plants and fungi that contain them, including magic mushrooms, peyote cacti, and so forth). For those of us more interested in psychedelics as historical and cultural phenomena, one way of categorising them are as substances and technologies that produce their profound alterations in conscious awareness in ways that are deeply sensitive to the context of their use—what in psychedelia's own history is dubbed the '[mind]set and setting' of their use (Hartogsohn, 2020). On this rendering we might consider the stimulant 3,4-Methyl enedioxymethamphetamine (MDMA) and the dissociative anaesthetic ketamine (at least, in high enough doses) as psychedelics, alongside the aforementioned serotonergic hallucinogens.

Having been near blanket-prohibited (even for research purposes) at the beginning of the 1970s, today psychedelic substances are on the verge of joining the arsenal of psychiatric medications in the Global North (see for example, Lykos Therapeutics, 2024). The past decade has witnessed the rise of a transnational, corporatised psychedelics industry, made up of psychedelic drug development companies, contract research organisations, venture capital-funded research trials, trade associations, philanthropic organisations, psychedelic therapy training organisations, large international conferences, and university-based research centres. The two primary research chemicals being medicalised are psilocybin—including in the treatment of depression, anxiety, obsessive-compulsive disorder (OCD), addictions, and anorexia nervosa—and MDMA, including in the treatment of post-traumatic stress disorder (PTSD) and social anxiety. The complex manoeuvring of actors in the psychedelic medicalisation space attests to the layers of stakes involved, including: tackling the growing global mental health burden; redeeming (the denigrated reputation of) these powerful, strange and/or sacred substances; reparations and reconciliation for Indigenous communities whose use of these substances has grounded and/or inspired how they have come to be used in Western scientific research and therapy; the 'thin end of the wedge' for broader access to psychedelics and thus community-based healing and 'cognitive liberty'; and the end of the racist and classist 'war on drugs'. In short, in the relatively brief period of the medicalisation of psychedelics, they have already promised a lot.

What follows is a contribution to existing debates in the sociology of addiction. As a whole new class of psychoactive substances being brought to the brink of medical availability, the addictiveness of psychedelics has become a pressing concern within medicine and public health. At the same time new identities of psychedelic user are coming into view, identities that have the potential to reconstellate understandings of the habitual use of psychedelics. Rather than adjudicate over claims about whether psychedelics are or are not addictive, this chapter considers how the social relations and knowledge claims making up psychedelic medicalisation speak back to drug addiction discourses, offering up new questions and provocations around addiction's more perennial themes of freedom, compulsion, and control (Reith, 2004; Rose, 1999; Valverde, 1998). My hope is to contribute to debates about the nature of addiction, supporting the framing of addiction as a kind of intimacy with—and through—pharmaceutical substances (Goodfellow, 2008; Keane, 2002).

Psychedelic medicalisation has in many ways thrown up challenges that are surplus to requirement in the medicalisation of new drugs. For instance, it has posed problems for research trial designs that 'control for' (often a codeword for 'minimise') all non-drug variables, such as the provision of a supportive container for the drug experience and the deployment of therapy alongside the drug. It has also inspired the latest round of discourse on 'cures' for mental illnesses, as well as the potential for optimisation, enhanced well-being, and self-actualisation—a continuation of psychedelics' role in biopolitical projects threaded through 1970s transpersonal and new age psychologies. The curative promise of psychedelics is reflected in recent cost-benefit and cost-effectiveness modelling (see for example, Marseille et al., 2020, 2022), extending the findings of clinical trials to demonstrate to healthcare payers that psychedelic therapy will be a worthwhile investment.

The claims around the effectiveness of psychedelics as mental health treatments have also been taken up by movements to decriminalise psychedelics and other psychoactive substances. In the United States, evidence from the early stage clinical trials that are paving the way for the medicalisation of psychedelics featured prominently in the campaigns of Decriminalize Nature, a community-based movement beginning in Oakland, California, in 2019 and spreading across US states since, which seeks to expand "access to entheogenic plants and fungi through political and community organizing, education and advocacy" (see https://www.decriminalizenature.org/about). Meanwhile, following the passing of a ballot initiative in November 2020, Oregon was the first US state to legalise the provision of what it called professional 'psilocybin services'. The corresponding statute needed to be careful not to frame these 'services' as mental health treatments, as psilocybin was not approved by the US Food and Drug Administration as a medication. The statute nevertheless justified the need for its psilocybin services by drawing on early stage clinical trial evidence, alongside calling attention to the high prevalence of 'mental illness' and the fact that "the Governor [of Oregon] has declared addiction as a public health crisis in this state" (see https://www.oregonlegislature.gov/bills_laws/ors/ors475A.html). Arguably the potency of medical authority, despite being based on a limited number of trials with mostly-small sample sizes, was working its own magic.

Throughout the current revival of scientific research, ascertaining that psychedelics are not addictive is important for their medicalisation. Psychedelics are not only regularly touted as non-addictive, but the contemporary clinical literature has elaborated through clinical trials and related research claims that psychedelics can treat drug addiction (dos Santos et al., 2016; Bogenschutz & Johnson, 2016). This has provided a rich arena to explore the social phenomenology of psychedelic-assisted addiction cessation. Mechanisms include increased neuroplasticity (Calder & Hasler, 2023) and psychological flexibility (Watts & Luoma, 2020), the loosening of prior expectations (Carhart-Harris & Friston,

2019), insights into oneself (Noorani et al., 2018), and even the kinds of collective effervescence being catalysed through their use in both naturalistic settings and clinical trials (Kettner et al., 2021; Noorani et al., 2023).

At the same time, the hype surrounding psychedelic therapy trial results is being increasingly contested and complicated. In the clinical trials research, there are growing signs of underreporting of adverse experiences (Breeksema et al., 2022; de Laportalière et al., 2023; Mustafa et al., 2024), criticisms of the incomplete descriptions of the psychological therapy or support that is being offered alongside the drug administration (Brennan et al., 2023), and concerns about relational harms that are made more likely by the suggestibility-enhancing nature of psychedelics (Carhart-Harris et al., 2015; Meikle et al., 2024). Taking a cue from the sociological subfield of agnotology, it might be helpful to distinguish between three kinds of ignorance that are in play as psychedelic research both drives, and is in turn resourced through, the medicalisation of psychedelic therapy, namely: ignorance as the sum of as-yet-unanswered questions about psychedelics and psychedelic therapy, an accompanying shadow that motivates yet further research; ignorance as the "lost realm" of counterfactual knowledge that would have been known had psychedelic researchers decided to research it; and ignorance as the product of a "deliberately engineered and *strategic ploy*"—clear manifestations of the incentive structures of corporatisation (Proctor, 2008, p. 3, emphasis original).

With knowledge (and ignorance!) production in full swing in today's psychedelic medicalisation, the transformation of psychedelic use from illicit activity into mental health intervention highlights many of the contingencies that enable and constrain what counts as 'drug' and what as 'medicine', how, when, and for whom. There are opportunities here for revisiting the question of the 'addictiveness' of psychedelics anew. In what follows, I will use the case study of the complex dynamics of psychedelic medicalisation to attend to assumptions behind how we think about addiction and the related concept of dependency, and explore the possibilities of (and difficulties in) articulating a non-moralising and anti-foundationalist approach to habitual drug use.

The Space Between Addiction and Dependence

As the psychedelic industry begins to take shape, questions over their addictive properties are returning. This is particularly so in the case of ketamine-assisted therapy, where the physiological grounds for such a claim are clearer (see Carroll et al., 2024), and there is concern that the medicalisation of ketamine for use in cases of depression and anxiety will herald a new wave of ketamine dependency (with iconic television show *Friends*' star Matthew Perry's death being a recent high-profile example, see Evans, 2023). Moreover, given the degree to which the boon of interest in psychedelics has stimulated research into related chemical structures, it is reasonable to expect that there will likely be a spate of novel, physically-addictive, psychedelic analogue molecules in the coming years.

With the classic hallucinogens, the question of addictiveness in a post-approval context is more curious. By and large, the epidemiological and pharmacological literatures buttressing the processes of psychedelic medicalisation emphasise the non-addictiveness of psychedelics (see for example, Perkins et al., 2021; Shalit et al., 2019). Nevertheless, the nature of psychedelic experiences invites consideration of the loci of activity of addiction that goes beyond the physical and even many measures of the behavioural. Speaking through a psychological register, is it possible to grow dependent upon the powerful and affectively-charged experiences psychedelics produce? Socially-speaking, may we come to rely upon the modes of communing psychedelics augment, from rave gatherings to deeply immersive forest walks? In a spiritual register, might we ache to return to states of interconnectedness and bliss? If addiction is defined as a narrowing of behaviour around psychedelic use to the detriment of the rest of one's life, each of these registers opens up narrative possibilities for how this could occur. Moreover, evidence drawn from self-selecting underground users, the rarefied participants of clinical trials, and forms of collective use that are strongly shaped by extended traditions of use, may not be applicable to the post-approval context of a sudden widespread availability of psychedelics as part of globalised cultures of health-improvement, meaning-seeking, and wellness-optimisation.

Some pro-medicalisation psychedelic advocates point to the extant distinction between 'addiction' and 'dependency' to argue that one can be dependent upon, but not addicted to, psychedelics. This distinction has its own history (see Müller, this volume) and has been the subject of debate in addiction science, where addiction has become construed as a mental disposition, while dependence a bodily disposition. For example, according to Szalavitz et al. (2021, p. 1990), "physical dependence is an ordinary biological consequence of taking certain medications for weeks or years—while addiction is continued drug use that persists in the face of negative experience" (see also West et al., 2024). I first heard this distinction articulated in the cultural politics of psychedelic medicalisation by Raquel Bennett, a respected US thought-leader in the ketamine-assisted therapy space. As profiled in a 2019 magazine article,

> [Bennett] doesn't consider herself addicted to ketamine because she feels no desire to take it between scheduled appointments. But she does feel dependent on the drug, in the same way that a person with high blood pressure takes medication for hypertension, [Bennett] says. (Underwood, 2019)

This reframes ketamine-assisted therapy—and any psychedelic therapy to which the same logical move is applied—as forms of maintenance therapy keeping clinical symptoms (in Bennett's case, her debilitating depression) at bay, rather than magic bullets that cure mental illness in a one-off manner.

Meanwhile, in my own ethnographic fieldwork on the rise of hype in psychedelic science and research communities during the period 2014–2022, I have witnessed a gradual movement—particularly since the heyday of psychedelic medicalisation hype, catalysed by academic journalist Michael Pollan's, 2018 bestselling book on psychedelic science and therapy, *How to change your mind: What the new science of psychedelics teaches us about consciousness, dying, addiction, depression, and transcendence*—away from the more extreme, 'one-and-done' claims that psychedelics will cure one's depression, OCD, PTSD and so on (see for example, Benson, 2022; Goldsmith, 2010). Instead, today one finds more measured suggestions around the embrace of the periodic use of psychedelics in the treatment of mental health conditions—that one may only need to 'trip' once a year, every three months, or perhaps once a month, to keep symptoms at bay. In turn, this has required shifts in the discursive framing of what psychedelics are doing, away from 'curing' and towards 'maintaining the neuroplasticity', the need for breaks 'from the daily grind', and/or much-welcomed reminders of certain timeless and infinite truths. Ethicists working in the psychedelic space have called for the continued provision of psychedelic therapy for people after their involvement in psychedelic clinical research trials end, pointing out that,

> it is not simply that the participants did not achieve the optimum possible benefit at the trial end date, but that the trial initiated but did not complete a process of psychological work—sometimes referred to as the *unfolding process*—that participants could not opt out of, but had to find external help in concluding. (Jacobs et al., 2024, p. 8, emphasis original)

The phenomenon of psychedelic therapy opening up "a process of psychological work" threatens to impact cost-effectiveness calculations, raising significant concerns for healthcare payers. At the time of writing, it was recently listed as a factor in the US Institute for Clinical and Economic Review's (ICER) interim report for healthcare payers, when discussing the corporation Lykos Therapeutics' (2024) clinical trial evidence for pairing MDMA with bespoke psychotherapy in the treatment of PTSD (Mustafa et al., 2024). Just months before Lykos' submission for MDMA-assisted psychotherapy as a new drug application is expected to receive its decision (in August 2024) from the US Food and Drug Administration, ICER's report concluded that the compiled clinical evidence was of "insufficient" quality, due to reasons including that the MDMA therapy was clearly creating new challenges for participants and, additionally, that these were suspected of being underreported.

Opening up the space between 'addiction' and 'dependency' can be useful as a pressure-release when psychedelic substances are being medicalised and there are doubts about psychedelic therapy's long-term efficacy, or ongoing questions about the addictive potential of the substances themselves—particularly apposite in the case of substances that have given rise to considerations of the centrality of 'set and setting' in determining drug effects. Claims of dependency might then be viewed along epistemic-economic axes as a bulwark against accusations of addiction, by functioning to smoothen and repair the processes of medicalising potentially-ineffective and/or addictive substances. Discursive shifts outwards from the narrow question of psychedelic addictiveness to enfold also possibilities of psychedelic dependency have agnotogenetic effects, raising more questions. When should someone be considered dependent on psychedelic substances or experiences? When should they be considered addicted? And does this depend on one's ability to afford professional psychedelic therapy, or otherwise curate the set and setting of their psychedelic use?

Moving Beyond Drug Foundationalism

I suggest psychedelic therapy makes a deeper, post-critical gesture, revealing and challenging a common assumption about the good life vis-à-vis drug use that is common to both addiction and dependency discourses. We could call this assumption 'drug foundationalism': that getting one's relationship to drugs right is fundamental in order to live well. The drug foundationalism of addiction is that drug abuse is considered the person's basic or 'ground' problem in need of solving. The drug foundationalism of dependency is that drug use is considered the body's basic regimen required in order for the individual to live well. Psychedelics reveal their trickster quality by troubling the very assumption undergirding both addiction and dependency—just as the trickster is the figure of the hinge, psychedelics enable another articulation, beyond either intervening through psychedelic medication use or intervening upon psychedelic drug abuse.

Unlike thinking about drug use as primary or foundational—whether in terms of 'presenting problems' or in terms of therapeutic interventions—the psychedelic revival's emphasis on enabling the "betterment of well people"—to quote Bob Jesse, a key behind-the-scenes player in the revival of psychedelic science in the US (Pollan, 2018, p. 45)—and the pursuit of wellness, curiosity and joy beyond 'curing illnesses' or 'healing suffering', suggests their use in a much less-foundationalist manner. Here we might ask, echoing anthropologist Aaron Goodfellow's (2008) interest in the relationship between humans and drugs, what new agencies and projects are made possible by the growing use of psychedelics as they forge new intimacies with those who take them, and thereby open up new pathways, labyrinths, and metaphorics (see Gearin, 2023) for exploration? This framing is not compatible with an articulation of the 'cure' of psychedelic therapies in terms of gaining what had been lacking. It fits better what anthropologist Patricia Kubala (2023, p. 482) describes—in terms of the language of Deleuze and Guattari's schizoanalysis—in relation to psychedelic therapies as "a completion of the process of desiring-production that is not arrested and reduced to pre-assigned ends." If psychedelic therapies are best understood as embracing unpredictable outcomes, perhaps via experiences both persuasive and weird (Davis, 2019), they become diametrically opposed to addiction recovery's normalising discourses.

More broadly, I suggest the revival of psychedelic therapies is forcing recognition that we both build our everyday practices of living and loving on drug regimens, *and* build drug regimens on top of our everyday practices of living and loving (see also Keane, 2002). This has been difficult to articulate in relation to other illicit drugs, but for various reasons—such as the privileged demographics of psychedelic and related drug-using communities advocating for psychedelic medicalisation today, the calling of attention to long-standing Indigenous and traditional use, the scientific evidence pointing at the non-addictive nature of psychedelics, and recent campaigns to normalise cannabis use—it is an increasingly vocal point within psychedelic-using communities in the Global North. Psychedelics—and drugs in general—might therefore be understood as components of wider technical operations, where there appears to be no necessary order in which drug versus non-drug interventions are to be deployed in the pursuit of healthy and flourishing lives.

The relevance of mental healthcare, and psychiatry in particular, may continue to wane unless it can engage at this level of creative technicity. As psychiatrist Kenneth Kendler (2012, p. 384) puts it in relation to his own discipline, "while you can worry about your theoretical reductions, where the world gives us causal traction is critical." Indeed, psychedelic therapies point to modes of care that evoke social psychiatry at its best:

collaborative, pragmatic, eclectic. Moreover, given their attentiveness to the set and setting of drug use, and their multiple putative mechanisms of action, psychedelic therapy may help to revivify social psychiatry at a time when there is a much deeper appreciation of the interacting effects of brain and experience upon one another, and multiple-vulnerability models suggest many inroads for therapeutic intervention (Aftab & Stein, 2022). Far from re-inspiring the "cult of immediacy" that historian Peter Sedgwick (1982, p. 124) argued resulted from the Laingian anti-psychiatry of the 1960s, today's rise of psychedelics as medical interventions may be pointing to the integration of psychedelics into a range of mental health care pathways.

Psychedelic Techné

Beyond mental health services *per se*, the explosion of the use of psychedelics both within and adjacent to therapy in the Global North partly flowing from the research hype, is flavouring wider cultural healing practices, creating what psychedelic anthropologists Nicolas Langlitz and Alex Gearin (2024) consider as new "forms of life". Coming straight from psychedelic therapy's toolbox, encouragements to 'trust, be open and let go' in the face of new experiences, or to submit to one's 'inner healing intelligence' as manifested through psychedelic consciousness, bring their own ethical imperatives and commitments. Moreover—and as distinct from being 'addicted to' psychedelics or even 'dependent upon' them—psychedelic users also describe coming to 'have a relationship with' the spirits and/or teachers that psychedelics embody and/or give reliable access to, suggestive of the widening appeal of complex neo-animist frameworks (Steinhardt, 2020). Such spirits and entities add to the psyche's ecological richness, as another 'part' or persona to fold into one's ecology of technical practices—to engage, dialogue, affect and be affected by. This speaks to enrichment, as opposed to the usual impoverishment associated with addiction—even if it can become burdensome or in turn lead to a thinning of relations if this relation (or these relations) become dominant.

In more formal terms, a psychedelic experience as delivered through psychedelic therapy might also be considered as something that can interrupt life, in providing life's punctuation—succeeding, preceding, and interceding upon one's life. Its own duration can be indexed both internally, insofar as the experience can feel eternal (or perhaps better stated, as if one is entering *into* eternity), and also in terms of the 'afterglow'—considered as an experienced mood elevation or high that appears to be correlated with markers of neuroplasticity in the emerging neuroscience (see Nardou et al., 2023)—for days or weeks post-use. And in cases where one is part of a tradition of psychedelic use, such as part of a(n intergenerational) community of practice, we might invert figure and ground, and frame the psychedelic experience as housing non-psychedelic life. Seen in these ways, the techné of psychedelic therapy does not just promise a discrete drug intervention that improves the quality of one's life, but rather so many ways of adding to, transforming, and multiplying it.

A non-foundationalist approach to psychedelics suggests framing them—and therein drugs in general—as techné, as overlapping and nested building blocks in the construction of flourishing. This offers a pastiche approach to healing, a 'whatever works' pragmatism. We might add psychedelics to the list provided by Leah Lakshmi Piepzna-Samarasinha (2018), a leading voice in the rise of the healing justice movement:

> When we asked folks what they did to stay alive. The answers were a rainbow femme quilt of femme emotional intelligence. Meds Netflix therapy prayer herbs change breakups fresh nails praying to the ancestors breaking bottles finding a friend you can be crazy with shutting down social media reaching out on social media groups that felt safe crying baths all the crystals shit talk. All little things that weren't so little.

A non-foundational approach also fits well with the idea that we are always-already-psychoactive, whether using drugs while on drugs, exercising on drugs, writing after drugs, dancing on, before, and after drugs, and so on. Such multiply-overlaid technical operations ironically trouble the very reductionist epistemologies of clinical trial methodologies that many claim are providing the justification for the wider 'psychedelicisation' of culture in the first place.

We need to keep open the question of how psychedelics heal. Consider the criticism levelled at psychedelic therapy research from within the broad 'critical psychiatry' camp, that it may only be working by getting people 'high' (Moncrieff, 2021), evocative of the drug soma in one of contemporary Anglophone psychedelia's seminal dystopian novels, *Brave new world* (Huxley, 2022, originally published in 1932). This fits with critical psychiatrist Joanna Moncrieff's (2008) preferred 'drug-centered model' of explanation, and may be tested by scientists currently working to trial non-psychoactive chemical analogues of psychedelics to assess the biomedically-oriented hypothesis that the subjective effects of psychedelics are incidental to their clinical efficacy (Olson, 2020). What risks being missed here is the extent to which the benefits of 'getting high' are medical or health effects, if they also, for instance, momentarily pull one out of rumination, obsessions and/or suicidal ideation, and/or show that such an experience (or the absence of experience-as-usual) is possible. Psychedelic therapy may instead pave the way to a broader cultural enjoyment of the reprieve of getting high, and combining that with other activities, times, places, people, and reminders that such states of mind can and do exist. It also reminds us that it is a question, if not a mystery, as to how one might cultivate such states by non-psychedelic means—or even again through the same means (as psychedelic experiences are far from predictable)—and of providing an experiential grounds for sharing and learning from and with others who also do so.

Indeed, this highlights how all techné is psychoactive, with the implication not of *equivalence* but of *specificity*. It offers a certain vision of personalised medicine, one which accords with the call for a "staunchly non-moralising attitude" towards psychedelics, bringing them into the realm of what Awais Aftab calls a "liberatory pharmacology" (Aftab, 2023). But does this depiction of the future of psychedelic use, as integrated into healing and the betterment of individuals' lives, really sidestep the dangers articulated in discourses of addiction? I suspect not. On the contrary, the rapid growth in psychedelic use may speak less to our addiction to specific acts or substances, and more to contemporary technology's capacity to 'addict' us to lifestyle identities themselves. The question of whether psychedelic use indexes new forms of addiction might then be reposed alongside analyses of today's technological capitalism, in which consumption practices are curated by algorithms that cater for 'what we are like' through analyses of 'what we like' (Lury & Day, 2019; see also Lacey et al., this volume). With attention itself serviced algorithmically and the production of knowledge (and ignorance) geared towards the success of emerging psychedelic commodity forms, we see the cultivation of new cultural archetypes: the entrepreneur microdosing for creativity who is also open to nootropics and cognitive enhancement apps; the healer on the unending journey to heal themselves who is also hungry to learn eclectic therapeutic and encounter group modalities; the seeker curious to plumb the depths of consciousness who is also into technologies and techniques for magnifying and extending their trips. Such psychedelic lifestyles can end up interfacing seamlessly with addiction recovery conceived as an unending journey, for instance in terms of limitless "shadow work" or as practices of vigilance demanded by the goal of abstinence (see for example, Cotogni & Cotogni, 2022; White, 2007).

Conclusion

The medicalisation of psychedelics may still collapse under its own weight—whether through sustained evidential scrutiny, the inability of psychedelic medicalisation entrepreneurs to find a way to turn a profit, or a widespread perception of medicalisation accelerating wider, illicit, psychedelic use, in turn generating a backlash. Even if so, the kinds of wider cultural reconfigurations that are weaving psychedelics as tools and teachers into complex webs of health, wellness, and meaning may well persist. Meanwhile, psychedelic normalisation builds on the call to justify and even celebrate psychedelic substance dependence as harmless, so long as the substances enable functioning or, even more, contribute to existing and new modes of flourishing (Hart, 2022).

Alongside ongoing scientific research programmes to determine whether psychedelics are addictive or can produce dependence, the substances are proving to be a useful case study for injecting some uncertainty into the very assumptions underlying these debates, pointing to ways of thinking about complex dependence, relationality and intimacy beyond the moralising strictures of drug foundationalism. On the one hand, perhaps the burgeoning of interest in psychedelic therapy might best be understood as fertile ground for algorithmic addiction, a new horizon for research into boundless addictions Yet on the other hand, perhaps it no longer makes sense to speak of addiction in relation to lives augmented by, and through, new habits of psychedelic use. It may be that the case study of psychedelic drugs, considered dangerous substances in need of prohibition half a century ago, today show us the myriad ways biomedical frameworks of addiction fail to capture the lived experiences of those enrolling psychedelics into projects aimed at meaning, connection, and transcendence.

References

Aftab, A. (2023). A psychopharmacology fit for mad liberation? *Asylum Magazine, 30*(1) https://asylummagazine.org/2023/03/a-psychopharmacology-fit-for-mad-liberation-by-awais-aftab/

Aftab, A., & Stein, D. J. (2022). Psychopharmacology and explanatory pluralism. *JAMAP sychiatry, 79*(6), 522–523. https://doi.org/10.1001/jamapsychiatry.2022.0470

Benson, D. (2022). Scott Shannon, MD—Psychedelics treating root causes. *Integrative Medicine: A Clinician's Journal, 21*(4), 22–25.

Bisbee, C. C., Bisbee, P., Dyck, E., Farrell, P., Sexton, J., & Spisak, J. W. (Eds.). (2018). *Psychedelic prophets: The letters of Aldous Huxley and Humphry Osmond*. McGill-Queen's University Press.

Bogenschutz, M. P., & Johnson, M. W. (2016). Classic hallucinogens in the treatment of addictions. *Progress in Neuro-Psychopharmacology and Biological Psychiatry, 64*, 250–258. https://doi.org/10.1016/j.pnpbp.2015.03.002

Breeksema, J. J., Kuin, B. W., Kamphuis, J., van den Brink, W., Vermetten, E., & Schoevers, R. A. (2022). Adverse events in clinical treatments with serotonergic psychedelics and MDMA: A mixed-methods systematic review. *Journal of Psychopharmacology, 36*(10), 1100–1117. https://doi.org/10.1177/02698811221116926

Brennan, W., Kelman, A. R., & Belser, A. B. (2023). A systematic review of reporting practices in psychedelic clinical trials: Psychological support, therapy, and psychosocial interventions. *Psychedelic Medicine, 1*(4), 218–229. https://doi.org/10.1089/psymed.2023.0007

Calder, A. E., & Hasler, G. (2023). Towards an understanding of psychedelic-induced neuroplasticity. *Neuropsychopharmacology, 48*(1), 104–112. https://doi.org/10.1038/s41386-022-01389-z

Carhart-Harris, R. L., & Friston, K. J. (2019). REBUS and the anarchic brain: Toward a unified model of the brain action of psychedelics. *Pharmacological reviews, 71*(3), 316–344. https://doi.org/10.1124/pr.118.017160

Carhart-Harris, R. L., Kaelen, M., Whalley, M. G., Bolstridge, M., Feilding, A., & Nutt, D. J. (2015). LSD enhances suggestibility in healthy volunteers. *Psychopharmacology, 232*(4), 785–794. https://doi.org/10.1007/s00213-014-3714-z

Carroll, A., Bayes, A., Montebello, M., Brett, J., Arunogiri, S., Saunders, J. B., & Loo, C. K. (2024). Drug dependence and prescribing ketamine for treatment-resistant depression in Australia and New Zealand. *Australian & New Zealand Journal of Psychiatry, 58*(10), 831–838. https://doi.org/10.1177/000486742412423

Cotogni, Z., & Cotogni, M. (2022). *Blue honey: Personal experiences using psilocybin for mental health in Aotearoa*. The National Library of New Zealand.

Davis, E. (2019). *High weirdness: Drugs, esoterica, and visionary experience in the seventies*. MIT Press.

de Laportalière, T. T., Jullien, A., Yrondi, A., Cestac, P., & Montastruc, F. (2023). Reporting of harms in clinical trials of esketamine in depression: A systematic review. *Psychological medicine, 53*(10), 4305–4315. https://doi.org/10.1017/S0033291723001058

dos Santos, R. G., Osório, F. L., Crippa, J. A., Riba, J., Zuardi, A. W., & Hallak, J. E. (2016). Antidepressive, anxiolytic, and antiaddictive effects of ayahuasca, psilocybin and lysergic acid diethylamide (LSD): A systematic review of clinical trials published in the last 25 years. *Therapeutic Advances in Psychopharmacology, 6*(3), 193–213. https://doi.org/10.1177/2045125316638008

Evans, J. (2023). Don't mention ketamine's addictiveness. *Ecstatic Integration*. https://www.ecstaticintegration.org/p/dont-mention-ketamines-addictiveness

Gearin, A. K. (2023). Moving beyond a figurative psychedelic literacy: Metaphors of psychiatric symptoms in ayahuasca narratives. *Social Science & Medicine, 334*, 116171. https://doi.org/10.1016/j.socscimed.2023.116171

Goldsmith, N. M. (2010). *Psychedelic healing: The promise of entheogens for psychotherapy and spiritual development*. Simon and Schuster.

Goodfellow, A. (2008). Pharmaceutical intimacy: Sex, death, and methamphetamine. *Home Cultures, 5*(3), 271–300. https://doi.org/10.2752/174063108X368328

Hart, C. L. (2022). *Drug use for grown-ups: Chasing liberty in the land of fear*. Penguin.

Hartogsohn, I. (2020). *American trip: Set, setting, and the psychedelic experience in the twentieth century*. MIT Press.

Huxley, A. (2022). *Brave new world*. DigiCat.

Jacobs, E., Murphy-Beiner, A., Rouiller, I., Nutt, D., & Spriggs, M. J. (2024). When the trial ends: The case for post-trial provisions in clinical psychedelic research. *Neuroethics, 17*(1), 3. https://doi.org/10.1007/s12152-023-09536-z

Keane, H. (2002). *What's wrong with addiction?* New York University Press.

Kendler, K. S. (2012). The dappled nature of causes of psychiatric illness: Replacing the organic–functional/hardware–software dichotomy with empirically based pluralism. *Molecular Psychiatry, 17*(4), 377–388. https://doi.org/10.1038/mp.2011.182

Kettner, H., Rosas, F. E., Timmermann, C., Kärtner, L., Carhart-Harris, R. L., & Roseman, L. (2021). Psychedelic communitas: intersubjective experience during psychedelic group sessions predicts enduring changes in psychological wellbeing and social connectedness. *Frontiers in Pharmacology, 12*, 623985. https://doi.org/10.3389/fphar.2021.623985

Kubala, P. (2023). Songs of life: Psychedelic-assisted psychotherapy and Deleuze and Guattari's 'desiring-production'. *Deleuze and Guattari Studies, 17*(4), 482–505.

Langlitz, N., & Gearin, A. K. (2024). Psychedelic therapy as form of life. *Neuroethics, 17*(1), 14. https://doi.org/10.1007/s12152-024-09550-9

Lury, C., & Day, S. (2019). Algorithmic personalization as a mode of individuation. *Theory, Culture & Society, 36*(2), 17–37. https://doi.org/10.1177/0263276418818888

Lykos Therapeutics. (2024). Lykos Therapeutics announces FDA acceptance and priority review of new drug application for MDMA-assisted therapy for PTSD. *PR Newswire*. https://www.prnewswire.com/news-releases/lykos-therapeutics-announces-fda-acceptance-and-priority-review-of-new-drug-application-for-mdma-assisted-therapy-for-ptsd-302058901.html

Marseille, E., Bertozzi, S., & Kahn, J. G. (2022). The economics of psychedelic-assisted therapies: A research agenda. *Frontiers in Psychiatry, 13*, 1025726. https://doi.org/10.3389/fpsyt.2022.1025726

Marseille, E., Kahn, J. G., Yazar-Klosinski, B., & Doblin, R. (2020). The cost-effectiveness of MDMA-assisted psychotherapy for the treatment of chronic, treatment-resistant PTSD. *PLoS One, 15*(10), e0239997. https://doi.org/10.1371/journal.pone.0239997

Meikle, S., Carter, O., & Bedi, G. (2024). Psychedelic-assisted psychotherapy, patient vulnerability and abuses of power. *Australian & New Zealand Journal of Psychiatry, 58*(2), 104–106. https://doi.org/10.1177/00048674231200164

Moncrieff, J. (2008). *The myth of the chemical cure*. Palgrave Macmillan.

Moncrieff, J. (2021). Psychedelics—The new psychiatric craze! *WordPress.com*. https://joannamoncrieff.com/2021/09/02/psychedelics-the-new-psychiatric-craze/

Mustafa, R. A., McQueen, B., Nikitin, D., Nhan, E., Zemplenyi, A., DiStefano, M. J., Kayali, Y., Richardson, M., & Rind D. M. (2024). 3,4-Methylenedioxymethamphetamine assisted psychotherapy for post-traumatic stress disorder: Effectiveness and value. Draft evidence report. *Institute for Clinical and Economic Review*. https://icer.org/assessment/ptsd-2024/#overview

Nardou, R., Sawyer, E., Song, Y. J., Wilkinson, M., Padovan-Hernandez, Y., de Deus, J. L., Wright, N., Lama, C., Faltin, S., Goff, L. A., Stein-O'Brien, G. L., & Dölen, G. (2023). Psychedelics reopen the social reward learning critical period. *Nature, 618*(7966), 790–798. https://doi.org/10.1038/s41586-023-06204-3

Noorani, T., Bedi, G., & Muthukumaraswamy, S. (2023). Dark loops: Contagion effects, consistency and chemosocial matrices in psychedelic-assisted therapy trials. *Psychological Medicine, 53*(13), 5892–5901. https://doi.org/10.1017/S0033291723001289

Noorani, T., Garcia-Romeu, A., Swift, T. C., Griffiths, R. R., & Johnson, M. W. (2018). Psychedelic therapy for smoking cessation: Qualitative analysis of participant accounts. *Journal of Psychopharmacology, 32*(7), 756–769. https://doi.org/10.1177/0269881118780612

Olson, D. E. (2020). The subjective effects of psychedelics may not be necessary for their enduring therapeutic effects. *ACS Pharmacology & Translational Science, 4*(2), 563–567.

Perkins, D., Sarris, J., Rossell, S., Bonomo, Y., Forbes, D., Davey, C., Hoyer, D., Loo, C., Murray, G., Hood, S., Schubert, V., Galvão-Coelho, N. L.,

O'Donnell, M., Carter, O., Liknaitzky, P., Williams, M., Siskind, D., Penington, D., Berk, M., & Castle, D. (2021). Medicinal psychedelics for mental health and addiction: Advancing research of an emerging paradigm. *Australian & New Zealand Journal of Psychiatry, 55*(12), 1127–1133. https://doi.org/10.1177/0004867421998785

Piepzna-Samarasinha, L. L. (2018). *Care work: Dreaming disability justice.* Arsenal Pulp Press.

Pollan, M. (2018). *How to change your mind: What the new science of psychedelics teaches us about consciousness, dying, addiction, depression, and transcendence.* Penguin Press.

Proctor, R. N. (2008). Agnotology: A missing term to describe the cultural production of ignorance (and its study). In R. N. Proctor & L. Schiebinger (Eds.), *Agnotology: The making and unmaking of ignorance* (pp. 1–33). Stanford University Press.

Reith, G. (2004). Consumption and its discontents: Addiction, identity and the problems of freedom. *The British Journal of Sociology, 55*(2), 283–300. https://doi.org/10.1111/j.1468-4446.2004.00019.x

Rose, N. (1999). *Powers of freedom: Reframing political thought.* Cambridge University Press.

Sedgwick, P. (1982). *Psychopolitics.* Pluto.

Shalit, N., Rehm, J., & Lev-Ran, S. (2019). Epidemiology of hallucinogen use in the U.S. results from The National Epidemiologic Survey on alcohol and related conditions III. *Addictive Behaviors, 89*, 35–43. https://doi.org/10.1016/j.addbeh.2018.09.020

Steinhardt, J. (2020). Teachers, friends, allies: What do we make of psychedelic animism? *Fieldsights.* https://culanth.org/fieldsights/teachers-friends-allies-what-do-we-make-of-psychedelic-animism

Szalavitz, M., Rigg, K. K., & Wakeman, S. E. (2021). Drug dependence is not addiction—and it matters. *Annals of Medicine, 53*(1), 1989–1992. https://doi.org/10.1080/07853890.2021.1995623

Tupper, K., & Labate, B. (2014). Ayahuasca, psychedelic studies and health sciences: The politics of knowledge and inquiry into an Amazonian plant brew. *Current Drug Abuse Reviews, 7*(2), 71–80.

Underwood, E. (2019). Listening to ketamine. *Knowable Magazine.* https://knowablemagazine.org/content/article/mind/2019/listening-ketamine

Valverde, M. (1998). *Diseases of the will: Alcohol and the dilemmas of freedom.* Cambridge University Press.

Watts, R., & Luoma, J. B. (2020). The use of the psychological flexibility model to support psychedelic assisted therapy. *Journal of Contextual Behavioral Science, 15*, 92–102. https://doi.org/10.1016/j.jcbs.2019.12.004

West, R., Cox, S., Notley, C. J., Du Plessis, G., & Hastings, J. (2024). Achieving consensus, coherence, clarity and consistency when talking about addiction. *Addiction, 119*(5), 796–798.

White, W. L. (2007). Addiction recovery: Its definition and conceptual boundaries. *Journal of substance abuse treatment, 33*(3), 229–241. https://doi.org/10.1016/j.jsat.2007.04.015

Part IV

Media, Political and Public Discourse

12

Addiction Discoveries: Hyping and Spinning the Superiority of Neuroscience

Matilda Hellman

Researchers have uncovered a previously unknown connection between the brain's basal ganglia and cerebellum, altering our understanding of motor learning and habit formation … This groundbreaking research has significant implications for understanding addiction … offering new potential targets for therapeutic interventions.
(Neuroscience News, 2024)

The citation above comes from *neurosciencenews.com*, an independent science news website focusing on neuroscience that has tasked itself to "scour news sources from universities, labs, news agencies, scientists, science publishers, and other science departments" (Neuroscience News, 2024). Together with communications offices at research organisations and different types of mass media outlets, science popularisation websites like *neurosciencenews.com* are the prime public mediators of

M. Hellman (✉)
Uppsala University, Uppsala, Sweden
e-mail: matilda.hellman@uu.se

B. M. Z. Cohen et al. (eds.), *Addiction and the Medicalisation of Conspicuous Behaviour*, The Politics of Mental Health and Illness,
https://doi.org/10.1007/978-3-032-06313-7_11

neuroscientific progress imageries. Their content details scientific findings by referencing specific brain mechanisms, framing them as groundbreaking and highlighting promising avenues for therapeutic advancements. In a cultural view on science communication, such neuroscience progress stories can be seen as a storytelling that furthers and upkeeps collective meaning-making (see Davies et al., 2019). They deliver glimpses of hope amidst a general awareness of the complexity of addiction, known to be deeply intertwined with mental health, poverty, and societal marginalisation. They can also be seen as part of a broader medicalisation of society, extending the influence of medical expertise and technologies (Goldberg, 2014; Satel, 2013).

In this chapter, I critically examine the popular discourse surrounding neuroscience progress. My aim is to further our understanding of the workings of addiction neurohype, which has recently faced criticism for disproportionate credibility claims, publicity, and resource allocation (see for example, Heather et al., 2022). Especially the brain disease model of addiction (BDMA) has been argued to effectively both medicalise and moralise addiction, shifting focus away from social policy and the sociocultural circumstances of substance use and addiction (Elam, 2015; Fraser et al., 2014; Kalant, 2015).

The popular neuro-narratives examined in this study are viewed as part of broader meaning-making processes designed to foster shared understandings (see Davies, & Horst, 2016). Drawing on the concepts of hype/hyping and spin/spinning as inevitable parts of science translation and popularisation, I explore how neuroscientific progress is given weight and relevance in the studied online genre (see Caulfield, 2018; Kamenova & Caulfield, 2015). Hype, characterised by exaggerated claims and inflated expectations, has become intertwined with neuroscience progress, particularly with the advent of technological innovations like neuroimaging and deep brain stimulation. It reflects a broader societal emphasis on neuroscience research as a means of addressing contemporary challenges (Caulfield, 2018, p. 560). Similarly, spin—the intentional orientation of messages to shape interpretation—plays a crucial role in crafting compelling narratives of neuroscientific progress (Kristensen, 2006). Attention-grabbing storytelling aids a widespread belief in scientific discoveries as gateways to a better future, often disregarding evidential deficiencies that do not serve the intended 'wow effect' (Boesman & Van Gorp, 2018; Boutron et al., 2019).

Hype and spin synergise to create engagement and a sense of legitimacy and credibility. Their pervasive presence highlights the need for critical scrutiny, especially given the difficulties of assessing the significance of scientific contributions solely based on online media content. By exploring textual expressions of hype and spin techniques, we gain insight into how language and discourse shape our understanding of scientific progress.

Hyping and spinning

Paul Ricoeur posits that language's act of reference goes beyond mere pointing to external objects or ideas. Rather, reference involves refiguration, where language reshapes our understanding of reality by mediating our relationship with the world (Ivic, 2009; Ricoeur, 1980, 2003). In the context of science and technology studies (STS), such reconfigurations are often viewed within research and innovation ecosystems that necessitate certain representations of science. Success in these systems may hinge on projecting compelling imageries of a science-shaped future (Bell et al., 2013; Roberson, 2020). The oversell of science contributions has been framed as direct responses to academic publication pressure and the commercialisation of science agendas (Caulfield & Condit, 2012; Nerlich, 2013), and explained in terms of various interdependent relationships between scientists, media, and the public (Moorhead et al., 2022; Soto-Sanfiel et al., 2023). Exaggeration and simplification in science communication are also linked to instrumental understandings of knowledge in law and policy (Jasanoff, 2014), as well as to the dynamics between scientists and the public (Pullman et al., 2013; Trench, 2011). Sociocultural entanglements, the literature suggests, often compromise moderation and nuance in presenting scientific results and contributions (Nerlich, 2013).

Researchers have sought to identify and demonstrate instances of spin and hype by comparing the representations and promotions of science findings with the original results. For instance, Bastian (2014) and Chiu et al. (2017) have highlighted spin by analysing the prevalence of excessively optimistic language in article abstracts. Similarly, a 2017 scoping review by Li et al. (2017) found that 39 percent of biomedical abstracts exhibited some degree of spin, while Lehmen et al. (2014) discovered that 75 percent of articles in the area of spine research contained inconsistencies between the main manuscript and the abstract. Some degree of hype and spin is of course necessary in all science communication. The narration of science, akin to journalism, relies on an author-reader awareness of connecting 'real-world events' with crafting a compelling story.

Empirical stories serve both referential and dialogic functions: the referential function relates to the accuracy of depicted events, while the dialogic function concerns how these events are mediated or packaged to the reader. The distinction between empirical truth and spin or storytelling format is artificial, yet necessary for understanding the communicative infrastructure and spin techniques involved in medicalisation (see for example, Polman, 2006). Doležel's concept pair of 'extension' and 'intension' captures this distinction. Extension pertains to the depiction of 'what is', such as stating ontological facts. It is the (truthful) description of how the study has progressed and the findings that have been generated. For example, it can be the informing statement that a researcher has conducted a study. Intension, on the other hand, involves the sense-making given to the discovery, crafting a story's 'wow factor' in terms of relevance and novelty for human progress and evolution. It can, for instance, be speculation regarding the study's contribution, such as "thanks to this discovery we might never have to worry about getting addicted to coffee again". Neurohype enables and requires hybrid worlds consisting of both the fictional and factual, with narrative formats and discursive techniques making it possible for these worlds to coalesce and make sense together (see Doležel, 1998, p. 187; Nerlich et al., 2016).

Neuroscience discovery stories

I performed a critical reading of addiction-related neuroscience progress stories, comprising online news items and opinion pieces with attention-grabbing headlines and images. These texts were sourced from various online platforms, including mainstream media and press releases from prestigious universities. Additionally, some texts originated from smaller local news outlets or health-related websites. These news items are typically found on search engine news pages, social media feeds, or as brief notices across online media outlets. Judging by the number of shares, likes, and comments, and the spread of singular press releases in different media outlets, it was evident that some of the texts had been widely circulated, potentially reaching a broad international audience through different kinds of media platforms (notices from larger universities were reposted up to ten times on Twitter (now renamed X); for an example, references and shares to the news item from Stanford University, as reported by Collins (see below), are available here: https://twitter.com/search?q=Stanford researchers say U.S. policies on drugs and addiction could use a dose of neuroscience&src=typed_query).

The original data collection was conducted in 2019, spanning the period from 2016 to 2019, using Google News (news.google.com, ticked for the US edition) with default search settings. Employing the search term 'addiction + brain', 670 texts were gathered from online sources primarily in the Anglophone world. Subsequently, additional items were incorporated into the dataset; other analyses of this material have been documented elsewhere (Hellman et al., 2022). For this study, 67 stories were selected from the original dataset, focusing on new neuroscience findings with references to addiction. In the winter of 2023–2024, an updated identical search was conducted retrieving 22 more recent news items on various neuroscience discoveries. These newer items adhere to similar reporting patterns and complement the older corpus, with references to some of these current items integrated into the analysis.

Even if the texts' sources, authors and themes varied in the material, the format, structure and content were homogenous and follow almost the exact same pattern in every news piece. In each of the items, a new neuroscience finding was presented as a game changer in solving addiction problems. The similarity in the story setup suggests that this material represents a 'hype and spin'-genre of its own (see Loughlin et al., 2013). I have intentionally excluded the identification of producers, senders and forces behind the texts from my discussion. My discussion concerns the hype and spin content that targets the average online news reader, who has no prior information on the original research that was reported.

The texts were analysed through identifying the contributing discursive elements when packaging the stories' references to 'what is' (hype/extension/sense) in a wrapping of 'what it means' (spin/intension/reference). The first round of reading led to the seven overlapping sense-making themes being re-ordered into four emplotment categories: namely, *temporality; connecting events and contexts; superior evidence*; and *asymmetries.* In the next section, I discuss how these traits show up as hype and spin.

Temporality

The material portrayed a transition from a less-informed past to a more informed future through references to the transformative nature of the reported discoveries. Neuroscience was presented as a pathway to acquiring more substantial and reliable evidence about addiction and to developing improved approaches for addressing addiction-related issues. It suggested that as more biomedical evidence accumulates, our understanding of addiction deepens, bringing us closer to grasping its true essence and facilitating the exploration of research questions previously deemed inaccessible.

In the material, the discoveries were presented as the results of systemic improvement of research techniques and rewarded after great diligence and systematics by the scholars involved. In an interview one researcher looks back at the work process: "we thought it was unlikely that we'd find a common [brain] circuit. But after much work and collaboration, we found something," and adds: "[i]t's exciting science" (Neuroscience News, 2023). A piece published in the commercial tech news service platform *Tech Times* explains that past studies have compared "brain functions of people obsessed with the Internet", but a new study provides further insights into what is *actually* happening in the brain (Navarro, 2016). "Researchers are now working to refine their understanding" by studying the neurological underpinnings of gambling, states a piece from the American Psychological Association (Sohn, 2023). The neuro-evidence thus brings us closer to a more precise and sophisticated knowledge than that of the past.

Emphasising the incomplete nature of prior knowledge underscored the transformative impact of the new brain-based discoveries. This framing aligns with a broader neurohype narrative, contrasting the strength and depth of neuroscience against the backdrop of past uncertainties and shortcomings. The implication is that further neuroscience discoveries are necessary to fully understand addiction and develop solutions to its myriad challenges.

In a Harvard-generated news piece, a study model of the brain reveals a new understanding of neuron diversity marking a moment of astonishment for scientists (Burrows, 2017). The dissemination of these revolutionary findings is justified by the discovery's impact on our presently underdeveloped understanding of neurons' diversity. Temporal markers like "then", "after", and "later" engage readers, involving them in the progress story (Ricoeur, 2003). By linking discovery contexts with their hypothetical uses, the collective is implicated in the events. This collective engagement fosters a sense of unity and solidarity, emphasising the importance of acting on newfound knowledge.

Connecting events and contexts

The studied news pieces often established connections between the events of a discovery and their societal implications, presenting these links as natural and direct. This spin tends to exclude alternative scenarios, focusing solely on potential implications (Doležel, 1998; Polman, 2006). Implications were achieved, for instance, by coupling laboratory findings with possible novel strategies for medication developments (see for example, University of Colorado Boulder, 2017). This type of association between discovery/extension and the implementation/intension does not step out of a certain sphere of medical and clinical epistemology—laboratories for scanning mice and laboratories for developing medical drugs are not totally different worlds, but rather they entail similar elements.

At times the discoveries' potential implications for societies were argued in connection to contexts, orders and societal spheres that were less obvious on closer scrutinisation. For example, the news agency *PBS Frontline's* piece on the ways in which new neuroscience discoveries can affect the length of prison time for US teens begins by temporal contrasting with a less-knowing past: "[i]n the 1990s, *before scientists had the tools to understand the teenage brain*", judges around the country would sentence thousands of adolescents to life in prison "without the chance for parole" (Tsiu, 2017, emphasis added). But now, the text continues, advances in brain science have proved that adolescent minds are fundamentally different from those of adults. Changes in the brain that occur during adolescence "make young people more impulsive, less able to make measured decisions and more susceptible to peer pressure" (Tsiu, 2017).

In the above example, the lack of mature cognitive reliability and resilience was accounted for via the new brain-based ontology of impulsive and easily addicted teens, presented as changing the future practices of the American legal system. This story setup substantiates Ricoeur's framework on science-making narration showing how heterogeneous elements—different spatial contexts of judges in courts, adolescents' brains, prison sentences, and so on—are brought together into a central thought of an intelligible whole orienting human societies towards new developmental pathways (see Ivic, 2019, p. 45). In the plot, the mapping of brain mechanisms becomes the crucial piece of information missing for changing the court system and the lives of young people who risk getting sentenced incorrectly. This is a great injustice that is spun as to be solved by neuroscience. Another example of when neuroscience is given extended societal use value is in a Stanford University piece on its value for US policies on drugs and addiction, which "could use a dose of neuroscience" (Collins, 2017). Here, neuroscience is—in a more general sense—stated to have the potential to "help shape more effective policies and save lives" (Collins, 2017). In an Australian news item, brain discoveries are presented as the basis for new treatment, making a distinction to old and less-good options that are "both ineffective and inaccessible' (Horton, 2017). Similarly, an article in the digital magazine *Undark* titled 'When addiction treatment fails, can a brain implant succeed?' (Madhusoodanan, 2024) prompts us to reconsider or question less effective and less precise methods from the past.

Superior evidence

Discursive models for claiming superior evidence involves affirming expressions of certainty that signify "we know that" or "we are now certain that". These differ from more arguing and suggestive expressions like "it's likely that" or "it's probable that" (see for example, Arner, 1959, p. 84). In the material, such confident evidence claims seemed to open up to social imageries of promising and precise medial applications. Small-scale laboratory discoveries were given decisive roles when segmented into a grand narrative of solving addiction problems. In a piece which originates from the University of Michigan Medical School, and reported extensively in many media channels, marijuana is stated to dampen the brain's emotional reward system and therefore the perceived 'emotional rush' related to using the drug (The Chronicle, 2017): "[w]e now have convincing evidence", states the item, "that regular marijuana use impacts the brain's natural response to [engaging in behaviours that feel rewarding and give us pleasure]. ... [T]his is likely to put individuals at risk for addiction." The rewarding feeling of marijuana and its potential addictive features are, in view of the neuroscientific mechanisms, reframed as a great new discovery with a study conducted with 108 people in their early 20s (see also Gavin, 2016; University of Michigan Health System, 2016). In this instance, hype amplifies claims of established facts, rendering them more ground-breaking compared to other approaches. The brain emerges as the primary and pertinent source of ontological insights.

The elevated status of brain observations enabled even seemingly insignificant findings to be spun as more convincing and revolutionary compared to the myriad of other forms of past knowledge. Future treatment precision is implied in the piece 'Cellular atlas of amygdala reveals new treatment target for cocaine addiction' (University of California, 2023), which is based on a study that tests and maps abstinence and other aspects of the brains of different group samples of outbred rats (12 rats, 19 rats, and so on) "with high and low cocaine addiction-like behaviors following prolonged abstinence" (Zhou et al., 2023, p. 1868). Another illustration of neuroscience's superior role in knowledge acquisition is evident in a podcast promotion that highlights that it will take the conversation to "the cellular level", discussing what "is actually happening in our brains" that triggers an addiction (Cengeri and Daniels, 2017). The cellular brain level inquiry is depicted as exposing what is 'actually happening' in human brains and bodies ("we know that"), not only as imagined or interpreted by humans through experiences, representations, senses, and so on. In comparison to previous and other types of research ("it's likely that"), neuroscience is presented as better explaining addiction and unravelling its essence. In fact, the idea of the superiority of neurological proof only functions properly when portrayed as an epistemic shift involving more accurate and precise future interventions. The comparative rejection is necessary as the new, precise and tidy knowledge—not the old, unclear and messy one —will solve the problems at hand. Images of linear progress validate neuroscience as a passage to new orders in which the problems may be solved.

In a piece published by *Live Science* (Miller, 2016), neuroscientists Nora Volkow and George Koob, directors of the National Institute on Drug Abuse and the National Institute on Alcohol Abuse and Alcoholism respectively, discuss their review on the stages of addiction in the brain, supporting the BDMA. They assert that this review not only aids in understanding addiction as a brain disease but also sheds light on its ontological workings. Similarly, *Science Daily* (2016) reports brain scans pinpointing the source of addictive craving to the right ventral striatum, a breakthrough attributed to functional magnetic resonance imaging (fMRI, typically used in the neurosciences for scanning the brain in search of potential abnormalities). These discoveries are portrayed as pivotal for understanding addiction. While the identified stages of addiction by Volkow, Koob, and colleagues may have been studied extensively in the past, the brain's status as a scientific object fosters hopes for a more clinically precise view of addiction as a treatable medical condition. The prevailing argument throughout the material emphasises that addiction can be better understood, defined, monitored, and treated with new technology and insights into brain function. For instance, it is reported about the Hayver Corporation's smartphone app addressing "the epidemic of drug addiction", that it can provide real-time insights into an addict's progress towards sobriety (PRWeb, 2017).

Additionally, neuroscience's evidence is portrayed as universal and generalisable, often expressed through metaphors and associations that gather various contexts under the same biological laws. For example, a report from *The Chronicle* (2017) suggests that all individuals are genetically hardwired to seek rewarding behaviours. This viewpoint suggests that biological factors govern addiction uniformly and can be targeted with universal treatments, such as targeting the oxytocin system (Horton, 2017).

Asymmetry

According to the main storyline of the analysed news items, superior brain-based evidence provides a more valid, reliable, and innovative foundation for developing new cures and treatment. This implies a path-breaking shift from merely describing and observing addiction to actively solving addiction problems. In a piece entitled 'It's the brain that has to be changed' (McCarron, 2017), neuroscience is claimed to be *the* domain for combatting and conceptualising addiction in the future. This broadens the implications: namely, that biomedical science can drive societal changes, as seen in the piece cited above regarding reevaluating juvenile sentencing due to brain predispositions.

The biopolitical emplotment of neurohype allows the story to proceed in ways that leave out complex circumstances and make the road to a solution more straightforward and applicable to the masses. In a *Live Science* report about stages of change in the addiction process within the brain, it is claimed that this understanding is essential for medical professionals to better treat people. The consequences are potentially great for the "20 million to 22 million people in the United States addicted to alcohol or other drugs" (Miller, 2016). Here, the relationship between the mapping of brain processes and the everyday lives of 20–22 million people entails an association between locations of plot. The proportional asymmetry is achieved in a combination of extensional statements (and objects) and intensional sense-making—between the world that has produced the finding reported upon and the world in which implication and change are claimed to occur.

The asymmetry between the little and the big entails a logic in social constructed ontology akin to that of a move "from causality to the constitute" (Haslanger, 1995, p. 100). For example, a story on the causal discovery of brain activity deficits that can be adjusted with the help of new non-addictive, nicotine-based treatments implies a sound constitute of help "for some of the 51 million people worldwide who suffer from the disease" (University of Colorado Boulder, 2017). It is a laboratory experiment with mice that have schizophrenic characteristics that underpins this claim. The sense-making of the small technical discovery in rodents is allowed to become a crucial part of an imagery of the lives of 51 million people taking a new and better turn.

These types of asymmetrical plot techniques figured in three (overlapping) formats: namely, asymmetry pertaining to scale, animal to human translation, and epistemic expansion (see also Hellman et al., 2022, pp. 53–55). The asymmetries in scale often entailed the assembling of groups and individuals as potential gainers from the new discoveries: in a *Huffington Post* piece, new insight into brain receptors is reported as a potential gain for not only the two million people in the US suffering from an opioid abuse disorder, but also for the five million Americans living with Alzheimer's disease and the more than 36 million Americans who are currently cigarette smokers. The article concludes: "[n]ew drugs that help with all three of these problems has the potential to affect the health of a lot of people in a significant way" (DiGiulio, 2017). In this case an association is formed between a small experiment with laboratory-developed molecular materials (for the original research, see Wang et al., 2017) and the enumeration of millions of people suffering from different kinds of complex mental health and addiction problems. Other examples are experiments with transcranial magnetic stimulation therapy, which is claimed to potentially offer help to "countless patients" with depression and substance dependence (Mohammad, 2017) and "the cerebellum of the brain" associated with future treatments for drug addiction (News Medical, 2017). The University of California study on outbred rats with cocaine addiction is implied to provide hope and help for "a major public health concern, associated with a rising number of overdose deaths and a high rate of relapse". The piece mentions that it is estimated that 4.8 million people in the US used cocaine in 2021, of which 1.4 million people "had a cocaine use disorder" (University of California, 2023).

The second type of asymmetry involves extrapolating findings from rodents to humans, a leap likely to be overlooked by readers. For instance, studies from the University of British Columbia suggest that insights from rats with brain injuries could inform treatments for human impulsivity in addiction (Technological Networks, 2018). As cited above, experiments on mice with schizophrenic traits, treated with nicotine, are proposed to lead to new nicotine-based therapies for millions worldwide (University of Colorado Boulder, 2017). Additionally, research on reducing drug cravings in addicted rats through vagus nerve stimulation is suggested to have implications for help efforts in human drug addiction (University of Texas at Dallas, 2017).

The third type of asymmetrical transaction materialises in epistemic expansions of the phenomenon of addiction by claims of the same brain mechanisms underpinning different types of problems; habits that are severe and harmful are used as metaphors or points of comparisons for habits that are more everyday-like and harmless. For example: 'Neuroscientist finds similarities in the brains of snack-lovers and drug-addicts' (Morgan, 2017), or 'Are you addicted to technology?' asks a book review in *The Guardian* (Bhutto, 2017) with the caption 'Half the developed world is addicted to something'. The latter text goes on to explain that internet connectivity behaviour (Facebook, gaming, and so on) is an addiction. It refers to research that reports that brain patterns of heroin users just after a hit and those of *World of Warcraft* 'addicts' starting up a new game are nearly identical.

The comparison between heroin use and playing *World of Warcraft* bridges the realms of video gaming and substance addiction, reshaping perceptions of behaviour and reality (Bhutto, 2017). Similarly, a study from Harvard Medical School suggests parallels between brain activations in response to monetary gains and cocaine use, implying similarities in addiction mechanisms (Brandt, 2017). Meanwhile, the *Boston Herald* highlights the neurobiological predisposition to 'love addiction', contrasting it with other forms of addiction (Braff, 2017). These neural observations serve to categorise diverse behaviours under the umbrella of addiction. The subjects with addicted brains—humans or lab rodents—are depicted as devoid of agency. Various addiction problems are lumped together as having identical characteristics, as exemplified in the above news piece suggesting that crisps are as addictive as hard drugs (Morgan, 2017).

Conclusions

In this chapter I have examined popular online texts that communicate neuroscience discoveries to the public. These messages not only assert a role in the addiction field but also influence our perception of human potential and societal challenges. The observations of the workings of hype and spin are summarised below, in Fig. 12.1.

This genre of media, constructed by various stakeholders (media professionals, university communication teams, scientists, and others), reinforces the notion of neuroscience as a solid and stable entity unaffected by its methodologies or other forms of inquiry. The temporal shift from a less-informed past creates a sense of a 'game-changing moment', facilitated by the brain's perceived superiority as a source of evidence.

The news items' attention-grabbing short information piece-formats do not allow for the notion of human 'addictive' bodies and minds also

Neurohype messages	*Spinning techniques*
• Neuroscience enhances our understanding of addiction; • Evidence at the cellular level is superior, more definitive and authoritative; • A more accurate ontology of addiction is emerging through its discovery in the brain; • Breakthrough findings are portrayed as transformative compared to traditional approaches to understanding addiction; • Established knowledge is reframed as new and revolutionary when validated by brain research.	• Coupling contexts: mapping brains will lead to profound changes in societal structures and policies; • Hope: shift from messy addiction realities to cleaner biomedically informed realities; • Shift: from describing to solving problem; • Logical asymmetries in: (1) scale; (2) translation between animals and humans; and (3) expansion of the various habits that are included under the umbrella idea of addiction.

Fig. 12.1 Hyping and spinning the neuroscience of addiction in popular online news items

being *made* in and through the making and production of science. An interesting condition is the cancellation of agency in the subjects that are carriers of the addicted brains. They become objects of interventions or objects of science. This is especially worrying since strong associations are made between contexts such as the 'laboratory' and 'world problems', or 'the brains of five laboratory rats' and 'the American opium crisis'. Aligning such associations into logical sequels or compositions are of special interest in understanding the hyping and spinning of science findings. The ways and logics in which we connect evidence to its adherent practice has been shown to have an impact on public perceptions of risk and facts (de Bruin and Bostrom, 2013; Kahan, 2017).

My analysis demonstrates how short online research discovery news pieces contribute to an ongoing collective cultural storytelling and sense-making of addiction through biomedicalisation discourse. The public's perception of science's utility and innovation hinges on various factors, including the accessibility of information, the packaging of results as solutions, and the cultural prestige of scientific fields. Neuroscience, in particular, enjoys positive perceptions of its potential usefulness, with human behaviours and habits increasingly framed in terms of brain mechanisms. Studies reveal that people are susceptible to exaggerated claims about neuroscience's applicability, regardless of their connection to reality (Raz & Thibault, 2019; van de Werff et al., 2016).

While certain metaphors, comparative constructions, and the significant impacts of small, hard science discoveries are well-known characteristics in biomedical texts (Fiszman et al., 2007), the precise mechanisms behind this phenomenon remain relatively unexplored. The ways in which the narrative of neuroscientific progress materialises in the material of this study offer us some insights into the imagined contribution of the epistemic project of addiction in the brain (see Hellman et al., 2022). The popular images of brain research on addiction unfold within a sociocultural framework made possible by the profound trust in this type of scientific production. A key premise for authority is the detachment and independence of science production from individuals' accounts, constructs, and social contexts (the position of which is the observation that "before we knew something, but now we know how it really is"). What is observed in the material is a popular cultural (bio)medicalising storytelling that is extending the influence and authority of neuroscience into everyday understandings.

My critical reading demonstrates how little information about complex science-making circumstances is revealed in the spinning of neuroscientific progress as ground-breaking discoveries. Discursively persuasive and influential elements come about through a 'logical asymmetry' between extensional claims and intensional connotations, both in temporal and spatial dimensions. The asymmetry is enabled both by the status of neuroscience and of the science discovery storytelling genre. The material indicates that a superior cultural position of neuroscientific knowledge enables and allows for both bold and simplified ideas of transition between the reference to discovery (extension) and its narrative and contextual sense-making (intension). Many circumstantial elements are bound to go unobserved to (quickly scrolling online) readers.

There are several contradictions hidden in the expansion stories in that they make generic claims while still covering specific problems as unique in their 'addictiveness'. Also, the solidness of the neuroscientific evidence can only function in a logical framework where the brain's plasticity plays a crucial role—solutions rely on the changeable nature of the brain, which is disregarded or excluded whenever the solidness of the evidence is claimed. Together with connecting the textual and narrative elements to speakers and sources, and to processes of transforming people into governable non-agentic subjects, these sorts of contradiction would be important tasks for future investigations.

References

Arner, D. (1959). On knowing. *The Philosophical Review, 68*(1), 84–92. https://doi.org/10.2307/2182548

Bastian, H. (2014). Science in the abstract: Don't judge a study by its cover. *PLoS*. https://absolutelymaybe.plos.org/2014/05/12/science-in-the-abstract-dont-judge-a-study-by-its-cover/

Bell, F., Fletcher, G., Greenhill, A., Griffiths, M., & McLean, R. (2013). Science fiction prototypes: Visionary technology narratives between futures. *Futures, 50*, 5–14. https://doi.org/10.1016/j.futures.2013.04.004

Bhutto, F. (2017). Irresistible by Adam Alter review—An entertaining look at technology addiction. *The Guardian*. https://www.theguardian.com/books/2017/apr/21/irresistible-by-adam-alter-review-technology-addiction

Boesman, J., & Van Gorp, B. (2018). Driving the frame: How news values, news pegs, and story angles guide journalistic frame building. In P. D'Angelo (Ed.), *Doing news framing analysis II* (pp. 152–174). Routledge.

Boutron, I., Haneef, R., Yavchitz, A., Baron, G., Novack, J., Oransky, I., Schwitzer, G., & Ravaud, P. (2019). Three randomized controlled trials evaluating the impact of "spin" in health news stories reporting studies of phar-

macologic treatments on patients'/caregivers' interpretation of treatment benefit. *BMC Medicine, 17*(105), 1–10. https://doi.org/10.1186/s12916-019-1330-9
Braff, D. (2017). You're gonna have to face it, you're addicted to love. *Boston Herald.* https://www.bostonherald.com/2017/07/16/youre-gonna-have-to-face-it-youre-addicted-to-love/
Brandt, C. (2017). Harvard research says investing and cocaine have the same effect to your brain. *University Herald.* https://www.universityherald.com/articles/68584/20170309/harvard-research-says-investing-and-cocaine-have-the-same-effect-to-your-brain.htm
Burrows, L. (2017). Multiregional brain on a chip. *Harvard John A. Paulson School of Engineering and Applied Sciences.* https://www.seas.harvard.edu/news/2017/01/multiregional-brain-on-chip
Caulfield, T. (2018). Spinning the genome: Why science hype matters. *Perspectives in Biology and Medicine, 61*(4), 560–571. https://doi.org/10.1353/pbm.2018.0065
Caulfield, T., & Condit, C. (2012). Science and the sources of hype. *Public Health Genomics, 15*(3–4), 209–217. https://doi.org/10.1159/000336533
Cengeri, R., & Daniels, P. (2017). This is your brain on drugs: How science explains addiction. *Vermont Public.* https://www.vermontpublic.org/programs/2017-07-25/this-is-your-brain-on-drugs-how-science-explains-addiction
Chiu, K., Grundy, Q., & Bero, L. (2017). 'Spin' in published biomedical literature: A methodological systematic review. *PLoS Biology, 15*(9), e2002173. https://doi.org/10.1371/journal.pbio.2002173
Collins, N. (2017). Stanford researchers say U.S. policies on drugs and addiction could use a dose of neuroscience. *Stanford University.* https://news.stanford.edu/2017/06/22/u-s-drug-policy-needs-dose-neuroscience/
Davies, S. R., Halpern, M., Horst, M., Kirby, D. A., & Lewenstein, B. (2019). Science stories as culture: Experience, identity, narrative and emotion in public communication of science. *Journal of Science Communication, 18*(5), 1–16.
Davies, S. R., & Horst, M. (2016). *Science communication: Culture, identity and citizenship.* Palgrave Macmillan.
de Bruin, B. W., & Bostrom, A. (2013). Assessing what to address in science communication. *Proceedings of the National Academy of Sciences, 110*(supplement_3), 14062–14068. https://doi.org/10.1073/pnas.1212729110

DiGiulio, S. (2017). A new type of drug could one day treat pain, memory loss and nicotine addiction. *HuffPost*. https://www.huffpost.com/entry/addiction-treatment-pain-memory-loss_n_59230253e4b03b485cb3742c

Doležel, L. (1998). *Heterocosmica: Fiction and possible worlds*. Johns Hopkins University Press.

Elam, M. (2015). How the brain disease paradigm remoralizes addictive behaviour. *Science as Culture, 24*(1), 46–64. https://doi.org/10.1080/09505431.2014.936373

Fiszman, M., Demner-Fushman, D., Lang, F. M., Goetz, P., & Rindflesch, T. C. (2007). Interpreting comparative constructions in biomedical text. In K. B. Cohen, D. Demner-Fushman, C. Friedman, L. Hirschman, & J. Pestian (Eds.), *Biological, translational, and clinical language processing* (pp. 137–144). Association for Computational Linguistics.

Fraser, S., Moore, D., & Keane, H. (2014). *Habits: Remaking addiction*. Palgrave Macmillan.

Gavin, K. (2016). Over time, marijuana use dampens brain response to reward. *University of Michigan*. https://www.michiganmedicine.org/health-lab/over-time-marijuana-use-dampens-brains-response-reward

Goldberg, D. S. (2014). Fatness, medicalization, and stigma: On the need to do better. *Narrative Inquiry in Bioethics, 4*(2), 117–123. https://doi.org/10.1353/nib.2014.0053

Haslanger, S. (1995). Ontology and social construction. *Philosophical Topics, 23*(2), 95–125.

Heather, N., Field, M., Moss, A. C., & Satel, S. (Eds.). (2022). *Evaluating the brain disease model of addiction*. Routledge.

Hellman, M., Egerer, M., Stoneham, J., Forberger, S., Männistö-Inkinen, V., Ochterbeck, D., & Rundle, S. (2022). *Addiction and the brain: Knowledge, beliefs and ethical considerations from a social perspective*. Palgrave Macmillan.

Horton, J. (2017). Hugs not drugs: The USyd researchers developing addiction treatment. *Honi Soit*. https://honisoit.com/2017/04/hugs-not-drugs-the-usyd-researchers-developing-addiction-treatment/

Ivic, S. (2009). Ricoeur's narrative theory applied to science. *Philosophical Papers and Review, 1*(3), 44–51.

Ivic, S. (2019). *Paul Ricoeur's idea of reference: The truth as non-reference*. Brill.

Jasanoff, S. (2014). Serviceable truths: Science for action in law and policy. *Texas Law Review, 93*, 1723.

Kahan, D. M. (2017). 'Ordinary science intelligence': A science-comprehension measure for study of risk and science communication, with notes on evolution and climate change. *Journal of Risk Research, 20*(8), 995–1016. https://doi.org/10.1080/13669877.2016.1148067

Kalant, H. (2015). Neurobiological research on addiction: What value has it added to the concept? *The International Journal of Alcohol and Drug Research, 4*(1), 53–59. https://doi.org/10.7895/ijadr.v4i1.196

Kamenova, K., & Caulfield, T. (2015). Stem cell hype: Media portrayal of therapy translation. *Science Translational Medicine, 7*(278), 278ps4–278ps4. https://doi.org/10.1126/scitranslmed.3010496

Kristensen, N. N. (2006). Spin in the media—The media in a (self-)spin? *MedieKultur: Journal of Media and Communication Research, 22*(40), 10. https://doi.org/10.7146/mediekultur.v22i40.1317

Lehmen, J. A., Deering, R. M., Simpson, A. K., Carrier, C. S., & Bono, C. M. (2014). Inconsistencies between abstracts and manuscripts in published studies about lumbar spine surgery. *Spine, 39*(10), 841–845. https://doi.org/10.1097/BRS.0000000000000290

Li, G., Abbade, L. P. F., Nwosu, I., Jin, Y., Leenus, A., Maaz, M., Wang, M., Bhatt, M., Zielinski, L., Sanger, N., Bantoto, B., Luo, C., Shams, I., Shahid, H., Chang, Y., Sun, G., Mbuagbaw, L., Samaan, Z., Levine, M. A. H., Adachi, J. D., & Thabane, L. (2017). A scoping review of comparisons between abstracts and full reports in primary biomedical research. *BMC Medical Research Methodology, 17*, 181. https://doi.org/10.1186/s12874-017-0459-5

Loughlin, M., Lewith, G., & Falkenberg, T. (2013). Science, practice and mythology: A definition and examination of the implications of scientism in medicine. *Health Care Analysis, 21*(2), 130–145. https://doi.org/10.1007/s10728-012-0211-6

Madhusoodanan, J. (2024). When addiction treatment fails, can a brain implant succeed? *Undark*. https://undark.org/2024/01/29/brain-implant-addiction/

McCarron, S. (2017). It's the brain that has to be changed. *The Martha's Vineyard Times*. https://www.mvtimes.com/2017/07/12/its-the-brain-that-has-to-be-changed/

Miller, S. G. (2016). Addiction changes brain biology in 3 stages, experts say. *Live Science*. https://www.livescience.com/53508-brain-disease-model-addiction.html

Mohammad, A. (2017). New brain stimulation therapy helps treat drug and alcohol addiction. *HuffPost*. https://www.huffpost.com/entry/new-brain-stimulation-therapy-treats-drug-and-alcohol_b_58af470ae4b02f3f81e4452d

Moorhead, L. L., Fleerackers, A., & Maggio, L. A. (2022). *"It's my job": A qualitative study of the mediatization of science within the scientist-journalist relationship., bioRxiv*, 2022–2008. https://doi.org/10.1101/2022.08.10.503486

Morgan, S. (2017). Proof that crisps are as addictive as hard drugs: Neuroscientist finds similarities in the brains of snack-lovers and drug-addicts. *Daily Mail*. https://www.dailymail.co.uk/health/article-4525270/Proof-crisps-addictive-hard-drugs.html

Navarro, A. (2016). Facebook addiction affects brain like cocaine, gambling: Study. *Tech Times*. https://www.techtimes.com/articles/136493/20160225/facebook addiction-affects-brain-like-cocaine-gambling-study.htm

Nerlich, B. (2013). Moderation impossible? On hype, honesty and trust in the context of modern academic life. *The Sociological Review, 61*, 43–57. https://doi.org/10.1111/1467-954X.12099

Nerlich, B., Elliott, R., & Larson, B. (2016). Communicating biological sciences: An introduction. In B. Nerlich, R. Elliott, & B. Larson (Eds.), *Communicating biological sciences: Ethical and metaphorical dimensions* (pp. 1–24). Routledge.

Neuroscience News. (2023). Addiction's common ground: A universal brain circuit revealed. *Neuroscience News*. https://neurosciencenews.com/addiction-brain-network-23971/

Neuroscience News. (2024). Brain pathway linking movement, addiction, and rewards discovered. *Neuroscience News*. https://neurosciencenews.com/addiction-reward-movement-dopamine-25523/

News Medical. (2017). Cerebellum can be responsible for brain alterations linked to drug addiction, research shows. *News Medical*. https://www.news-medical.net/news/20170223/Cerebellum-can-be-responsible-for-brain-alterations-linked-to-drug-addiction-research-shows.aspx

Polman, J. L. (2006). True stories, storied truth: Stitching narrative and logico-scientific discourse together in an age of "spin". In S. A. Barab, K. E. Hay, & D. T. Hickey (Eds.), *The Proceedings of the 7th international conference of the learning sciences, volume 2* (pp. 557–563). International Society of the Learning Sciences.

PRWeb. (2017). Announcing the launch of Hayver to address the epidemic of drug addiction and alcoholism with a revolutionary verification technology to keep up to 90% of people clean. *PRWeb*. https://www.prweb.com/releases/announcing_the_launch_of_hayver_to_address_the_epidemic_of_drug_addiction_and_alcoholism_with_a_revolutionary_verification_technology_to_keep_up_to_90_of_people_clean/prweb14503185.htm

Pullman, D., Zarzeczny, A., & Picard, A. (2013). Media, politics and science policy: MS and evidence from the CCSVI trenches. *BMC Medical Ethics, 14*(6), 1–9. https://doi.org/10.1186/1472-6939-14-6

Raz, A., & Thibault, R. T. (Eds.). (2019). *Casting light on the dark side of brain imaging*. Academic.

Ricoeur, P. (1980). Narrative time. *Critical Inquiry, 7*(1), 169–190.

Ricoeur, P. (2003). *The rule of metaphor: The creation of meaning in language*. University of Toronto Press.

Roberson, T. M. (2020). Can hype be a force for good? Inviting unexpected engagement with science and technology futures. *Public Understanding of Science, 29*(5), 544–552. https://doi.org/10.1177/0963662520923109

Satel, S. (2013). *Brainwashed: The seductive appeal of mindless neuroscience*. Basic Books.

Science Daily. (2016). New study reveals how the brain processes social rewards. *Science Daily*. https://www.sciencedaily.com/releases/2016/08/160830131205.htm

Sohn, E. (2023). How gambling affects the brain and who is most vulnerable to addiction. *Monitor on Psychology, 54*(5). https://www.apa.org/monitor/2023/07/how-gambling-affects-the-brain

Soto-Sanfiel, M. T., Chong, C. W., & Latorre, J. I. (2023). Hype in science communication: Exploring scientists' attitudes and practices in quantum physics. *arXiv preprint arXiv:2311.07160*. https://doi.org/10.48550/arXiv.2311.07160

Technological Networks. (2018). Brain injury causes impulsivity in rats. *Technological Networks*. https://www.technologynetworks.com/neuroscience/news/brain-injury-causes-impulsivity-in-rats-288503

The Chronicle. (2017). Marijuana dampens emotional rush, study finds. *The Chronicle*. https://www.chroniclenewspaper.com/news/local-news/marijuana-dampens-emotional-rush-study-finds-MTCN20170528170529996

Trench, B. (2011). Scientists' blogs: Glimpses behind the scenes. In S. Rödder, M. Franzen, & P. Weingart (Eds.), *The sciences' media connection—Public communication and its repercussions* (pp. 273–289). Springer Netherlands. https://doi.org/10.1007/978-94-007-2085-5_14

Tsiu, A. (2017). How brain science is changing how long teens spend in prison. *Frontline*. https://www.pbs.org/wgbh/frontline/article/how-brain-science-is-changing-how-long-teens-spend-in-prison/

University of California. (2023). Cellular atlas of amygdala reveals new treatment target for cocaine addiction. *University of California*. https://www.uni-

versityofcalifornia.edu/news/cellular-atlas-amygdala-reveals-new-treatment-target-cocaine-addiction
University of Colorado Boulder. (2017). Nicotine normalizes brain activity deficits that are key to schizophrenia. *Medical Xpress*. https://medicalxpress.com/news/2017-01-nicotine-brain-deficits-key-schizophrenia.html#google_vignette
University of Michigan Health System. (2016). Marijuana use dampens brain's response to reward over time, study finds. *Science Daily*. https://www.sciencedaily.com/releases/2016/07/160706114407.htm
University of Texas at Dallas. (2017). Potential way to reduce drug cravings: Vagus nerve stimulation therapy. *Science Daily*. https://www.sciencedaily.com/releases/2017/01/170123162315.htm
van de Werff, T., Slatman, J., & Swierstra, T. (2016). Can we "remedy" neurohype, and should we? Using neurohype for ethical deliberation. *AJOB Neuroscience, 7*(2), 97–99. https://doi.org/10.1080/21507740.2016.1189978
Wang, Z. J., Deba, F., Mohamed, T. S., Chiara, D. C., Ramos, K., & Hamouda, A. K. (2017). Unraveling amino acid residues critical for allosteric potentiation of (α4) 3 (β2) 2-type nicotinic acetylcholine receptor responses. *Journal of Biological Chemistry, 292*(24), 9988–10001.
Zhou, J. L., de Guglielmo, G., Ho, A. J., Kallupi, M., Pokhrel, N., Li, H. R., Chitre, A. S., Munro, D., Mohammadi, P., Carrette, L. L. G., George, O., Palmer, A. A., McVicker, G., & Telese, F. (2023). Single-nucleus genomics in outbred rats with divergent cocaine addiction-like behaviors reveals changes in amygdala GABAergic inhibition. *Nature Neuroscience, 26*(11), 1868–1879. https://doi.org/10.1038/s41593-023-01452-y

13

Social Media, Dark Patterns and Contemporary Discourses of Addiction

Cherie Lacey, Ian Goodwin, and Antonia Lyons

It's like having a slot machine in my pocket.
(Tristan Harris, cited in Bosker, 2016)

Nearly three decades ago, Edward Tufte—professor of computer science at Yale University—wryly observed that "there are only two industries that call their customers 'users': illegal drugs and software" (Computer Literacy Bookshops, 1995). It was the mid-1990s and Tufte was telling his interviewer about his recently acquired Macintosh computer; the professor was eager to finish up the interview so he could get back to his new machine. Thirty years on, however, and this quote has entered our cultural vernacular, appearing, for example, in

C. Lacey (✉) • I. Goodwin • A. Lyons
Waipapa Taumata Rau/University of Auckland, Auckland, New Zealand
e-mail: cherie.lacey@auckland.ac.nz; ian.goodwin@auckland.ac.nz; antonia.lyons@auckland.ac.nz

B. M. Z. Cohen et al. (eds.), *Addiction and the Medicalisation of Conspicuous Behaviour*, The Politics of Mental Health and Illness,
https://doi.org/10.1007/978-3-032-06313-7_12

the popular Netflix documentary about the harmful impacts of social networking, *The Social Dilemma* (Orlowski, 2020), and printed on t-shirts or coffee mugs and sold—ironically?—by Instagram stores. Tufte's quip about 'users', made in passing to a postgraduate reporter for a small university magazine, now strikes us as uncannily prescient of a culture which has become, according to many, 'addicted' to our digital devices.

In this chapter, we examine the ways in which social media use is framed using dominant discourses of addiction in popular culture and contemporary research. We explore how these discourses of addiction are drawn upon by different actors, including the technology industry, whistleblowers, users of platforms, lawyers and lawmakers, and others, and consider the ideological work that they achieve. We critically interrogate the ways in which these dominant understandings of addiction function according to neoliberal logics, including individualising and pathologising users of social media and placing responsibility on them to manage their 'addiction', while overlooking systemic issues—including platforms and apps that are deliberately designed to keep users engaged for as long as possible. We show how whistleblowers draw on discourses of addiction to describe 'addictive' design features of social media platforms, particularly 'dark patterns' and other manipulative design techniques. Such framing of social media use is essential to understanding the phenomenon of so-called social media addiction that pervades media and other forms of popular culture, as well as in users' own accounts of their social media habits. We conclude by considering how contemporary hegemonic discourses of social media addiction do extraordinary ideological work: they reinforce individual-level framing of habitual and compulsive use of platforms, and sustain the status quo, which includes supporting dominant platform capitalist business models that prioritise profit-making above all else (Srnicek, 2017).

Discourses of Social Media Addiction

The word *addiction* originally referred to a relationship of debt between two parties. Its origins come from ancient Rome, when someone who owed money could be assigned over (*addictus*) to a creditor and become what was effectively a 'debt slave' (Rosenthal & Faris, 2019). A peasant may, for example, be 'addicted' to a wealthy landowner, forced to work to pay off their debt. In this sense, addiction might be considered a form of relationality that is marked by a kind of structural indebtedness. This same kind of enslavement economy can be identified in contemporary social media business models, which rely on users to pay with their personal data in order to use a service (Zuboff, 2019). This exchange—personal data for service use—is both powerfully imbalanced and what keeps the two parties tethered. It is also a business model that is fundamentally built on continual and habitual user engagement.

In describing their platforms and business models, social media companies conspicuously do not draw on discourses of addiction—although this is the language used by whistleblowers when they expose the practices and tactics of these companies, as we describe more fully below. Instead, they design new apps or create new affordances that are intended to help individuals manage their own use. Interestingly, the 'fixes' designed by tech firms are almost always framed in positive terms, and most often draw on the discourse of well-being or wellness to describe their functionality, such as Google's 'Be Internet Awesome' or Apple's 'Attentive'.

Yet, despite these efforts, it is increasingly common to come across the term 'social media addiction' in the media and mass culture. Popular discourse uses phrases and terminology from dominant medical understandings of addiction, which function to align social media use with more general understandings of being addicted to highly addictive substances (for example, tobacco, caffeine, methamphetamine) or (negative) behaviours (for instance, gambling). For example, as at the time of writing, there are many millions of TikTok videos that address topics such as 'social media detox' and 'social media addiction', and are tagged with "I'm a TikTok addict". Concerns about pervasive social media use have led to public declarations of social media 'detoxes' and "digital detox experiments" (Bosker, 2016), not to mention the influx of digital well-being apps to help people 'manage' their digital 'dosage'. Hundreds of thousands of parents now send their children to digital detox camps to help them break what they consider to be a harmful digital habit (Khalil, 2019).

Similarly, these ideas around social media 'addiction' have been taken up by a broad range of researchers, who also draw on dominant discourses of addiction to describe their investigations into people being addicted to their digital devices and their social media feeds. A burgeoning field has developed that investigates *nomophobia* (an abbreviation of 'no mobile phobia')—a term coined in 2008 which means "a fear of becoming incommunicable, separated from the mobile phone and losing connection to the Internet" (León-Mejía et al., 2021, p. 1). Reviews of studies suggest that the prevalence of nomophobia ranges from six to 79 percent (Banerjee et al., 2023; Bhattacharya et al., 2019; León-Mejía et al., 2021), suggesting this is a relatively common phenomenon. The language used to describe nomophobia is the language of medicine and addiction, with researchers describing people as *suffering* from the *problem* or *condition*, and as a result experiencing anxiety and other negative emotions. One review of the research concludes that nomophobia "negatively affects personality, self-esteem, anxiety, stress, academic performance, and other physical and mental health problems" (Rodríguez-García et al., 2020). Similarly, some argue that prolonged social media use is due to an individual having an "addictive personality", or traits such as high sensation-seeking (see Chen et al., 2022). Other studies have argued that individuals who suffer from screen addictions have "maladaptive cognitions", such as a "ruminative cognitive style, feelings of self-consciousness, low self-worth, a depressogenic cognitive style, low self-esteem, and social anxiety" (Davis, 2001). This research, which functions to medicalise behaviour related to engaging with the online world, can be seen as providing some validation and legitimacy for people whose excessive use disrupts their lives and everyday functioning. However, the language of addiction also reduces complex systems and structures down to individuals and their behaviour, obscuring more structural aspects that encourage (and require) such behaviour.

Users of social media platforms also draw on discourses of addiction when they describe their own experiences and practices. Research with young people shows they talk about their phone and social media use as "like an addiction" (Conroy et al., 2022). Adorjan and Ricciardelli (2021) undertook discussions with 115 Canadian teenagers about their use of digital media as well as media portrayals that suggested young people are addicted to devices and platforms. They found that the teenagers actively embraced the addiction label, and ironically positioned themselves as addicted "despite a felt sense of debased agency in relation to the power of the algorithms and affordances of the technologies mediating their use" (Adorjan & Ricciardelli, 2021, p. 45). They viewed feeling addicted as not simply arising from the technologies *per se* but also from peer group and sociality requirements. This is consistent with the notion that engagement with social media is a necessary requirement for young people to take part in civic and social life (boyd, 2014; Dobson et al., 2018).

Platforms and Devices that Are Addictive-by-Design

Since 2018, a growing body of tech-insider 'whistleblowers' have exposed the techniques used by designers to keep users 'hooked' (Eyal, 2012, 2014) to their products, such as the bottomless feed, the pull-to-refresh mechanism, variable rewards, or the auto-play function. These figures draw on addiction discourses to describe both how these techniques were developed (using insights from addiction research), and how specific features were implemented within apps and platforms to keep users continually engaged and on their devices and platforms. These whistleblowers have successfully garnered widespread media attention in an attempt to inform everyday users on the 'addictive-by-design' business model used by many tech firms, including Meta, X (formerly Twitter), Snap Inc., and Discord. For example, Aza Raskin, former Mozilla employee and the designer responsible for the infinite scroll mechanism, told a BBC journalist (Andersson, 2018),

> [m]any designers were driven to create addictive app features by the business models of the big companies that employed them … It's as if they're taking behavioural cocaine and just sprinkling it all over your interface and that's the thing that keeps you like coming back and back and back.

This use of a medicalised notion of addiction—comparing apps to cocaine—reinforces a view of behaviour as beyond users' control or agency, and frames it instead as a consequence for individuals. Similarly, in the same year (2018), *The Guardian* compared techniques used by tech firms to those used by the gambling industry, constructing them as manipulative and predatory, with potentially significant consequences for users:

> social media platforms are using the same techniques as gambling firms to create psychological dependencies and ingrain their products in the lives of their users. These methods are so effective they can activate similar mechanisms as cocaine in the brain [and] create psychological cravings. (Busby, 2018)

In this way, social media are described using an addiction discourse, with framings around 'psychological dependencies' and comparisons to drugs (cocaine) and behaviours known to be addictive (gambling). However, the emphasis here shifts from individual behaviour to technology firms—specifically, to the ways in which technology and behavioural design combine to create apps and devices that are intended to encourage prolonged and habitual use. Most prominently, many journalists have included tech addiction as part of a broader 'techlash' movement that critiques the likes of Meta (formerly Facebook) and Amazon for being "BAADD"—that is, "too big, anti-competitive, addictive and destructive to democracy" (Smith, 2018). With the benefit of a few years' hindsight, it appears that the media's engagement with these whistleblowers from 2016 onwards was crucial in beginning the process of shifting the emphasis away from individual pathology to addictive-by-design business models—while also validating the experiences of many users who felt anxious, worried, depressed, or guilty about their social media habits.

At the same time as such popular developments unfolded, academic researchers in fields such as science and technology studies and critical design studies have sought to understand the ways in which digital technologies and interface design leverage human psychology to encourage habitual use (Lacey et al., 2023; Luguri & Strahilevitz, 2021). A crucial figure in the development of 'behavioural design', as it has come to be known, is the experimental psychologist B. J. Fogg, who founded Stanford University's notorious Persuasive Tech Lab (now rebranded as the Behavior Design Lab) in 1998. The lab earned a cult-like following among entrepreneurs and engineers hoping to master Fogg's principles of behaviour design—a euphemism for what sometimes amounts to building software that nudges us towards the habits a company seeks to instil. Students studied the psychology of behaviour change, such as how clicker training for dogs and the bottomless bowl—among other methods of conditioning—can 'inspire' app design as a means for conditioning human behaviour. For example, rewarding someone with an instantaneous 'like' after they post a photo on a social media platform can reinforce the action, and potentially shift it from an occasional to a daily activity. Students also learned that the most successful sites and apps 'hook' users by tapping into deep-seated human needs, such as social approval and fear of exclusion. Harris (see Bosker, 2016) refers to these as 'hijacking techniques'—digital versions of pumping sugar, salt, and fat into junk foods in order to induce bingeing or compulsive use. Alumni of Fogg's programme include the founders of vape device Juul, Instagram, LinkedIn, and Snapchat (Samrai, 2020).

One major branch of this broader movement of behavioural design is the study of 'dark patterns' of interface design, or user-experience (UX) design. The term 'dark patterns' was coined by UX designer Harry Brignull (2010) on the website www.deceptive.design, which catalogues instances where established design patterns and user behaviours are exploited to manipulate or deceive users for the benefit of the product owner. Mathur et al. (2019, p. 2) summarise dark patterns as "interface design choices that benefit an online service by coercing, steering, or deceiving users into making decisions that, if fully informed and capable of selecting alternatives, they might not make." These design techniques are often deployed to undermine user autonomy, to encourage the user to spend more money or share more personal data, or to spend more time on a platform than they intended. There are hundreds of examples of dark patterns, but common ones include instances of 'interface interference', such as when the user finds it difficult to close out of an app's interstitial advert because the 'x' close function is too hard to find (or so small you accidentally click on the ad itself and are redirected to another website), or the 'roach motel' whereby a service makes it very easy to subscribe to, but difficult to cancel. An emerging area of dark patterns scholarship looks at the relationship between interface design and prolonged or habitual—and what has also been called 'addictive'—social media use (European Data Protection Board, 2022; Mildner et al., 2023), although there is still relatively little on this topic to date.

Dark Patterns and Social Media: A Gap in our Research and Understanding

Mildner et al. (2023) point out that, despite a growing interest in unethical design practices across numerous domains, there is a gap in research on dark patterns on social networking platforms. Most of the attention so far has been on e-commerce websites, where a growing corpus of dark patterns has been catalogued (Mathur et al., 2019). This research shows that many dark patterns are domain-specific, and so the dark patterns thus far documented in domains like online shopping cannot be wholesale applied to social networking sites (SNS). This is because the dark patterns that are used in social media interfaces need to be highly satisfying to the user, given their purpose is to keep users on the platform for as long as possible, rather than, say, to extract more money from the user—something we discuss in more detail below. To date, the small amount of work that has been conducted on social media dark patterns has focused on specific elements only (such as the account deletion process), with the exception of Mildner and colleagues' recent research (also see Montag et al., 2019). Given their popularity and domination of social space online, it seems clear that there is now an "urgent need to deepen our understanding of how SNSs harm their users through unethical design practices" (Mildner et al., 2023). In particular, Mildner et al. (2023) argue, platform interfaces that encourage *excessive* use of social media should be examined, with a view towards regulating platform design. Terms such as harm, excessive use, and unethical design do point towards an addiction framing here, although it is not explicitly used. In line with previous dark patterns scholarship that emphasises the undermining of user autonomy, this research suggests 'addictive-by-design' features encourage users to spend more time on social media than they originally intended.

In an effort to understand how SNSs use dark patterns, Milder and colleagues (2023) identified a number of "engaging strategies" used by platforms to keep users on the site for as long as possible. One particularly powerful technique in engaging strategies appears to be *variable rewards*. Delivering rewards at random has been proved to quickly and strongly reinforce behaviour. A key part of how Instagram and X's design hooks users is by routinely delivering variable rewards as part of the everyday user experience. Messages, photos, and 'likes' appear on no set schedule, so users check for them compulsively, as they are never sure when they'll receive that dopamine-activation prize (see also Lempke, 2021). Also, as Eyal has pointed out, variable rewards work affectively through creating a craving. "Feedback loops are all around us", he explains, "but predictable ones don't create desire" (cited in Cox, 2017). Variable rewards are therefore one of the most powerful dark patterns that have thus far been documented, allowing social media apps to hook millions of users. This is perhaps because research shows that levels of dopamine surge when people are expecting a reward, and so introducing variability creates a focused state, which in turn suppresses the area of the brain associated with judgement and reasoning, while activating the areas of the brain associated with wanting and desire (Courtwright, 2019; Lempke, 2021). In highlighting the ways in which dark patterns affect neurotransmitters such as dopamine, as well as brain activity and desire, this research draws on biomedical notions of addiction. This shifts agency from the user—even the desire is created by the platform—and relocates the issue as one built into the platforms and systems themselves.

Another dark pattern technique that appears highly relevant to social media is *endless scrolling*. This technique is drawn from what, in behavioural psychology, is known as the bottomless bowl experiment. The 'bottomless bowl' refers to a study that found that people eat 73 percent more soup out of a self-refilling bowl than out of regular ones, without realising they have consumed extra (see Dominus, 2023). This insight has informed how social media feeds are structured, so that the user never reaches the end of content delivery, and therefore, like endlessly refilling bowls of soup, consumes more without realising it and takes longer before feeling 'satiated'.

The *pull-to-refresh mechanism* is another technique, borrowed from slot machines, to keep people online and swiping to obtain new content for as long as possible (see Schüll, 2012a). The designer who created the pull-to-refresh mechanism—first used to update Twitter feeds in 2010—is Loren Brichter. Since then, the pull-to-refresh mechanism has become one of the most widely emulated features in apps; as Brichter himself admits, "the downward-pull action is … as intuitive as scratching an itch" (Lewis, 2017). Writing in *The Guardian,* Paul Lewis notes that the pull-to-refresh feature "appears to serve a psychological function—after all, slot machines would be far less addictive if gamblers didn't get to pull the lever themselves" (Lewis, 2017). The personalised algorithms of social media are also designed to deliver *more of what you like,* such that users are given more and more of the content that they specifically desire on the platform, which reinforces the affective cravings created through techniques like variable rewards.

Social media dark patterns such as these induce a specific affective-cognitive state in users that has been described in research on other forms of addictive behaviours, such as gambling. In Schüll's study (2012a, p. 19), gamblers described this state (or the 'zone') as being in "a trance, you're on autopilot" and "like a magnet, it just pulls you in and holds you there". Similarly, the memoirist Mary Sojourner has described video gambling as a "trancelike preoccupation in which perpetuating the trance was reward enough" (2010, p. 149). Here it is not the chance of winning to which people become addicted; rather, it is the "world-dissolving state of subjective suspension and affective calm they derive from machine play" (Schüll, 2012a, p. 19). This research and scholarship therefore suggests that social media users become 'addicted' to the state of affective calm produced within the zone of interaction, and that continuously checking social media feeds fulfils a need or craving that is deliberately created by the platforms. Although companies and some dark pattern researchers do not explicitly draw on addiction discourses, their terminology reinforces a view of creating compulsive needs and behaviours. Such framings reinforce an individualistic view of the system: the individual has needs and desires that can be fulfilled by the system (even though the system created these). These framings also work to obscure the business models of the platforms and the broader environment in which they operate.

Social Media Business Models and Their Implications

The predominant business model of social media platforms involves growing the user base as aggressively as possible, without requiring users to pay a fee for the use of the application, and then retaining and monetising users' personal data and attention. The amount of data collected from users can be vast, and can often include data from other sites and apps. Social media companies sell this data to third parties for advertising, and they are reliant on advertising revenue. As a result of this process, social media developers have a keen interest in designing their online platforms with the goal of keeping users occupied on their platform for as long as possible in order to extract more data, and then creating algorithms that process this data in real-time in order to tune feeds in ways that align content specific to users' interests. Any increase in the amount of data gathered tends to increase revenues, due to more effective micro-targeting of customised ads. As Schüll has pointed out, "Facebook, Twitter, and other [social media] companies use methods similar to the gambling industry to keep users on their sites ... In the online economy, revenue is a function of continuous user attention—which is measured in clicks and time spent" (cited in Busby, 2018).

Antonia Lyons et al. (2023) have argued that social media platforms go beyond simply placing advertising content in front of users. Rather, they "are designed to generate, analyse and apply vast amounts of personalised data in an effort to tune flows of online content" to "influence their [users'] affects, moods, emotions and desires in order to increase profits". This tuning of affect and desire includes the use of dark patterns to shape users' behaviour. For example, alcohol companies have been found to employ online techniques that have implications for promoting misinformation on social media that exploit cognitive biases in information processing, and that lead to increased sales of alcohol products and increased drinking (Petticrew et al., 2020). This has been argued to have health consequences, including driving people towards online purchase and the delivery of harmful products (Lyons et al., 2023). Meta (then Facebook) whistleblower Frances Haugen has previously commented that "Facebook has realized that if they change the algorithm to be safer, people will spend less time on the site, they'll click on less ads, [and] they'll make less money" (cited in Sullivan, 2021).

While social media companies deploy a business model that relies on prolonged and attentive use, when it comes to people who are struggling with excessive engagement with social media they enthusiastically support the notion that such 'addictive' behaviour is an affliction of a relatively small handful of individuals who are weak of will or morally compromised (Frank & Nagel, 2017)—recall the 'maladaptive cognitions' approach. This shifts the blame away from their platforms, how they are designed, and how much revenue and profit they generate, and onto individual users themselves. Compulsive users are framed as people who are unable to resist their internal impulses—an age-old public relations strategy deployed previously by industries such as tobacco and vaping, gambling, and fast food (Courtwright, 2019; Schüll, 2012b). One of the most visible ways social media companies do this is through the introduction of digital well-being tools such as Apple's Screentime or App Limits, which enable (or 'empower') the user to take control of their own 'time-on-device'.

This individualised approach to prolonged, problematic social media use is consistent with what L. Ayu Saraswati (2021, p. 5) calls the "neoliberal logic of social media". Indeed, prioritising the responsibilities of the individual as a consumer of goods and services over any structural or contextual factors in play is a key aspect of the broader neoliberal project of societal reform. As Saraswati suggests, neoliberalism is "a political-economic ideology and practice that promotes individualism, consumerism, deregulation, and transferring state power and responsibility to the individual" (2021, p. 279). While there is a strong sense of individuals being able to exercise freedom through market choice, Wendy Brown (2005, p. 44) argues neoliberal subjects are equally "controlled through their freedom"—freedom comes with the obligation to choose how to best invest in the self. This suggests, as Saraswati (2021, p. 40) argues, that neoliberalism comes to influence how we do almost everything on social media, including how we practice subjectivity, the forms our political activism takes, how we think about embodied issues like pain, suffering, and healing, and how we share emotions on social media.

The specific realm of 'social media addiction' has become a key frame within which such forms of power play out. The entrepreneurial approach to subjectivity that neoliberalism fosters extends, increasingly, into dominant business discourses as social media companies respond to techlash critiques by encouraging individuals to monitor their own 'time-on-device', as well as proffering *personalised* solutions that may be necessary due to problems of social media overuse. The manipulation of user-affect here does not solely relate to personalising content feeds to drive desire and longing, but also to personalised feelings of guilt or shame that a user experiences when their social media use extends beyond 'proper', accepted, or even ideal use (Gil, 2023). The fault, or error, is internalised. The business model that structures and encourages overuse necessarily fades into the background, as model neoliberal subjects must be "extremely autonomous, highly rational, and ever-alert masters of themselves and their decisions; constant contingency management is the task" (Schüll, 2012b). The risk of compulsive and continuous social media use, like all everyday risks in neoliberal society, is presented within a framework that emphasises the necessity of making a seemingly never-ending set of choices. Or, to put it another way, "[m]odern individuals are not merely 'free to choose' … but *obliged to be free*, to understand and enact their lives in terms of 'choice'" (Rose, 1999, p. 87; emphasis original).

Under such circumstances, discourses of social media addiction drive towards the occlusion of social media platforms' business models and political practices. Nevertheless, the business structures and political practices of platform owners remain consistent with the characterising features of the commercial determinants of health (CDOH), defined by Kickbusch et al. (2016) as "the strategies and approaches used by the private sector to promote products and choices that are detrimental to health". With this logic in mind, Zenone et al. (2023) argue that social media companies in the twenty-first century should be placed alongside the likes of fast food, tobacco, gambling and other health-harming industries as a key area of concern for public health. According to Zenone et al. (2023), social media platforms' drive towards ever higher levels of engagement, which we have analysed in terms of developing 'dark patterns' which could be argued to "elicit addictive behaviours and retain user attention for advertisement views", with high engagement in turn leading to mental health problems, particularly among young people (Khalaf et al., 2023). However, recognition of social media as a CDOH goes against what has been the prevailing trend in thinking about compulsive and excessive social media use, even in the current age of the techlash. As Zenone et al. (2023) point out, social media-related public health concerns remain too often attributed to the decisions or actions of users, or considered by-products of platform usage rather than design features. The role of social media platforms themselves, and the rationale of the companies that design them, is rarely considered. Still today, the bulk of research tends to focus on user's motivations and psychiatric profiles rather than on the social media platforms with which they engage.

Conclusions: Discourses of Addiction and 'Real' Addictive Behaviours

Our focus in this chapter has been on the ways in which discourses of addiction have been used by various groups to convey particular understandings of social media platforms, systems, and users. The term 'social media addiction' has emerged as a key ideological battlefield of our era, where the tussle is between those who position addiction as an individual problem and those who see it as a deliberate and malicious business model; users themselves appear caught in between, adopting the term 'addict' when it feels like it fits, but also internalising the guilt and shame that tends to come with the term (for further examples, see chapters in this volume from Arntsen and Campbell; Brossard et al.; Taylor). We need to ask who benefits from framing addiction as an individual problem and who benefits from seeing it as a systemic problem. The fact that different parties—from Big Tech to whistleblowers, legislators and popular media—are so invested in this notion of social media 'addiction' shows there is something quite significant at stake.

This chapter has attempted to understand how the term 'social media addiction' operates as an ideological battlefield, and identify some of the stakes in this ground. We are aware that there is a simultaneous medical debate occurring about whether social media use constitutes a 'real' addiction. 'Smartphone addiction' is not currently recognised in official medical diagnostic manuals such as the World Health Organization's (2022) *International classification of diseases* (ICD) or the American Psychiatric Association's (2022) *Diagnostic and statistical manual of mental disorders* (DSM). With respect to the general debate on the addictive nature of excessive engagement with online content, it is noteworthy that 'gaming disorder'—as a specific form of 'internet addiction'—has been included in the latest ICD (World Health Organization, 2022). This means that a first form of internet addiction is now recognised as an official health condition (Darvesh et al., 2020).

Whether or not social media addiction is classified as a 'disorder' that can be diagnosed, the medical discourse of addiction continues to pervade much of our public discourse, and it has powerful, real-life impacts and effects. For example, this discourse is used within the justice system (Stokel-Walker, 2024); as we write, in the US, Match Group—the maker of popular dating apps Tinder, Hinge and The League—are being sued for deliberately 'addicting' users to their apps. The lawsuit claims that Match Group's app designs "transform users into gamblers locked in a search for psychological rewards that Match make elusive on purpose" (Allyn, 2024). The lawsuit claims that the apps are deliberately designed to "turn users into 'addicts'" (Allyn, 2024). Other lawsuits that target addictive dark pattern design—particularly in online gaming—are reportedly on the rise (Wilde, 2024).

It is important that we critically examine the dominant discourses of social media addiction now, as tech companies are coming under increasing pressure by state legislators to account for the harm caused by their platforms (European Data Protection Board, 2022; Paul, 2024). Although there has not been the space to look too closely at the legislative landscape in this chapter, the arguments being made by Big Tech rely heavily on the neoliberal injunction of 'correct' self-management, which—as we signalled earlier—is lifted directly from the tobacco and gambling public relations playbook. The hegemonic, highly individualising discourses of social media addiction work ideologically to obscure the economic, political, and technological systems that underpin all social media platforms, and which rely on, at the most constitutive level, a relationship of dependency (*addictus*) in order to operate. This unsettles all notions of user choice and agency in this context. It also highlights the importance of identifying and understanding addiction discourses and how they function across many areas of contemporary society.

References

Adorjan, M., & Ricciardelli, R. (2021). Smartphone and social media addiction: Exploring the perceptions and experiences of Canadian teenagers. *Canadian Review of Sociology, 58*(1), 45–64. https://doi.org/10.1111/cars.12319

Allyn, B. (2024). Maker of Tinder, Hinge sued over 'addictive' dating apps that puts profits over love. *NPR*. https://www.npr.org/2024/02/14/1231513991/tinder-hinge-match-group-lawsuit

American Psychiatric Association. (2022). *Diagnostic and statistical manual of mental disorders* (5th ed.) (text rev.) American Psychiatric Association. https://doi.org/10.1176/appi.books.9780890425787

Andersson, H. (2018). Social media apps are 'deliberately' addictive to users. *BBC*. https://www.bbc.com/news/technology-44640959

Banerjee, I., Robinson, J., Kashyap, A., & Sathian, B. (2023). Nomophobia: An emerging problem. *Nepal Journal of Epidemiology, 13*(3), 1285–1287. https://doi.org/10.3126/nje.v13i3.58932

Bhattacharya, S., Bashar, M. A., Srivastava, A., & Singh, A. (2019). NOMOPHOBIA: NO MObile PHone PhoBIA. *Journal of Family Medicine and Primary Care, 8*(4), 1297–1300. https://doi.org/10.4103/jfmpc.jfmpc_71_19

Bosker, B. (2016). The binge breaker. *The Atlantic*. https://www.theatlantic.com/magazine/archive/2016/11/the-binge-breaker/501122/

boyd, d. (2014). *It's complicated: The social lives of networked teens*. Yale University Press.

Brignull, H. (2010). Deceptive patterns [website]. www.deceptive.design.

Brown, W. (2005). *Edgework: Critical essays on knowledge and politics*. Princeton University Press.

Busby, M. (2018). Social media copies gambling methods 'to create psychological cravings'. *The Guardian*. https://www.theguardian.com/technology/2018/may/08/social-media-copies-gambling-methods-to-create-psychological-cravings

Chen, B., Chen, M., Wu, Y., & Wu, Y. T. (2022). The relationship of social media addiction with internet use and perceived health: The moderating effects of regular exercise intervention. *Frontiers in Public Health, 10*, 854532. https://doi.org/10.3389/fpubh.2022.854532

Computer Literacy Bookshops. (1995). Interview with Edward R. Tufte. *Computer Literacy Bookshops*. https://kkh.ltrr.arizona.edu/kkh/dendro/PDFs.Tufte/Edward%20R.%20Tufte%20%2D%2D%20CLB%20Interview%20 1994-1997.pdf

Conroy, D., Chadwick, D., Fullwood, C., & Lloyd, J. (2022). You have to know how to live with it without getting to the addiction part: British young adult experiences of smartphone overreliance and disconnectivity. *Psychology of Popular Media, 12*(4), 471–480. https://doi.org/10.1037/ppm0000425

Courtwright, D. (2019). *The age of addiction: How bad habits became big business*. Belknap Press.

Cox, T. (2017). How to create addictive content (that people love). *Yellowstep: B2B Marketing Performance*. https://blog.yellowstep.co.uk/how-to-create-addictive-content

Darvesh, N., Radhakrishnan, A., Lachance, C. C., Nincic, V., Sharpe, J. P., Ghassemi, M., Straus, S. E., & Tricco, A. C. (2020). Exploring the prevalence of gaming disorder and internet gaming disorder: A rapid scoping review. *Systemic Reviews, 9*, 68. https://doi.org/10.1186/s13643-020-01329-2

Davis, R. (2001). A cognitive-behavioral model of pathological internet use. *Computers in Human Behavior, 17*(2), 187–195. https://doi.org/10.1016/S0747-5632(00)00041-8

Dobson, A. S., Carah, N., & Robards, B. (2018). Digital intimate publics and social media: Towards theorising public lives on private platforms. In A. S. Dobson, B. Robards, & N. Carah (Eds.), *Digital intimate publics and social media* (pp. 3–27). Palgrave Macmillan. https://doi.org/10.1007/978-3-319-97607-5_1

Dominus, L. (2023). In search of 'finity' in the face of the endless online landscape. *The Michigan Daily.* https://www.michigandaily.com/opinion/in-search-of-finity-in-the-face-of-the-endless-online-landscape/

European Data Protection Board. (2022). Guidelines 3/2022 on dark patterns in social media platform interfaces: How to recognise and avoid them. *EDPB.* https://edpb.europa.eu/our-work-tools/documents/public-consultations/2022/guidelines-32022-dark-patterns-social-media_en

Eyal, N. (2012). Want to hook your users? Drive them crazy. *TechCrunch.* https://techcrunch.com/2012/03/25/want-to-hook-your-users-drive-them-crazy/

Eyal, N. (2014). *Hooked: How to build habit-forming products.* Random House.

Frank, L. E., & Nagel, S. K. (2017). Addiction and moralisation: The role of the underlying model of addiction. *Neuroethics, 10*(1), 129–139. https://doi.org/10.1007/s12152-017-9307-x

Gil, R. (2023). *Perfect: Feeling judged on social media.* Wiley.

Khalaf, A., Alubied, A., Khalaf, A. M., & Rafaey, A. (2023). The impact of social media on the mental health of adolescents and young adults: A systematic review. *Cureus, 15*(8), e42990. https://doi.org/10.7759/cureus.42990

Khalil, S. (2019). Parents are sending their technology-addicted kids to digital detox bootcamp. *news.com.au.* https://www.news.com.au/lifestyle/parenting/kids/parents-are-sending-their-technologyaddicted-kids-to-digital-detox-bootcamp/news-story/8d7f16a0250ccb8cd88b99d1c38ac693

Kickbusch, I., Allen, L., & Franz, C. (2016). The commercial determinants of health. *The Lancet Global Health, 4(12), e895–e896.* https://doi.org/10.1016/s2214-109x(16)30217-0

Lacey, C., Beattie, A., & Sparks, T. (2023). Clusters of dark patterns across popular websites in New Zealand. *International Journal of Communication, 17,* 3164–3188.

Lempke, A. (2021). *Dopamine nation: Why our addiction to pleasures is causing us pain.* Penguin Random House.

León-Mejía, A. C., Gutiérrez-Ortega, M., Serrano-Pintado, I., & González-Cabrera, J. (2021). A systematic review on nomophobia prevalence: Surfacing results and standard guidelines for future research. *PloS one, 16*(5), e0250509. https://doi.org/10.1371/journal.pone.0250509

Lewis, P. (2017). 'Our minds can be hijacked': The tech insiders who fear a smartphone dystopia. *The Guardian*. https://www.theguardian.com/technology/2017/oct/05/smartphone-addiction-silicon-valley-dystopia#:~:text=It%20is%20the%20possibility%20of,design%20features%20in%20modern%20technology

Luguri, J., & Strahilevitz, L. J. (2021). Shining a light on dark patterns. *Journal of Legal Analysis, 13*(1), 43–109. https://doi.org/10.1093/jla/laaa006

Lyons, A., Goodwin, I., Carah, N., Young, J., Moewaka Barnes, A., & McCreanor, T. (2023). Limbic platform capitalism: Understanding the contemporary marketing of health-demoting products on social media. *Addiction Research & Theory, 31*(3), 178–183. https://doi.org/10.1080/16066359.2022.2124976

Mathur, A., Acar, G., Friedman, M., Lucherini, E., Mayer, J., Chetty, M., & Narayanan, A. (2019). Dark patterns at scale: Findings from a crawl of 11k shopping websites. *Proceedings of the ACM Conference on Human-Computer Interaction, 3*(CSCW), 1–32. https://doi.org/10.1145/3359183

Mildner, Y., Savino, G., Doyle, P. R., Cowan, B. R., & Malaka, R. (2023). About engaging and governing strategies: A thematic analysis of dark patterns in social networking services. *Proceedings of the 2023 CHI Conference on Human Factors in Computing Systems*, 1–15. https://doi.org/10.1145/3544548.358069

Montag, C., Lachmann, B., Herrlich, M., & Zweig, K. (2019). Addictive features of social media/messenger platforms and freemium games against the background of psychological and economic theories. *International Journal of Environmental Research and Public Health, 16*(14), 2612. https://doi.org/10.3390/ijerph16142612

Orlowski, J. (Director). (2020). *The Social Dilemma* [film]. Exposure Labs.

Paul, K. (2024). Zuckerberg tells parents of social media victims at Senate hearing: 'I'm sorry for everything you've been through'. *The Guardian*. https://www.theguardian.com/us-news/2024/jan/31/tiktok-meta-x-congress-hearing-child-sexual-exploitation

Petticrew, M., Maani, N., Pettigrew, L., Rutter, H., & Van Schalkwyk, M. C. (2020). Dark nudges and sludge in big alcohol: Behavioral economics, cognitive biases, and alcohol industry corporate social responsibility. *Milbank Quarterly, 98*(4), 1290–1328. https://doi.org/10.1111/1468-0009.12475

Rodríguez-García, A. M., Moreno-Guerrero, A. J., & Lopez Belmonte, J. (2020). Nomophobia: An individual's growing fear of being without a smartphone—A systematic literature review. *International Journal of Environmental Research and Public Health, 17*(2), 580. https://doi.org/10.3390/ijerph17020580

Rose, N. (1999). *Powers of freedom: Reframing political thought.* Cambridge University Press.

Rosenthal, R. J., & Faris, S. (2019). The etymology and early history of 'addiction'. *Addiction Research & Theory, 27*(5), 437–449. https://doi.org/10.1080/16066359.2018.1543412

Samrai, Y. (2020). How Stanford profits off addiction. *The Stanford Review.* https://stanfordreview.org/how-stanford-profits-tech-addiction-social-media/

Saraswati, L. A. (2021). *Pain generation: Social media, feminist activism, and the neoliberal selfie.* New York University Press.

Schüll, N. D. (2012a). *Addiction by design: Machine gambling in Las Vegas.* Princeton University Press.

Schüll, N. D. (2012b). Gambled away: Video poker and self-suspension. *Anthropology Now, 4*(2), 1–13. https://doi.org/10.1080/19492901.2012.11728356

Smith, E. (2018). The techlash against Amazon, Facebook and Google—and what they can do. *The Economist.* https://www.economist.com/briefing/2018/01/20/the-techlash-against-amazon-facebook-and-google-and-what-they-can-do

Sojourner, M. (2010). *She bets her life: A true story of gambling addiction.* Seal Press.

Srnicek, N. (2017). *Platform capitalism.* Wiley.

Stokel-Walker, C. (2024). Can a lawsuit make social media less 'addictive'? Politicians are about to find out. *BBC.* https://www.bbc.com/future/article/20240626-can-a-law-make-social-media-less-addictive

Sullivan, M. (2021). Facebook is harming our society: Here's a radical solution for reigning it in. *The Washington Post.* https://www.washingtonpost.com/lifestyle/media/media-sullivan-facebook-whistleblower-haugen/2021/10/04/3461c62e-2535-11ec-8831-a31e7b3de188_story.html

Wilde, T. (2024). Lawyer warns game developers about 'unlawful game design' as 'dark patterns' lawsuits rise. *PC Gamer.* https://www.pcgamer.com/gaming-industry/dark-patterns-in-games-gdc-2024/

World Health Organization. (2022). *ICD-11: International classification of diseases.* World Health Organization.

Zenone, M., Kenworthy, N., & Maani, N. (2023). The social media industry as a commercial determinant of health. *International Journal of Health Policy and Management, 12*, 6840. https://doi.org/10.34172/IJHPM.2022.6840

Zuboff, S. (2019). *The age of surveillance capitalism: The fight for a human future at the new frontier of power*. PublicAffairs.

14

The Instrumentalization of the Concept of 'Gambling Addiction': A Discourse Analysis of German Parliamentary Debates

Gerd Möll

How society defines the problem of gambling addiction and what measures are taken to deal with it depends on the specific knowledge about the problem that is generated and disseminated in the prevailing scientific, public (media) and political discourses. A number of studies have examined the discursive construction of so-called 'problematic' and 'pathological' gambling behaviour and its changes over time (Castellani, 2000; Ferentzy & Turner, 2013; Reichertz, this volume; Reith, 2007, 2018; Schmidt, 1999, 2012; Wilcox, 2021). Previous research has also pointed to the importance of political actors in the discursive construction of the concept of problem gambling (Markham & Young, 2015; Matilainen, 2017; Tammi, 2014). However, there is a lack of research on how gambling addiction is understood as a social problem in parliamentary debates (Miller et al., 2015). This is a serious research gap, as it is the political discourses that contribute significantly to the definition of this

G. Möll (✉)
Institute for Advanced Study in the Humanities, Essen, Germany

B. M. Z. Cohen et al. (eds.), *Addiction and the Medicalisation of Conspicuous Behaviour*, The Politics of Mental Health and Illness,
https://doi.org/10.1007/978-3-032-06313-7_13

problem area, the groups affected and the moral judgements involved (Goedecke et al., 2023; Selin, 2022).

Parliamentary debates are a comparatively visible part of the political discourse in democratically constituted societies and thus a suitable object of study. In the case of gambling addiction, these debates influence public opinion about the specific issues, causes and consequences of problem gambling and thus contribute to the institutionalisation of the knowledge order in this field of practice. In turn, the discursively constructed order of knowledge (Keller, 2011b; Keller et al., 2013) has a crucial impact on which measures are considered and selected to deal with gambling addiction, as well as which institutions are legitimised as having responsibility for it (Conrad & Barker, 2010).

The majority of contributions to the scientific and public debate on gambling focus on the question of which measures are suitable for combating the problem of gambling addiction. Gambling addiction is seen as a phenomenon whose existence can no longer be denied and whose extent can be demonstrated in regular empirical surveys (Bundeszentrale für gesundheitliche Aufklärung, 2010). Using the example of the parliamentary discourse on gambling in Germany, the following discussion will substantiate the thesis that the fight against gambling addiction is indeed generally placed in the foreground by the participants in the political discourse. In reality, however, this intention often serves as a pretext for pursuing completely different goals.

Methodology

The main steps in the study of German parliamentary discourse on which this chapter is based (Möll, 2021) was the collection of data (the corpus building), the selection of specifically identified discourse for further investigation, and the detailed analysis of this data. The examination of the parliamentary documents was based on the analysis proposed by Schetsche (2014) for the study of social problems, as well as on the sociological discourse analysis of knowledge (Keller, 2011a, 2011b). Most of the parliamentary documents were investigated through the use of content analysis. Selected documents or parts of documents were also analysed by hermeneutic methods (Hitzler et al., 1999).

The *federal parliament* (the *Bundestag*) and the sixteen *state parliaments* are the central organs of German legislation. As these institutions traditionally (also) address the public, it was possible to comprehensively analyse the perception of gambling-related problems as expressed directly by the members of the parliaments. This analysis was based on the relevant plenary and committee documents as well as government inquiries and legislative proposals. The information systems of the state parliaments and the Bundestag—which are freely accessible and searchable on the internet—provided access to parliamentary documents relevant to the project study. The search for documents was mainly based on the terms 'Glücksspiel' (gambling), 'Glücksspielsucht' (gambling addiction), 'Spielhallen' (gaming halls), 'Spielbank' (casino), 'Sportwetten' (sports betting), and 'Lotterie' (lottery).

Although the term 'gambling addiction' did not feature prominently in parliamentary discourse until the mid-1980s, it seemed advisable to consider earlier debates on gambling. It was assumed that knowledge of the arguments for and against commercial gambling that were put forward in the early stages of the debates in the Federal Republic of Germany (that is, the country of West Germany, before Germany was reunified in 1990) could clarify the current discussion on gambling. Therefore, the corpus of gambling-related documents in the state parliaments of Bavaria, North Rhine-Westphalia, Schleswig-Holstein, Berlin and Hesse as well as in the Bundestag for the period between the foundation of the respective parliaments after the end of the Second World War and the year 2019 were systematically examined. A total of around 2,000 documents with a volume of approximately 7,000 pages were viewed. The analysis focused on the plenary debates and hearings that represent key themes in the German gambling discourse and are particularly relevant to the field of gambling addiction. Specifically, these themes were the relicensing of casinos, the regulation of gaming halls and gambling machines, the liberalisation of the (online) gambling market, and the introduction of a multi-venue exclusion programme.

Relevant rulings by the Federal Constitutional Court, administrative courts and the European Court of Justice have repeatedly had a significant influence on the parliamentary debate on gambling and gambling addiction. It was therefore inevitable to include key court decisions in the body of the texts to be examined. The study also included the minutes of the Conference of Minister-Presidents when important decisions on the regulation of gambling were on the agenda.

The analysis of parliamentary hearings on gambling-related issues proved to be extremely informative. The positions of gambling experts and interest groups presented at these hearings provided a helpful overview of relevant discourse positions beyond the parliamentary parties. Parliamentary hearings are also a place to observe which individuals and groups of actors are allowed to participate in the social discourse at all.

Results: Morality, Medicalisation and Money

The discourse on gambling in the parliaments of the Federal Republic of Germany were characterised early on by a post-prohibition orientation. However, there have always been counter-movements in favour of bans or at least significant restrictions on gambling. The resulting disputes usually took place within the framework of two opposite positions: namely, a 'gambling-critical' and a 'gambling-friendly' strand of discourse. The gambling-critical position primarily emphasised the *social threats* posed by commercial gambling. The issues at stake ranged from Christian morality to urban planning ideals, from the state monopoly on gambling to the mental health of gamblers and society. In contrast, the gambling-friendly camp defined gambling services as a normal *consumer good*, and preferred to focus on defending the liberties of gambling providers and consumers. Using the term 'consumer' expresses the liberal view that freedom involves the right to consume and that citizens are consumers in a market.

As a result of this bipolar constellation of discourses, ambivalence emerged in the parliamentary debates on the regulation of commercial gambling. For a long time, there was a tendency towards permissiveness, although this never meant the end of state control. This trend has given way to an ongoing struggle between permissive and restrictive positions, which has ultimately led to the liberalisation of online gambling markets and the introduction of new forms of control over gamblers.

The Moral Side of Gambling and the Re-Authorisation of Casinos

The first clash between the two opposing gambling discourses took place just a few years after the end of the Second World War. The scene was the Bavarian state parliament, where the re-authorisation of casinos in Bavarian health resorts was on the agenda. Critics of casinos saw Christian morality and the work ethic in danger. One Catholic delegate, for example, described the revenue casinos generated for the state as "sinful money with a dark, sinister, demonic power attached to it" (Weber, 1952, p. 8287, English translation by the author). Representatives of Protestant asceticism saw casinos as "a mockery of honest work made flesh" (Bausch, 1952, p. 8289, English translation by the author). The dangers of addiction were also cited by casino opponents. However, this was still without any pathological connotations. Though there was occasional talk of gambling addiction, most parliamentarians spoke of a "passion for gambling", "gambling mania", or even the "gambling devil" which led people to gamble uncontrollably and to financial ruin.

Those in favour of casinos pointed to the tax revenue they would generate. This would be essential for (post-war) reconstruction and could be used for housing. At the same time, it was pointed out that nowhere in the world had it been possible to enforce an effective ban on public gambling; unauthorised gambling behind closed doors had always existed despite such bans. The causes of this situation were localised in the "urge to play" and "enjoyment of playing". From this, it was concluded that a responsible government would never ask itself whether gambling should be officially organised at all (or not). Rather, the question was whether the existing gambling instinct could only be pursued in "forbidden gambling dens" or whether it would better to take place in "state-licensed and strictly monitored casinos".

The idea that every "decent citizen" must have the right to do what they want with their own money, including giving away their fortune to someone else through gambling, was also emphasised in the pro-gambling discourse. However, this discourse strand considered gambling immoral if it was either carried out in an excessive manner and in disregard of social obligations, or if it was carried out in morally dubious, illegal places. Even though casinos were eventually re-licensed and fiscal and freedom arguments came to the fore, moral reservations about excessive forms of gambling have by no means disappeared, even on the part of gambling advocates.

Medicalising Gambling Addiction as a Means of Dealing with Urban Planning Problems

Since the mid-1970s, the ever-increasing proliferation of amusement arcades in German city centres has been the subject of a debate about the curse or blessing of this gambling institution. The first part of society to be confronted with the problems associated with gaming halls were the urban centres. In many cities, the rapid growth of the number of gaming halls was seen to contradict the prevailing model of a lively and attractive city centre. This led to social and economic unease being expressed by various stakeholders. Parliamentarians cited not only the reactions of shopkeepers as evidence of the problems associated with the proliferation of amusement arcades, but also the negative attitudes of large sections of the population towards gambling. Although the parliamentary actors themselves no longer spoke of "sin" in connection with gambling, they nevertheless revived this moral interpretation by invoking the "voice of the people". This meant that gaming halls were defined as a source of problems not only from an urban planning perspective, but also from a moral and socio-political perspective. However, the basic right to freedom of trade and of profession meant that gaming halls could not simply be banned. From an urban planning point of view, it was a kind of 'serendipity' that the issue of gambling addiction came to the fore in Germany in the early 1980s and could be used in the fight to reduce the number of gaming halls.

With the publication in 1980 of the third version of the *Diagnostic and statistical manual of mental disorders* (the DSM-III)—a classification system published by the American Psychiatric Association that includes descriptions, symptoms and other criteria for mental disorders—the socially deviant act of excessive gambling became a disease. 'Pathological gambling' was categorised as an "impulse control disorder", yet nothing was mentioned about the causes of this 'disease' (see American Psychiatric Association, 1980, pp. 291–293). However, this was due to the general nature of the DSM, which only classifies mental disorders, but neither explains their development nor guides their treatment (Paris and Phillips, 2013; Rüppel, 2022). The diagnosis was based on a checklist of behavioural symptoms. Endeavouring to gain social recognition as a discipline, this form of descriptive diagnosis had the advantage for psychiatry that it did not have to rely on ideas about the nature and causes of mental illness that were difficult or impossible to prove (Rantala & Sulkunen, 2012). From a therapeutic point of view, the classification systems were associated with the fact that it remained unclear on which therapy-relevant causes the clinical pictures designed could have been based. However, even if the corresponding diagnoses are merely based on a list of symptoms and behavioural consequences, they claim to be able to differentiate between normal and pathological behaviour (see also Reichertz, this volume).

It is remarkable that an attentive look at the moral theological writings of the nineteenth century—which dominated the public discourse on problem gambling at the time, at least in America and England—can reveal something striking: in today's specialist scientific interpretations of pathological gambling, the assessments of moral theologians shine through with great clarity (Bernhard, 2007; Bernhard et al., 2010). All the criteria that have found their way into modern medical literature obviously have historical precursors. The morally saturated writings of past centuries—which lamented the dark and diabolical aspects of gambling—have found echoes in modern medicine and psychiatry. What was once described as a moral problem has thus become a medical-psychiatric problem. In other words, the medical-psychiatric terminology used to describe and diagnose pathological gambling is based on moral judgments (Bernhard, 2007; Cohen et al., this volume).

In Germany, the thesis of pathological gambling was formulated by the Bremen psychologist Gerhard Meyer using the example of gambling machines. This view, reinforced by relevant articles in popular magazines, quickly found resonance in some state parliaments. In various hearings, the parliamentarians were confronted with the internal scientific controversies about the appropriateness of the concept of gambling addiction. However, the parliamentarians were only moderately inspired or even impressed by the scientific discourse. Only occasionally did they attempt to take up the criticism of the concept of addiction levelled by certain scientists.

Basically, there was no debate between the parliamentary groups on the concept of addiction. Initially, there was still an alternative discourse that saw the social problem not in the "supposed gambling addiction", but above all in the threat to civil liberties posed by the gambling addiction discourse. However, even in the context of this discourse—which focused on the right to free development of the personality and freedom of occupation—the concept of gambling addiction was adopted after initial criticism. The notion of addiction thus found its way into the parliamentary gambling discourse quite quickly and with little resistance. Even though official health institutions have moved away from the 'addiction' term because of its pejorative connotations, the use of the term has usually been retained in the speeches of parliamentarians, although "pathological gambling" and "problem gambling" are also occasionally used.

As a result, gambling addiction was recognised as a social problem to which policymakers had to respond. The argument of combating gambling addiction now could be used to justify restrictive gambling policies against the much lamented "flood of gaming halls". This led, for example, to a significant increase in the amusement tax for slot machines. The phrase "flood of gaming halls", which appeared more and more frequently in parliamentary debates from 1987 onwards, popularised a term used in the context of natural disasters and usually associated with the occurrence of an uncontrollable threat. Even more clearly, the term "amusement arcade nuisance" (in German, *Spielhallenunwesen*), also found in the debates, resonated with "what constitutes the core content of the problem claim: the judgement of unworthiness of the state of affairs so designated" (Schetsche, 2014, p. 112).

However, the efforts to close down gaming halls by pointing to the risks of gambling addiction were not particularly successful. On the one hand, the arcade industry found ways to counteract all strategies aimed at making the operation of an arcade financially unattractive. On the other hand, the state became increasingly accustomed to the revenues generated by the operation of gaming halls. As a result, many attempts to restrict the gaming hall market have been half-hearted and the concept of gambling addiction has lost much of its public appeal.

Fighting Addiction as an Argument for Guaranteeing Gambling as a Source of Government Revenue

With the ruling of the Federal Constitutional Court in March 2006, the German state monopoly on sports betting (namely, the licensed betting provider Oddset) came under considerable pressure. During the court proceedings, the phenomenon of gambling addiction unexpectedly received renewed attention, as the legislature had turned to the argument of player protection in the fight to uphold this monopoly (Reichert, 2019). Of all the arguments put forward in favour of the state monopoly, this was the only one to be accepted by the Federal Constitutional Court (Reichert, 2019, p. 288).

However, as the constitutional judges did not consider the consistent orientation of the monopoly towards the fight against addiction to be a given, the federal states (or, if applicable, the federal government) were called upon to enact a constitutionally compliant regulation by the end of 2007. From the point of view of the constitutional judges, two alternatives were possible: either a state monopoly strictly oriented towards the goal of actively combating gambling addiction, or a legally standardised and controlled license for private betting companies. The Constitutional Court's ruling was the beginning of a debate that soon went beyond sports betting. The regulatory model for commercial gambling of all kinds was up for discussion.

It was the northernmost federal state in Germany, Schleswig-Holstein, where the debate about the future of commercial gambling was most intense and which ultimately played a pioneering role in the liberalisation of the gambling market. The parliamentary debates argued either for maintaining the state gambling monopoly or for opening the gambling market to private (internet) providers. The argument in favour of maintaining the state gambling monopoly, which represented the gambling-critical point of view and was put forward by members of the Social Democratic Party, was as follows: due to its lack of profit orientation, the state is in a much better position than private companies to successfully combat the problem of gambling addiction. On the other hand, the legalisation of private operators interested in increasing their profits would not only lead to an increase in the supply of gambling, but also to a greater number of gambling addicts. Furthermore, it was feared that the increase in revenues from the gambling market would be at the expense of gambling addicts and their families. The social normalisation of gambling and the associated invitation to excessive spending, it was argued, must not be encouraged. Despite these justified concerns about the disintegrative effects of gambling, the aim was not to ban gambling, but rather to restrict its supply under state control, while strictly observing the protection of players and young people and resolutely combating the criminal activities that accompany it.

The arguments of the proponents of opening the market to private gambling service providers, representing the pro-gambling strand of the Christian Democratic and Liberal Party discourse, can be summarised as follows: maintaining the state gambling monopoly neither solves the problem of gambling addiction nor ensures that state revenues from gambling can be used for public welfare purposes. Since blocking the internet is neither possible nor desirable, the relevant gambling services must be legalised. A regulated license for private gambling service providers has the advantage that the state gains control over the previously unregulated and illegal parts of the gambling market. The controlled autonomy of the industry results in higher government revenues from gambling taxes and concession fees, which can also be used for addiction prevention purposes. In addition, private gambling service providers can also be obliged to effectively combat gambling addiction. This is particularly true in the online market, they argued, where competition will ensure sufficient player protection.

The differences between the competing discourse strands relate primarily to the favoured form of gambling regulation. At the centre of the debate was the question of whether a state monopoly on gambling was superior to a private-sector form of regulation. Although this debate was fuelled by competing visions of social and economic order, the various discourse positions felt compelled to integrate the problem pattern of gambling addiction into their respective arguments and thus to use it for their preferred solutions. However, it was never just a question of how to prevent and effectively combat gambling addiction, but rather also a problem of how the state would secure revenue from taxes and duties on the gambling business.

The Gaming Hall Industry Is Presented as a Pioneer in the Fight Against Gambling Addiction

At the beginning of the debate on gambling addiction in the 1980s, the gaming hall industry and the parliamentary representatives of the pro-gambling side of the debate tried to deny or at least play down the phenomenon. Twenty years later, when amusement arcades once again became the focus of political debate (mainly because of a reform of federalism, in which regulatory competences were shifted to the federal states), a completely different picture emerged. Several parliamentarians now recognised the industry as one of the key players in the fight against addiction. It was proposed that their role is to "channel" the so-called "natural gaming instinct" of the population and thereby prevent the emergence of an illegal market.

For this reason, the attractiveness of gambling machines should not be unduly restricted in terms of limits on stakes, losses and winnings. Accordingly, gaming halls were presented not as part of the problem but as part of the solution, whose positive effects should not be hindered by excessive regulation. This view was underpinned by the assertion that it was not the games on offer that were the cause of the development of a 'gambling addiction', but rather pathological structures in the player's personality. It was therefore necessary to strengthen the operators in their responsibility to recognise, avoid and prevent abuse. The focus here was on the training of staff in gambling venues with regard to the early detection of players at risk. There is now even a joint venture between three arcade operators (namely, Löwen Entertainment, Löwen Play and

Schmidt.Gruppe) to provide such training also for gaming hall staff of other operators. In this way, revenue is generated from dealing with a problem that the industry itself helped to create. More important than the financial return, however, is the gain in legitimacy that is sought with this offer, as the gaming hall industry can be presented as a committed fighter against gambling addiction.

A specific feature of the German debate on gaming halls, in contrast to international discussion on this issue, is that the gambling industry talks much less about 'responsible gambling' and much more about the quality of the products they offer. For years, the associations of the gaming hall industry have been strongly promoting the 'certification' of their member companies. Certification is based on quality management philosophy and is conducted by independent auditing organisations. The aim is to formalise operational processes and procedures in the organisation of a gaming hall in order to protect players. At the same time it is intended to help differentiate them from illegal gambling operators. Parliamentarians representing the pro-gambling discourse have commented favourably on this initiative. Ultimately, the quality argument (and thus the documented intention to actively participate in addiction prevention) helps to counteract parliamentary criticism of the gaming hall industry, even though no evidence has yet been produced to prove the effectiveness of the measures initiated (Hayer et al., 2020). This form of preventing addiction turns out to be more of a "productive fiction" (Schulz & Müller, 2019) than an empirically verified fact.

Extensive Social Control of Gamblers

In the course of securing state revenues from gambling and solving urban development problems, parliaments have already adopted a number of measures to regulate land-based (offline) gambling. In this context, the instrument of exclusion of gamblers from gambling venues has recently become particularly important. The exclusion of a player (whether by self-exclusion or third-party exclusion) requires that access to gaming halls is strictly controlled. Each player will have to present an identity document at the entrance in order to check whether they are listed in the file of banned participants. Together with the introduction of a player card—which is required to unlock and play a slot machine—this is the first building block of a new control regime that will make anonymous gambling in legal venues impossible.

In particular, the introduction of self-exclusion placed the affected gamblers in a paradoxical situation, as it was assumed that, despite their addiction problem, they were capable of self-critical reflection on their gambling behaviour. This paradox seemed to be solvable in terms of time because, at least in 'moments of sudden insight', it was assumed that the gambler should be able to make a responsible decision. However, the limitations of these preventive measures are obvious. For example, research from Lischer et al. (2016) has shown that prohibited and high-risk gamblers switch to alternative gambling services in large numbers. A recent empirical study on the increase in illegal gambling in Germany confirms this finding (Trümper, 2021).

The development of comprehensive control strategies will be driven by the new Interstate Treaty on Gambling (the *Glücksspielstaatsvertrag*; see for example, https://www.idnow.io/glossary/gluecksspielstaatsvertrag-glustv/), which came into force in July 2021 and allows online gambling under certain conditions. Licensed gambling platforms will be obliged to closely monitor their customers' gambling behaviour. Not only does this include setting deposit limits for all players, but the new monitoring regime also requires platform operators to use software to identify "problem gambling" (Becker, 2022). Information will be collected not only on pathological and problem gamblers, but on the entire population of gamblers. On the pretext of combating gambling addiction, it has become possible to control the gambling activities of a large part of the population whose gambling behaviour was previously inconspicuous.

Discussion

The history of the parliamentary discourse on gambling addiction in Germany can be read as a history of the instrumentalization of this problem for a wide variety of interests. The *social construction* of gambling addiction (Berger & Luckmann, 1966; Keller et al., 2013) has contributed to solving other problems alongside legitimising certain institutional interests and the measures derived from them. In the field of urban development, this can be traced back to the early 1980s when the concerns of the city planners were justified with addiction policy arguments (Becker, 2016). Subsequently, the argument of combating gambling addiction has been used to legitimise the enforcement of certain forms of gambling regulation. Initially, this was used to justify the preservation of the state gambling monopoly. The argument of player protection and addiction prevention is now being used to justify the legalisation of online gambling by private operators.

In addition, the gambling industry has not only adopted the addiction-related directives passed by parliaments, but has also tried to claim a leading role in the field of addiction prevention. In doing so, the state is ceding to the private sector the competence it has long claimed for itself in the fight against addiction. However, despite the risks associated with gambling, the aim is always to maintain it as a source of revenue for the state.

Against this background, there is much to be said for not taking the widely postulated objectives of player protection and addiction prevention at face value. Rather, it seems more realistic to assume that the measures in question are less about protecting players from the dangers of gambling than about protecting political and economic interests from the threats posed by the behaviour of certain types of players (for a similar line of argumentation regarding addiction prevention in general, see Dollinger, 2006). However, it is not only economic and regulatory interests that are protected by the reference to the fight against gambling addiction, but also an important component of social reality: namely, the moral order.

The negation of meritocratic principles inscribed in gambling and the associated "profanation of money" (Bjerg, 2009) challenge essential components of the moral order. Gambling is not only played *for* money—as in the lottery, where the dream of winning big plays a key role (Lutter, 2010)—but also *with* money. This is especially true of slot machines, where money is usually the means, rather than the ends, of gambling (Reichertz et al., 2008; Schüll, 2012). However, this profanation of money does not only challenge the socially accepted relationship between effort and reward, between labour and its wage, and between performance and gratification. It also challenges the role of money as the sublime object of desire in capitalism. Especially for those gamblers who do not primarily play for but with money, and especially for those who are classified as problem gamblers, there is always a risk that money will be de-sublimated, making it impossible for them to "function as an ordinary capitalist subject" (Bjerg, 2009, p. 47).

Political science research claims that historically there has been a 'de-moralisation' of gambling and correspondingly permissive regulatory consequences (Euchner et al., 2013). Even if this claim were limited to the declining effectiveness of Catholic and Protestant morality, it would be difficult to agree with. It is true that hardly anyone speaks of 'sin' in connection with gambling any more. At the same time, however, the careless handling of money is regarded in psychiatric diagnostic manuals—and not only there—as an unmistakable characteristic of problem and pathological gamblers. It is precisely this misbehaviour that is repeatedly attested to excessive gamblers. The corresponding medical and psychiatric expertise serves to reinforce the moral ideal of the self-responsible consumer as a foil for criticism. Thus, a distinction is made between pathological and non-pathological cases, depending on the number of diagnostic criteria met by the individual concerned, with some being denied participation in gambling and others being allowed to participate (in a controlled manner). This classification suggests that moral criteria for evaluating gambling are still valid, but they are covered by the postulate of protecting gamblers. At the same time, these moral criteria help to secure the existing social order (see also Schetsche, 2013).

Outlook

In the parliamentary discourse on gambling, the relationship between individual freedom and social control of gamblers has always been ambivalent. It is worth noting that this relationship has changed in favour of a new form of control, not least because of the liberalisation of gambling markets. On the one hand, it appears that gamblers are being encouraged to work continuously on their ability to control themselves. However, not only have opportunities been created that make 'self-controlled' gambling behaviour more likely (for example, time-limited self-exclusion or options for self-defined wagering limits). At the same time, structural measures (for instance, internet blocking and restrictions on slot machines) make it more difficult or impossible to access certain gambling services or to engage in high-risk forms of gambling. Following Mark Elam (in this volume) these measures could be described as 'disarming innovations'.

Nevertheless, it is still largely an open question as to what the future form of gambling control in Germany will look like and what implications this will have for gamblers and their gambling behaviour. In order to find an instructive answer, it is necessary to go beyond the level of discourse and to clarify how and by whom social control is institutionally implemented, how the affected gamblers and gambling companies react, and what obstacles and evasive manoeuvres can be observed. For example, legal gambling hall operators have recently called for the withdrawal of disarming innovations that limit the winnings and losses or reduce the speed of play, because many players have switched to illegal operators who not only do not care about player protection and addiction but also do not pay taxes. It remains to be seen whether this demand will be successful.

For the time being, the only thing that seems clear is that no homogeneous and consistent control regime is likely to emerge in the foreseeable future, as the regulation of gambling is a contested field in which state and private actors fight for recognition of their position in the discourse as a guideline for action. As a result, there is always the possibility that, as in the past, the fight against 'gambling addiction' will be used as a pretext for other intentions, with the aim of protecting society and its normative structures from so-called problem or addicted gamblers rather than, more generally, players from the risks of gambling.

References

American Psychiatric Association. (1980). *Diagnostic and statistical manual of mental disorders* (3rd edn.) American Psychiatric Association.

Bausch, P. (1952). Bundestagsprotokoll der 193. Sitzung am 14. Februar 1952. https://www.bundestag.de/protokolle

Becker, T. (2016). *Verfügbarkeit und Sucht beim Automatenspiel.* Peter Lang Verlag.

Becker, T. (2022). Algorithmen zur Früherkennung von glücksspielgefährdeten Spielern. *Beiträge zum Glücksspielwesen, 1*, 22–23.

Berger, P. L., & Luckmann, T. (1966). *The social construction of reality: A treatise in the sociology of knowledge.* Anchor Books.

Bernhard, B. J. (2007). The voices of vices: Sociological perspectives on the pathological gambling entry in the *diagnostic and statistical manual of mental disorders. American Behavioral Scientist, 52*(1), 8–32. https://doi.org/10.1177/0002764207304869

Bernhard, B. J., Futrell, R., & Harper, A. (2010). "Shots from the pulpit": An ethnographic content analysis of United States anti-gambling social movement documents from 1816–2010. *UNLV Gaming Research & Review Journal, 14*(2), 2.

Bjerg, O. (2009). Too close to the money: A theory of compulsive gambling. *Theory, Culture & Society, 26*(4), 47–66. https://doi.org/10.1177/02632764091049

Bundeszentrale für gesundheitliche Aufklärung. (2010). *Glücksspielverhalten in Deutschland 2007 und 2009: Ergebnisse aus zwei repräsentativen Bevölkerungsbefragungen.* BZgA.

Castellani, B. (2000). *Pathological gambling: The making of a medical problem.* State University of New York Press.

Conrad, P., & Barker, K. K. (2010). The social construction of illness: Key insights and policy implications. *Journal of Health and Social Behaviour, 51*(1), 567–579. https://doi.org/10.1177/0022146510383495

Dollinger, B. (2006). Prävention: Unintendierte Nebenfolgen guter Absichten. In B. Dollinger & J. Reithel (Eds.), *Aktivierende Sozialpädagogik. Ein kritisches Glossar* (pp. 145–154). VS Verlag für Sozialwissenschaften. https://doi.org/10.1007/978-3-531-90353-8_10

Euchner, E.-M., Heichel, S., Nebel, K., & Raschzok, A. (2013). From 'morality' policy to 'normal' policy: Framing of drug consumption and gambling in Germany and the Netherlands and their regulatory consequences. *Journal of European Public Policy, 20*(3), 372–389. https://doi.org/10.1080/13501763.2013.761506

Ferentzy, P., & Turner, N. E. (2013). *The history of problem gambling: Temperance, substance abuse, medicine, and metaphors.* Springer. https://doi.org/10.1007/978-1-4614-6699-4

Goedecke, K., Spångberg, J., & Svensson, J. (2023). License to gamble: Discursive perspectives on the 2019 reregulation of the Swedish gambling market. *Critical Gambling Studies, 4*(2), 16–29. https://doi.org/10.29173/cgs157

Hayer, T., Brosowski, T., & Meyer, G. (2020). Multi-venue exclusion program and early detection of problem gamblers: What works and what does not? *International Gambling Studies, 20*(3), 556–578. https://doi.org/10.1080/14459795.2020.1766096

Hitzler, R., Reichertz, J., & Schröer, N. (Eds.). (1999). *Hermeneutische Wissenssoziologie: Standpunkte zur Theorie der Interpretation.* Universitäts Verlag Konstanz.

Keller, R. (2011a). *Diskursforschung: Eine Einführung für SozialwissenschaftlerInnen* (4th ed.). VS Verlag für Sozialwissenschaften. https://doi.org/10.1007/978-3-531-92085-6

Keller, R. (2011b). *Wissenssoziologische Diskursanalyse: Grundlegung eines Forschungsprogramms* (3rd ed.). VS Verlag für Sozialwissenschaften. https://doi.org/10.1007/978-3-531-92058-0

Keller, R., Knoblauch, H., & Reichertz, J. (Eds.). (2013). *Kommunikativer Konstruktivismus: Theoretische und empirische Arbeiten zu einem neuen wissenssoziologischen Ansatz.* Springer VS. https://doi.org/10.1007/978-3-531-19797-5

Lischer, S., Auerbach, S., & Schwarz, J. (2016). *Die Spielsperre im Kontext des Spielerschutzes.* Hochschule Luzern.

Lutter, M. (2010). *Märkte für Träume: Die Soziologie des Lottospiels.* Campus.

Markham, F., & Young, M. (2015). "Big gambling": The rise of the global industry-state gambling complex. *Addiction Research & Theory, 23*(1), 1–4. https://doi.org/10.3109/16066359.2014.929118

Matilainen, R. (2017). *Production and consumption of recreational gambling in twentieth-century Finland.* Academic dissertation, University of Helsinki.

Miller, H. E., Thomas, S. L., Smith, K. M., & Robinson, P. (2015). Surveillance, responsibility and control: An analysis of government and industry discourses about "problem" and "responsible" gambling. *Addiction Research & Theory, 24*(2), 163–176. https://doi.org/10.3109/16066359.2015.1094060

Möll, G. (2021). *Mit Geld spielt man nicht! Glücksspiel und »Glücksspielsucht« im parlamentarischen Diskurs* [You don't gamble with money! Gambling and 'gambling addiction' in parliamentary discourse]. Transcript Verlag. https://doi.org/10.14361/9783839460719

Paris, J., & Phillips, J. (2013). *Making the DSM-5: Concepts and controversies.* Springer. https://doi.org/10.1007/978-1-4614-6504-1

Rantala, V., & Sulkunen, P. (2012). Is pathological gambling just a big problem or also an addiction? *Addiction Research & Theory, 20*(1), 1–10. https://doi.org/10.3109/16066359.2011.552819

Reichert, R. (2019). Der Glücksspielstaatsvertrag als Werkzeug des Spielerschutzes. In A. Wöhr & M. Wuketich (Eds.), *Multidisziplinäre Betrachtung des vielschichtigen Phänomens Glücksspiel* (pp. 287–314). VS Springer. https://doi.org/10.1007/978-3-658-24972-4_18

Reichertz, J., Niederbacher, A., Möll, G., Gothe, M., & Hitzler, R. (2008). *Jackpot: Erkundungen zur Kultur der Spielhallen.* VS Verlag für Sozialwissenschaften.

Reith, G. (2007). Gambling and the contradictions of consumption: A genealogy of the "pathological" subject. *American Behavioural Scientist, 51*(1), 33–55. https://doi.org/10.1177/0002764207304856

Reith, G. (2018). *Addictive consumption. Capitalism, modernity and excess.* Routledge. https://doi.org/10.4324/9780429464447

Rüppel, J. (2022). *Die Biomarkerisierung der Depression: Eine Soziologie psychiatrischer Wissensproduktion.* Campus. https://doi.org/10.12907/978-3-593-44979-1

Schetsche, M. (2013). Pathologization as strategy for securing the Wirklichkeit: The example of paranormal experiences. In M. Dellwing & M. Harbusch (Eds.), *Krankheitskonstruktionen und Krankheitstreiberei: Die Renaissance der soziologischen Psychiatriekritik* (pp. 271–286). Springer VS. https://doi.org/10.1007/978-3-531-18784-6_11

Schetsche, M. (2014). *Empirische Analyse sozialer Probleme: Das wissenssoziologische Programm.* Springer VS. https://doi.org/10.1007/978-3-658-02280-8

Schmidt, L. (1999). *Psychische Krankheit als soziales Problem: Die Konstruktion des »Pathologischen Glücksspiels«.* Leske+Budrich. https://doi.org/10.1007/978-3-322-97456-3

Schmidt, L. (2012). Glücksspielsucht. Aufkommen der Problemdefinition und anhaltende Kontroversen. *Soziale Probleme, 22*(1), 40–66.

Schüll, N. D. (2012). *Addiction by design: Machine gambling in Las Vegas.* Princeton University Press. https://doi.org/10.1515/9781400834655

Schulz, J., & Müller, R. C. (2019). Glücksspiel und Werbung—Zwei klärungsbedürftige Politica. *Frankfurter Allgemeine Sonntagszeitung,* 23 June, V2.

Selin, J. (2022). Parliamentary debates on gambling policies as political action: An interpretive political analysis. *Critical Gambling Studies, 3*(1), 24–34. https://doi.org/10.29173/cgs85

Tammi, T. (2014). The form and transformation of gambling policy. In R. Pauliina (Ed.), *Gambling in Finland* (pp. 71–85). Gaudeamus.

Trümper, J. (2021). *Einblicke in den illegalen Glücksspielmarkt 2021: Feldstudie*. VDAI Verlags- und Veranstaltungsgesellschaft mbH.

Weber, J. (1952). Bundestagsprotokoll der 193. Sitzung am 14. Februar 1952. https://www.bundestag.de/protokolle

Wilcox, S. (2021). A genealogical analysis of the medical model of problem gambling. *Critical Gambling Studies, 2*(1), 97–107. https://doi.org/10.29173/cgs72

15

Aesthetic Pathologisation: Cinema, Psychiatry and Sex Addiction

Baptiste Brossard and Benjamin Hemmings

While sociologists and anthropologists have largely studied the history of norms surrounding mental health through their presentation in medical and psychological texts, less has been done to investigate how mental health categories, representations, and practices discreetly diffuse beyond the articulated arguments of professional specialists. What about the images, sounds, innuendos, intonations, and colours that suggest more than they tell? What about the textures of everyday normativity or, to use Fanon's (1961, p. 10) inspiring formula, "all these aesthetic expressions of respect for the established order"?

In light of the mass diffusion of psy-discourses in Western cultures since the late twentieth century (Cohen, 2016; Harbusch, 2022; Rose,

B. Brossard (✉)
University of York, York, UK
e-mail: baptiste.brossard@york.ac.uk

B. Hemmings
Deakin University, Melbourne, VIC, Australia
e-mail: Ben.Hemmings@anu.edu.au

B. M. Z. Cohen et al. (eds.), *Addiction and the Medicalisation of Conspicuous Behaviour*, The Politics of Mental Health and Illness,
https://doi.org/10.1007/978-3-032-06313-7_14

1996), critical mental health research should be more concerned with the *aestheticised* forms of pathologisation in social life. This claim applies well to the case of sexual excess—an expression we use to denote situations where the quantity of one's sexual thoughts, emotions, and activities are socially deemed problematic—which has been increasingly captured in the last decades by the popular category of 'sex addiction' (Reay et al., 2013). Sexuality has long been subject to social control (Foucault, 1977, 1985), as a wealth of medical measurement tools, representations, and categories have come to differentiate proper and improper sexual activities, thereby *medicalising and psychologising* these activities (Flore, 2020; Keane, 2004; Taylor, 2019). But how have these categories, associated representations, and practices 'translated' into cultures? What aesthetic forms have come into being in relation to these normative understandings of life?

The study of films is one way to 'probe' societies from this perspective. Because filmmakers are not traditional 'moral entrepreneurs' (Becker, 1963), they rarely promote articulated norms; rather, they often convey vaguely normative portrayals of some medical or psychological issues, both via scripts and the stylised means of expression that cinema affords—editing, camera movement, sounds, sets, or costume design. Further, as we will show, the discourses of medicine, psychology, and cinema never perfectly coincide; they instead obey different temporalities and stakes. For instance, the *International classification of diseases* (ICD) has included a sub-section on 'nymphomania' since the late 1980s (World Health Organization, 1989, p. 219), but this category—well-known in psychiatry at least since the nineteenth century—was mainly present in films in the 1950s and 1960s. Similarly, 'sex addiction' entered the *Diagnosis and statistical manual of mental disorders* (DSM; American Psychiatric Association, 1987) in 1987 but was then quickly replaced by 'hypersexuality' in 1994 (American Psychiatric Association, 1994), though the notion of sex addiction has been a recurrent theme on screens since the early 1990s. Thus, the changing relations between the fields of psychiatry and mass culture (Scull, 2015, pp. 351–357) embody a *productive discrepancy* whose various clashes and rapprochements generate a space of narrative and emotional possibilities (Brossard et al., 2023).

This chapter explores how sexual excess has been depicted in Western films since the 1930s. After laying some theoretical and methodological bases, we identify five ideal-typical narratives of sexual excess unevenly related to contemporaneous psychiatric classifications. Then, we turn to cinematographic techniques, such as sound, editing, and camera movements. We show that the Western cinematographic treatment of sexual excess has shifted over the twentieth century from *scripting* the negative *consequences* of excessive sexuality to *framing* the *anticipation* of sexual activities—that is, developing an aesthetic that problematises *desire itself*.

The Sociological Significance of Film

What does film tell us about the societies in which they are produced? This link between 'cinema' and 'society' has long been theorised and explored in the social sciences, from the Frankfurt School to British Cultural Studies (Kellner, 2002). However, the study of movies has often been confined to specialist fields, and examinations in non-specialised areas remain far from commensurate with the magnitude of this cultural phenomenon, especially in the field of mental health where films have the capacity to convey powerful representations of emotions, healing, and human psychology.

To establish such a link between cinema and society, sociologists have tended to reason either synchronically or diachronically. Synchronically, some have associated characters, plots, and messages found in one or several films with certain traits of a given society—trying to identify 'backstage cultural assumptions' (Bergesen, 2016). For instance, Wonser and Boyns (2016) interpret zombie films as mirroring contemporary anxieties surrounding autonomy and selfhood, while Benshoff and Griffin (2009) describe how mainstream cinema reproduces gender, class, and racial stereotypes. Diachronically, others have analysed the evolution of films over time to reveal certain social transformations, such as Hansen and Magnussen (2018) with the history of business or Buffet (2017) with that of Cold War propaganda. Films can also be used, alongside interviews with concerned people, to critically examine social narratives circulating about a given phenomenon, such as Heney's (2022) research on cinema and self-harm. Underlying these approaches lies an epistemological assumption that cinematographic variations and regularities are not random, that we can find in films some patterns whose very occurrence expresses something about the social world.

From this perspective, films might be taken as a kind of magnifying glass that reflects, exaggerates, and distorts certain aspects of the societies in which they are produced *through variable forms of influence*. In addition to partially mirroring the cultures in which they emerge, cinematographic productions may also echo the social dynamics to be found in microcosms such as Hollywood which are male-dominated, wealthy circles, situated in global centres of power. Finally, they may reflect how these microcosms draw connections with various external sources of expertise, as demonstrated by Khitrov (2020). Thus, as we will see, film directors seem to have abundantly mobilised psychiatric, psychological, and self-help literature to portray sexual excess—film director Steve McQueen, who originally wanted to shoot his 2011 film *Shame* in London, even moved its production to New York as he met "some kind of specialist in the field [of sex addiction, who] happened to be in New York" (Calautti, 2011).

Ultimately, films depicting sexual excess should be seen as part of this configuration where several fields strive to define what such excess looks like (Brossard et al., 2023), including the mass media (Reay et al., 2013), religious groups, self-help movements (Irvine, 1995), psychology, and psychiatry (Flore, 2020). In this context, cinematographic production teams are influenced by these fields while simultaneously maintaining relative independence from them. Therefore, in this chapter, we pay attention not only to the content of films but also to their shifting alignment with variable contexts and sources of expertise.

Methodology

Using the Internet Movie Database (IMDb), a large online database referencing more than 500,000 items, we introduced the keywords 'sex addiction', 'sex addict', and 'nymphomania', and only included films in which (a) one of the actors is characterised by the number of sexual activities they strive to achieve and (b) this excessiveness is a structuring element of the plot. This latter criterion raises a critical point. It is common in fiction for male characters to be sexually excessive (according to our definition above) without this excess constituting a structuring part of the plot; for instance, in James Bond films, where sexual endeavours—despite potentially leading to some inconveniences—remain peripheral to the main plot (namely protecting the interests of the British state). Masculine sexual excess is often 'unmarked' (Zerubavel, 2018). A certain sense of normalcy—more specifically, a *non-problematisation*—surrounds intense masculine sexuality, especially when the concerned characters are successful in their activities or hold prestigious statuses (on masculinity in cinema, see Bruzzi, 2013). Thus, our method oriented us towards *problematised* forms of sexual excess.

Another methodological challenge of using IMDb is that it gives primacy to the selection of its users—that is, popular movies, almost all Anglophone, and mainly produced in the US. The non-Anglophone films that were included were predominately made by directors of international renown, such as François Truffaut, Pedro Almodóvar, and Lars von Trier. Reflecting the social dynamics at play in the construction of the 'mainstream' in the globalised industry of cinema, our study investigated the mainstream representations of sexual excess in the West.

Our sample counted 54 films from 1932 to 2019 (the films can be found here: https://letterboxd.com/georgsimmel/list/films-analysed-for-framing-desire-cinema). We aimed at reaching 'saturation'—namely, the point where adding new data would not generate new insights for each decade studied, given that few movies were found in the 1940s and 1950s and that some productions of other decades were quite repetitive (such as romantic comedies in the 1990s and 2000s). Each co-author watched half of the films, documenting how sexual excess was scripted and framed.

To unravel these documents, our first axis of analysis concerned *narratives*: researching how certain themes, characters, and stories were articulated into recurrent patterns, tracking the emergence of certain ideal-typical figures (Olesen, 2020), and how they were either rewarded or punished, agreeing with Getz (2016) and Smith (2012) that the fate of characters tends to express normative relations to the social order. Second, we examined how sexual excess was *framed* through music, photography, costume design, and postproduction effects, turning to these techniques that introduce allusions, 'subtexts' (Martin-Jones, 2006), and symbolism (Llinares, 2009) evoking more than they enounce.

The Decline of 'Screenwriting Punishments'

The analysis of plots led us to identify five recurrent models of interaction between sexually excessive and non-sexually excessive characters to whom specific personality traits and modes of action were attributed. These ideal-typical relationships peak in certain decades—which we will indicate—but may be found in other periods; they are obvious in certain movies but sometimes appear in hybrid forms, hence our allusion to the Weberian notion of ideal-type (Swedberg, 2018).

Throughout this succession of ideal-typical relationships, several shifts can be observed. There is a gendered shift at first: whereas most sexually excessive characters were women, from the 1980s onwards, they are progressively 'replaced' with men, then mainly labelled as 'sex addicts'. Another transformation is the decline of *screenwriting punishments*: whilst plots often 'punish' sexually excessive characters, the gravity of these punishments decreases, and, towards the end of the twentieth century, sexually excessive characters merely struggle for their well-being, professional position, and conjugal peace.

Self-Serving Women and Idealists (1930s)

The first relationship model opposes *self-serving women*, who have sex with men to gain material advantages, and *idealist men*, who fall in love with these women, blinded by their romantic idealism. Epitomised by *Red-headed woman* (1932) and *Baby face* (1933), this model dominated Pre-Code Hollywood—that is, the era preceding 1934 when, mirroring the increasing permissiveness of the 'Roaring Twenties' (Wouters, 2004), the quasi-absence of censorship enabled film directors to delve into sexual topics. This model reflects that even if sexuality had already received significant medical interest and political control—the concept of paraphilia, coined in 1930, focused on atypical sexual practices rather than their intensity and frequency (Giami, 2015)—medical categorisations at the time indiscriminately grouped homeless people, 'criminals', sex workers, and 'perverts' within the same categories (De Block & Adriaens, 2013). Thus, in medicine, as in cinema, sexuality did not appear as a *hermetic area of deviance.*

Many films of this time are marked by the vicissitudes provoked by the 1929 economic crisis. Male figures frequently struggle to maintain or boost their social standing. Often foregrounded is the risk of losing their partner if unsuccessful. In this context, self-serving women seek out men to increase their economic comfort and social status, maintaining complete control over their sexual desire and exhibiting a coldly manipulative demeanour. Conversely, men are portrayed as unable to resist these women's charms, unwittingly falling for any seduction. They desire and love without agency, lacking free will, and consequently have less accountability. Above all, they do not need to use their sexuality for social mobility.

In this model, women who are not sexually excessive are less ambitious; they wish to remain in their social/sexual place. Married, they do not seek men other than their husbands. Single, they do not pursue men of a higher social status. The present model is illustrated by *Red-headed woman* (1932) and *Baby face* (1933), both of which tell the story of ambitious women escaping their modest circumstances by seducing wealthier men. In both films, signs of wealth are displayed immediately after the first sexual encounter, with the characters discarding their modest house dresses in favour of fur-lined coats and luxury cars.

Such ambitions come at a cost: screenwriting punishments. On the one hand, their romantic naiveté may have led some manipulated men to experience serious troubles, such as trying to kill themselves (*Baby face,* 1933) or being shot (*Red-headed woman,* 1932). On the other hand, for these self-serving women, few happy endings exist. They are often 'put in their place' upon realising the harm they caused or fall victim to terrible tragedies, such as in *The Story of Temple Drake* (1933), wherein a female character who seems to enjoy having casual sex is kidnapped and raped before the viewer can find out more about her.

Nymphomaniacs and Reasonable Men (1950s)

The second model contrasts the figure of the nymphomaniac woman, disturbed by her overwhelming sexual drive, with that of the rational man trying to preserve some sense of order. This model dominated in the 1950s and 1960s, when censorship (Benshoff & Griffin, 2009) and sexual conservatism (Wouters, 2004) were at their peak. Nymphomania was increasingly presented as a *disease,* coinciding with a moment in the late 1940s (ICD-6: World Health Organization, 1948) and the early 1950s (DSM-I: American Psychiatric Association, 1952) when medical classifications began to dissect 'sexual deviation' from a psychopathological perspective. However, these specifications were more concerned with the objects of desire than their quantity. Therefore, although not strictly following the course of medical knowledge, with the figure of the nymphomaniac, sexual excess was nevertheless—and later than in medicine—*cinematographically medicalised.*

It is not just sexuality troubling nymphomaniacs but also the general failure of reason. As a character in *Spellbound* (1945) tells a psychiatrist, "I hate men, I loathe them", ambivalently articulating a seductive and aggressive attitude. Nymphomaniacs are systematically associated with alcohol consumption, smoking, and suicidal tendencies. They are poor timekeepers and mercurial, afflicted by bouts of melancholy that leave them struggling with everyday tasks. In contrast, men and 'normal' women are depicted as reasonable, responsible, and in step with the expectations attached to their social status, maintaining this order disrupted by the nymphomaniac. Again, excessive sexuality expresses some discrepancy with one's social position, some discomfort that is embodied as nymphomaniacs are filmed displaying nervous body language, like constantly adjusting their garments. They are often desperate, oriented to a psychiatrist; a dramatic example is *Birds in Peru* (1968), where Adriana agrees with her husband that he should kill her if she 'falls ill' again.

Screenwriting punishments flow quite naturally from this type of script due to the risk associated with the behaviour of sexually excessive characters. In *The Chapman Report* (1962), which illustrates the famous Kinsey studies of sexual behaviours among the US population, the 'nymphomaniac' character appears five times: namely, (1) she wakes up late; (2) she is late to a meeting, busy seducing the delivery boy; (3) she is abused by the friends of a man she has sex with, a jazz musician; (4) she bewilders the researcher by narrating her sexual perdition; and (5) she kills herself.

Emancipated People and 'Squares' (1970s)

Around the 1970s, when psychiatry was increasing the number of official categories labelling sexual deviance and reinforcing its assessment of sex through quantity (too much or too little), most film productions took a different route. Aligning with the 'expressive revolution' (Wouters, 2004), a third model emerged, portraying *de-medicalised* sexual excess as a path towards both personal and political emancipation.

In this model, sexually excessive characters are still marginal, but they are portrayed in a more positive light. They are the vanguard of the new society to come—a society in which religious and moral repression will collapse, allowing sexuality to become a part of self-expression. In contrast to these characters are the 'squares', who abide by customs, monogamous marriage, reluctance towards atypical sexual practices, and, sometimes, to pleasure itself. While sexually excessive characters act in a straightforward manner—they want to have sex, so they have sex—'squares' suffer from their own repression, with some of them secretly fantasising about joining the ranks of the emancipated people.

This model was reinforced in the 1960s by the rise of low-budget, independent films that delved into niche genres like 'sexploitation' (Williams, 2008, p. 9, p. 91). For example, in *The Tale of The Dean's Wife* (1970), characters range between the sexually 'open' and politically progressive students and academics, and the more conservative 'squares'.

Two possibilities for turning 'squares' into 'emancipated' characters are shown: a prudish student bangs her head and suddenly becomes obsessed with sex, and students put LSD in the Dean's bottle to drag him into a compromising orgy. It only takes one step—a substance, a shock, a click—to turn off the repression in which 'squares' live, initiating a journey towards self-fulfilment (see *Emmanuelle,* 1974). Unlike the previous models, plots in this vein do not revolve around the essential distinction between excessive and non-excessive sexuality but around the porosity of this distinction.

However, even self-proclaimed 'progressive' films, such as *Supervixens* (1975) —whose trailer promises a "blunt attack on modern sexual morality"—or the psychedelic *Spermula* (1975) severely 'punish' sexual excess, with tragedies ranging from individual death to the destruction of an extra-terrestrial civilisation. The glorified seducer of *The Man Who Loved Women* (1977) dies by falling out of his hospital bed trying to catch a glimpse of a nurse's legs, while the previously mentioned Dean in *The Tale of The Dean's Wife* (1970), once recovered from his LSD trip, commits suicide. Screenwriting punishments still lurk in the background.

One-Sided and Multi-Faceted Characters (1990s)

The fourth model appeared in an era that has sometimes been called the sexual counter-revolution, characterised by the alignment of the neoliberal agenda with family moralism (Cooper, 2017) in the context of the AIDS epidemic and increased mass distribution of pornography through the development of videocassettes and discs. In this model, 'sex addicts' are one-dimensional roles, interacting only in relation to their sexual urges, as opposed to having well-rounded personalities.

It also coincided with significant changes in the psychiatric approach to sexual excess. In the DSM-III-R (American Psychiatric Association, 1987), 'sex addiction' was added as a sub-division of 'sexual dysfunction not otherwise specified' before being excluded in the DSM-IV (American Psychiatric Association, 1994), which instead favoured the classification of 'hypersexual disorder'. In 1994, the ICD-10 included 'excessive sexual drive' as a diagnostic item of 'compulsive behaviour' (World Health

Organization, 1994, p. 177). Thus, in the 1990s, psychiatry intensively revised its standards of sexual excess, accompanied by the multiplication of self-help groups around the globe that contributed to diffusing its perspectives (Irvine, 1995). It was in this context that 'sex addiction' almost immediately made it onto the screen.

Whereas sex addicts constantly bite their lips, inappropriately touch the opposite sex, and speak in innuendo, non-sexually excessive characters in this model are strikingly complex: they hesitate, they want sex to be meaningful, and their temptations are moderated by carefulness. They are *mindful*. Their desire is *elusive*. Viewers discover more facets of their personalities through doubts that excessively sexual characters cannot grasp, stuck in their static attraction to sex. On the other hand, much like 'nymphomaniacs', sex addicts are unable to fulfil the expectations associated with their status, not because they are incapable but because their passion for sex makes them too frivolous for such efforts. This is the case in *There Goes the Neighborhood* (1992): Marty, a real estate agent who has not sold a house in three years, acts as a burden to the neighbourhood through his frequent visits to (relatively more complex and subtle) neighbours accompanied by inappropriate touching. His character has comedic value only.

Three common plotlines of the 1990s fit with the present model. First, some films include a sexually addicted secondary character, often relatively insignificant, such as in *Color of Night* (1994), where Sondra is just another patient to be treated, or in the character of Marty in *There Goes the Neighborhood* (1992). Second, sex comedies, from *Screwballs* (1983) to *American Pie* (1999), revolve around the reduction of certain characters' purposes to their sexual drives, which generate repetitive comic situations. Third, sexuality can come with a form of mysticism. For instance, *Delta of Venus* (1995) and *Eyes Wide Shut* (1999) portray the wanderings of a hesitant central character who reflects on themselves navigating among variously over-sexualised people: a nymphomaniac child, an African psychic, and numerous sex workers.

This model signalled the decline of screenwriting punishments. Unlike in previous models, one-sided sexually excessive characters are less likely to be killed or lead others to be killed; rather, they are condemned to suffer indefinitely from their incompleteness, their superficiality, or their blind obsession, unless they commit to therapy.

Self-Deceptive Addicts and Healthy People (2000s–2010s)

The last model constitutes the overwhelmingly dominant narrative of sexual excess since the 2000s. A main character, addicted to sex and unable to lead their life, is either unaware of or unwilling to confront their inner problems. This contrasts with other characters who look happier, healthier, and more sensible precisely because their thoughts and lives are not as centred around sex. The emergence of this model coincides with the diffusion of 'sex addiction' as a popular psychological category (Brossard et al., 2023), while mainstream psychiatry turned to other frameworks—particularly 'compulsive sexual behaviour disorder', now endorsed by both the ICD-11 (World Health Organization, 2019) and DSM-5 (American Psychiatric Assocation, 2013). In addition, broader factors—such as the increased accessibility of pornography through the internet—came to influence the psychological approach to sexual excess, including porn addiction (Taylor, 2019). In this context, some scenarios clearly illustrate the psychological—rather than psychiatric and biomedical—stance toward sex addiction, exemplified in films like *Sex, Lies & Obsession* (2001) and *Cyber Seduction* (2005), indicating the cinematographic *psychologisation* of sexual excess.

The narratives of *Black Snake Moan* (2006), *Choke* (2008), *Thanks for Sharing* (2012), *Don Jon* (2013), and *Sleeping with Other People* (2015) all explore the inner conflicts awakened by sex addiction. Typically, these conflicts disrupt a potential romantic union with another character. Conversely, non-addicts are portrayed from the very beginning of the film as having *understood* the benefits of commitment to a monogamous relationship with moderate sexual activity.

Many films of this period adapted the romantic comedy genre, in which relations are usually disrupted by external elements, such as family reluctance (à la *Romeo and Juliet*), to rather centre their plot on intra-individual issues. For instance, both *Choke* (2008) and *Shame* (2011) extend this narrative and stage their main characters' physical inability to have sexual intercourse with someone they *genuinely* love. In this model, 'sex addicts' do not *realise* how unhealthy their relationships are. They often struggle with their past, using sex as an escape, never *truly* knowing themselves. Therefore, the turning point of these plots is when they come to the *realisation* that their excessive sexual life is not *really* what they strive for. Self-deception, which was attributed to non-sexually excessive characters in the first model, now underlies excessive sexuality.

Therapy has the potential, so to speak, to 'save' sex addicts from screenwriting punishments. Indeed, instead of being killed, committing suicide, or experiencing some dramatic event, as in previous models, the present model highlights the possibility of recovery, echoing the contemporary diffusion of the 'recovery narrative' in the Global North (Woods et al., 2019). 'Working on themselves', sexually excessive characters may be able to engage in a traditional relationship and the associated 'healthy' lifestyle, embodying such change in every aspect of their lives—for example, by cleaning their apartment, throwing away their porn collection, or paying attention to their physical health and appearance. Sex addicts are less punished for their deviant attitudes and behaviours on screen and more rewarded for 'recovering' to conformity, which often serves as the happy ending of many such films.

The Aesthetic of Moderation

Although narratives involving sexual excess seem to have taken a less moralistic turn throughout twentieth-century cinema, in that sexually excessive characters face fewer 'screenwriting punishments'—as well as sexual activities becoming more and more graphically displayed on the screen (Williams, 2008)—cinematographic effects tell a different story. As plot resolutions involve increasingly fewer tragic consequences for sexually excessive characters, the *framing* of their desire is intensified. A range of effects have come to colour what happens on screen when a character deemed sexually excessive is attracted to someone, interacts with this person, and eventually has intercourse with them. These sights, sounds, colours, effects, props, and staging all problematise such desires in a non-narrative way. Thus, whereas some argue that aesthetics should remain out of the scope of sociology (Sutherland & Feltey, 2013, p. 6), we suggest that, much like figures of speech in novels or intonations in theatre, in the mundane aesthetics of cultural productions lie some of the most subtle expressions of social normativity.

Sonic Disorders

In cinematic depictions of sexual excess, sound and music emphasise moments of sexual tension. Often, the overall volume of the soundtrack increases to match the rising intensity of these situations. In addition, the sexualisation of interactions is frequently accompanied by three musical shifts. First, music can be 'exoticised', either through borrowing songs from African, Latino-American, or Caribbean repertoires (generally with intense percussions), or in 'exoticising' an existing soundtrack, such as introducing Latin sonorities into jazzy songs. Such 'exoticisation', which taps into the old association between sensuality and the Orient, decreased from the 1990s onward. Second, *dissonances* can be introduced—for instance, a psychedelic solo in rock soundtracks or atonal themes within classical music—evoking a loss of control. This technique goes as far as superposing two soundtracks, as in the gay bar scene in *Shame* (2011). Sexualisation is thus framed as a loosening of *both* interactional and musical conventions. Third, especially after the 1990s and in films using the notion of 'sex addiction', soundtracks play with the *register of authenticity.* In *Don Jon* (2013), for example, heavy electronic music gives rhythm to Jon's porn-watching routine, while classical music accompanies his more conventional relationship with Barbara. This insinuates an association between the artificiality of sounds and that of the social situation. Such an association is reinforced when Jon begins a relationship with Esther, his real 'true' love. No music plays when they make love, leaving the viewer with the faint sounds of suburban nightlife—leaves rustling and nocturnal insects chirping.

Sound design became widely used after the 2000s as a way of problematising desire and sexual excess, especially through the inclusion of 'non-diegetic' sounds (that is, sounds whose source is not shown on-screen). Sound signifies the emotions of a character, signalling and intensifying their mood. In *Black Snake Moan* (2006), moments preceding sex are heralded by the rattle of a snake—maybe a biblical reference?—while other noises reverberate. In *Thanks for Sharing* (2012), white noise builds in moments of sexual 'craving', combined with out-of-focus, handheld, shaky camera shots. Through sound, the desire to engage in sexual encounters is associated with a form of social/sonic disconnection from the 'normal' rhythm and atmosphere of everyday life.

Fragmented Editing

Over time, the studied movies began to increasingly problematise excessive desire with the help of editing techniques, such as *rhythmic montage* and the *inclusion of intrusive images*. Some films frame 'traditional' relationships (following a step-by-step dating process, monogamous, and turned towards the possibility of marriage) as slow-paced, whereas excessive sexuality is portrayed as rapid, mirroring the fleetingness of sexual partners and the ephemerality of their pleasure. In *Shame* (2011), Brandon's sex life is characterised by fast edits, emphasising his pursuit of quick raptures but also his disconnection from his countless, nameless sexual partners. Yet, moments spent with Marianne, with whom he desires to have more than a causal relationship, are markedly longer, highlighting slower embraces, foreplay, and the clumsiness that comes with their undressing.

Repetitiveness in montage can be used in two ways. First, routines can be shown as disrupted by sexual excess. In *Auto Focus* (2002), Bob's sanitised routine—work, church, and family dinners—is interrupted by his new lifestyle, as he foregoes family dinners for attending orgies. Here, sexual excess unsettles the social/visual order of life, presenting this engagement in sexual excess and these desires as incongruent with normal social and familial life. Second, scenes can be edited at a repetitive tempo to express the monotony in which sexually excessive characters are stuck. The beginning of *Shame* (2011) illustrates this: wake up, commute to work, have sex with a sex worker, wake up, masturbate in the shower, commute to work, and so forth. Montage, therefore, helps frame sexual excess against pleasure; as such, an editing strategy enshrines sexual encounters to be another quotidian aspect of Brandon's life.

The final editing technique we analysed consists of 'flashes'. When sexually excessive characters feel some desire, they are increasingly shown experiencing short excerpts of previous sexual encounters, visualising naked bodies or fantasising about anticipated intercourse. This practice began with *The Labyrinth of Sex* (1969) and *The Man Who Loved Women* (1977) as a technique evoking *nouvelle vague* films, which influenced the increasing deployment of visual effects in film montages (Marie, 2003). For instance, in *Choke* (2008), when Victor looks at a woman, the camera blinks, and she becomes topless, then it blinks again, and her clothes reappear. Insertions can also be more literary. When Sylvia gets hit on the head in *A Dirty Shame* (2004), the letters W-H-O-R-E and then V-A-G-I-N-A flash. When Sylvia gets hit on the head again, becoming a sexual introvert, we see the lettering N-E-U-T-E-R and then N-O-R-M-A-L instead. These flashes insinuate that excessively sexual characters' problematic relationship with sexuality comes with an unfocused mental life constantly shaken by intrusive thoughts.

Problematising Focus

Three types of camera movements were frequently employed in the movies under study. First, to mirror the sexual obsessions of their characters, some directors insidiously oriented their cameras to suggestive body parts. In *Cyber Seduction* (2005), once high-school student Justin sees a pornographic website for the first time, he becomes disinterested in his swimming lessons and instead fixates on women in their bathing suits, which is portrayed through camera zoom-ins. These techniques evoke a character's obsessional and out-of-control intentions.

Second, close-ups can highlight micro-gestures, such as nervous hands and blank expressions, which add an element of discomfort to a character's construction. In *Color of Night* (1994), Sondra—labelled a nymphomaniac—is presented through frequent close-ups of her restless, nervous hands, framing her as continuously struggling against her desires. *Black Snake Moan* (2006) goes further, as in moments of sexual craving, Rae writhes on the ground, fighting against herself; close-ups zoom in on her hands as they claw at her skin and twisting body as she repeats the word "no". This effect conveys that beyond the actual disturbances induced by sexual activities, sexually excessive characters are acted up by some deeper malaise.

Third, camera shaking can be utilised either to evoke craving symptoms—literally trembling—or to underscore the authenticity of certain relationships over others. The former is well illustrated in *Thanks for Sharing* (2012) when Adam breaks five years of sexual sobriety with a sex worker in his hotel room: this relapse interrupts the visual/social order of the movie with unstable camera movements. The latter option appears in both *Shame* (2011) and *Don Jon* (2013). In these films, 'meaningless' sexual encounters are shot through a stabilised camera, using sleek movements, whereas 'authentic' encounters occur through a slightly trembling, slightly imperfect handy cam; here, the shaky camera expresses a sense of realism. In sum, unstable camera movements can convey either the disturbance of excess or the authenticity of love—two ways of framing normalcy and deviance.

Deviant Set and Costume Design

Sexually excessive characters often stand out by their distinguishable appearances, as if their problems would materialise in their self-presentation, which includes costume and make-up. Additionally, settings can also mark the problematisation of sexual life. From *Written on the Wind* (1956) to *Bitter Moon* (1992), sexually excessive women wear more ostentatious colours and textures. In addition to being less covered than others, they also stand out by their relatively extravagant clothing, including attention-catching lipstick and leopard patterns. Tellingly, clothing changes once the characters themselves change. In *Black Snake Moan* (2006), once 'recovered', Rae no longer dresses in a ripped t-shirt with a gun and confederate flag motif; she then dons a conservative dress with floral patterns bought in a middle-aged women's shop. Her mentor, Lazarus, introduces the outfit as 'proper'.

In the case of sexually-excessive men, costume operates on a different level in their degree of preparedness. Whereas in *Thanks for Sharing* (2012) and *I Am a Sex Addict* (2005), Neil and Caveh, respectively, become cleaner and more attentive to their appearance as they 'recover', Cameron and Brandon, respectively in *Sex, Lies & Obsession* (2001) and *Shame* (2011), abandon their slick self-presentation when they commit to a potentially long-term relationship. Brandon goes to his only regular date tousled and wearing colours, while Cameron returns home from a therapy session wearing a modest, family-man brown pullover. The time for classy suits and leather jackets is over! Hence, clothing symbolises both self-care and conformity in recovery and the superficiality of seductive appearances.

Finally, set designs colour the material circumstances in which sexually excessive characters carry out their transgressions. The problematic dimension of sexual encounters is often reflected in dirtiness. For example, *Choke* (2008) introduces Victor's addiction through one sex scene on a filthy bathroom floor while his Sex Addicts Anonymous meeting continues in the background, and then a second scene with a nurse in his mother's care home among dirty bathtubs and hospital beds. A palette of dark greens and greys accentuates this mucky atmosphere. Only with Victor's dream partner do colours become brighter. A similar evocation operates in *Addicted to Fresno* (2015), where Shannon compulsively has sex anywhere (a car, an unclean hotel room, or an alleyway) with anyone (such as a hotel guest with a prominent mullet). Set designs thus reinforce the impression of a link between excessive sexuality and a pervasive dirtiness, even when the life of a character might otherwise appear quite sanitised. In the 2010s, films such as *Saint Nicholas* (2018) or *Don Jon* (2013) drifted away from this aesthetic, portraying sexual encounters in an evocation of mainstream pornography, immoderately choreographed in well-arranged rooms, with exaggeratedly sexualised bodies and outfits. In sum, sexual excess tends to be staged in places that, through their aesthetic—too dirty or too sanitised—present the resulting encounters as being associated with dirtiness or the stereotypes carried by pornography.

Conclusion

From the early twentieth century to the present, mainstream Western cinema has shifted in its treatment of sexual excess. In more recent films, designated 'sex addicts' are relatively less punished and condemned in the narratives. They are less stigmatised, discriminated against, injured, or killed. Nonetheless, such desires and attractions are increasingly *framed* through various cinematographic effects to *feel* dissonant, dirty, unhealthy, shaky, and inauthentic. Through sounds, movements, colours, and shapes, sexually excessive characters are shown undergoing a pathological experience, embodying it as if by a sort of *aesthetic normativity*, evocative of what Foucault called a 'stylisation of existence' (Foucault, 1985).

Such transformation must be understood in light of the changing relationship between the field of cinema and that of psychiatry and, later, psychology. In the 1930s, cinema and medicine did not conceive of sexuality as a specific field of deviance and stayed relatively independent in their formulation of sexual excess. In the 1950s, scripts came closer to the psychiatric framing of sexual excess as illness. It was at this point that the figure of the 'nymphomaniac'—a category known for at least a century—quite brutally emerged on the screen. 1970s cinema distanced itself from the psychiatric approach, surfing the 'sexual revolution'. However, both fields re-joined in the 1990s around the notion of 'sex addiction', although this concept soon became privileged in psychology and abandoned by official psychiatric nosology (Brossard et al., 2023). Finally, 2000s and 2010s cinema further elaborated on this addiction to sexual excess, following a more psychology-inspired than strictly psychiatric stance.

Although the increased visibility of sexual encounters in contemporary cinema has sometimes been considered indicative of a 'sexualisation of culture' (Attwood, 2009), our study leads to a mixed conclusion. To be sure, contemporary films display more and more flexible stories in terms of mores and sexual orientation; and sexual scenes are more explicit. However, we argue that cinematographic effects reintroduced new forms of pathologisation. Evoking Wouters' (2004) concept of informalisation, sex might be less hidden, less 'ruled', less scripted, but more tacit expectations came to weigh on the realisation of its authenticity. This is why sociologists and anthropologists of mental health need to go beyond the study of specialised, professional arguments; in liberal societies that tend to celebrate their own open-mindedness—in which social norms surrounding sexuality and mental health might appear quite loose—enduring forms of pathologisation might survive in the most seamless refinements of *aesthetics*.

Acknowledgements The research project discussed in this chapter was supported by a 2018 grant from the Social Sciences and Humanities Research Council of Canada (Grant No. 435-2018-0729, principal investigators: Nicolas Moreau, Dahlia Namian and Baptiste Brossard; research coordinators: Mélissa Roy and Emmanuelle Larocque). We are grateful to James Chouinard and Mary Lou Rasmussen for their insightful feedback on an earlier version of this text. Special thanks are also extended to the editors of this volume, Bruce Cohen, Martin Harbusch and Jo Reichertz, for their help with the finalisation of this chapter.

References

American Psychiatric Association. (1952). *Diagnostic and statistical manual: Mental disorders*. American Psychiatric Association.

American Psychiatric Association. (1987). *Diagnostic and statistical manual of mental disorders* (3rd Rev. ed.) American Psychiatric Association.

American Psychiatric Association. (1994). *Diagnostic and statistical manual of mental disorders* (4th ed.) American Psychiatric Association.

American Psychiatric Association. (2013). *Diagnostic and statistical manual of mental disorders* (5th ed.) American Psychiatric Association.

Attwood, F. (Ed.). (2009). *Mainstreaming sex: The sexualization of western culture*. Bloomsbury.

Becker, H. S. (1963). *Outsiders: Studies in the sociology of deviance*. Free Press.

Benshoff, H., & Griffin, S. (2009). *America on film: Representing race, class, gender, and sexuality at the movies*. Wiley-Blackwell.

Bergesen, A. (2016). How to sociologically read a film. *The Sociological Quarterly, 57*(4), 585–596. https://doi.org/10.1111/tsq.12151

Brossard, B., Roy, M., Brown, J., Hemmings, B., & Larocque, E. (2023). On the social existence of mental health categories: The case of sex addiction. *Social Problems, 72*(1), spad024. https://doi.org/10.1093/socpro/spad024

Bruzzi, S. (2013). *Men's cinema: Masculinity and mise-en-scène in Hollywood*. Edinburgh University Press.

Buffet, C. (Ed.). (2017). *Cinema in the Cold War: Political projections*. Routledge.

Calautti, K. (2011). Michael Fassbender and director Steve McQueen expose Shame. *CBR*. https://www.cbr.com/michael-fassbender-and-director-steve-mcqueen-expose-shame/

Cohen, B. M. Z. (2016). *Psychiatric hegemony: A Marxist theory of mental illness*. Palgrave Macmillan.

Cooper, M. (2017). *Family values: Between neoliberalism and the new social conservatism*. Princeton University Press.

De Block, A., & Adriaens, P. (2013). Pathologizing sexual deviance: A history. *Journal of Sex Research, 50*(3–4), 276–298. https://doi.org/10.1080/00224499.2012.738259

Fanon, F. (1961). *The wretched of the Earth*. Grove Press.

Flore, J. (2020). *A genealogy of appetite in the sexual sciences*. Palgrave Macmillan.

Foucault, M. (1977). *Discipline and punish: The birth of the prison*. Penguin Books.

Foucault, M. (1985). *The history of sexuality, volume 2: The use of pleasure*. Pantheon Books.

Getz, G. (2016). Transmission of ideology through film: The cinematic construction of gendered domination in Mr. Deeds Goes to Town. *The Sociological Quarterly, 57*(4), 654–674. https://doi.org/10.1111/tsq.12155

Giami, A. (2015). Between DSM and ICD: Paraphilias and the transformation of sexual norms. *Archives of Sexual Behavior, 44*(5), 1127–1138. https://doi.org/10.1007/s10508-015-0549-6

Hansen, P., & Magnussen, A. (2018). Making sense of business and community in Hollywood films, 1928–2016. *Business History Review, 92*(2), 307–337. https://doi.org/10.1017/S000768051800003X

Harbusch, M. (2022). *Troubled persons industries: The expansion of psychiatric categories beyond psychiatry*. Springer.

Heney, V. (2022). *Our stories, our selves: Fictional representations of self-harm*. (Doctoral thesis),. University of Exeter.

Irvine, J. M. (1995). Reinventing perversion: Sex addiction and cultural anxieties. *Journal of the History of Sexuality, 5*(3), 429–450.

Keane, H. (2004). Disorders of desire: Addiction and problems of intimacy. *Journal of Medical Humanities, 25*, 189–204. https://doi.org/10.1023/B:JOMH.0000036637.03254.38

Kellner, D. (2002). The Frankfurt School and British Cultural Studies: The missed articulation. In J. T. Nealon & C. Irr (Eds.), *Rethinking the Frankfurt*

School: Alternative legacies of cultural critique (pp. 31–49). State University of New York Press.
Khitrov, A. (2020). Hollywood experts: A field analysis of knowledge production in American entertainment television. *The British Journal of Sociology, 71*(5), 939–951. https://doi.org/10.1111/1468-4446.12775
Llinares, D. (2009). Idealized heroes of 'retrotopia': History, identity and the postmodern in Apollo 13. *The Sociological Review, 57*(1), 164–177. https://doi.org/10.1111/j.1467-954X.2009.01823.x
Marie, M. (2003). *The French new wave: An artistic school.* Blackwell.
Martin-Jones, D. (2006). No literal connection: Images of mass commodification, US militarism, and the oil industry, in The Big Lebowski. *The Sociological Review, 54*(1), 133–149. https://doi.org/10.1111/j.1467-954X.2006.00641.x
Olesen, T. (2020). The Whistleblower hero in cinematic dramatization. *The Sociological Review, 69*(2), 414–433. https://doi.org/10.1177/0038026120928880
Reay, B., Attwood, N., & Gooder, C. (2013). Inventing sex: The short history of sex addiction. *Sexuality & Culture, 17*, 1–19. https://doi.org/10.1007/s12119-012-9136-3
Rose, N. (1996). *Inventing our selves: Psychology, power, and personhood.* Cambridge University Press.
Scull, A. (2015). *Madness in civilization: A cultural history of insanity, from the Bible to Freud, from the madhouse to modern medicine.* Princeton University Press.
Smith, S. (2012). Scripting sexual desire: Cultural scenarios of teen girls' sexual desire in popular films, 2000–2009. *Sexuality & Culture, 16*(3), 321–341. https://doi.org/10.1007/s12119-012-9126-5
Sutherland, J.-A., & Feltey, K. (2013). Introduction. In J.-A. Sutherland & K. Feltey (Eds.), *Cinematic sociology: Social life in film* (pp. 6–23). Sage.
Swedberg, R. (2018). How to use Max Weber's ideal type in sociological analysis. *Journal of Classical Sociology, 18*(3), 181–196. https://doi.org/10.1177/1468795X17743643
Taylor, K. (2019). Pornography addiction: The fabrication of a transient sexual disease. *History of the Human Sciences, 32*(5), 56–83. https://doi.org/10.1177/0952695119854624
Williams, L. (2008). *Screening sex.* Duke University Press.
Wonser, R., & Boyns, D. (2016). Between the living and undead: How zombie cinema reflects the social construction of risk, the anxious self, and disease pandemic. *The Sociological Quarterly, 57*(4), 628–653. https://doi.org/10.1111/tsq.12150

Woods, A., Hart, A., & Spandler, H. (2019). The recovery narrative: Politics and possibilities of a genre. *Culture, Medicine, and Psychiatry, 46*(2), 221–247. https://doi.org/10.1007/s11013-019-09623-y
World Health Organization. (1948). *International classification of diseases-6*. World Health Organization.
World Health Organization. (1989). *International classification of diseases-9*. World Health Organization.
World Health Organization. (1994). *International classification of diseases-10*. World Health Organization.
World Health Organization. (2019). *International classification of diseases-11*. World Health Organization.
Wouters, C. (2004). *Sex and manners: Female emancipation in the West 1890–2000*. Sage.
Zerubavel, E. (2018). *Taken for granted: The remarkable power of the unremarkable*. Princeton University Press.

Publisher Correction to: Addiction and the Medicalisation of Conspicuous Behaviour

Bruce M. Z. Cohen, Martin Harbusch, and Jo Reichertz

Publisher Correction to: B. M. Z. Cohen et al. (eds.), *Addiction and the Medicalisation of Conspicuous Behaviour*, The Politics of Mental Health and Illness, https://doi.org/10.1007/978-3-032-06313-7

The book had been inadvertently published with an error, which was later corrected.

The first chapter of the book, "*Introduction: Pathologising Pleasure?*", had been incorrectly placed in the front matter, whereas it should have appeared as Chapter 1. The book was subsequently updated with the correct chapter sequence, and the Table of Contents was revised to reflect these changes.

The updated version of this book can be found at https://doi.org/10.1007/978-3-032-06313-7

B. M. Z. Cohen et al. (eds.), *Addiction and the Medicalisation of Conspicuous Behaviour*, The Politics of Mental Health and Illness,
https://doi.org/10.1007/978-3-032-06313-7_16

Index

B. M. Z. Cohen et al. (eds.), *Addiction and the Medicalisation of Conspicuous Behaviour*, The Politics of Mental Health and Illness,
https://doi.org/10.1007/978-3-032-06313-7

C

FSC
www.fsc.org
MIX
Papier | Fördert gute Waldnutzung
FSC® C083411

Kolibri 360 GmbH
Ferdinand-Jühlke-Straße 7
99095 Erfurt, Deutschland
produktsicherheit@kolibri360.de